BECOMING RAW

The Essential Guide to
RAW VEGAN DIETS

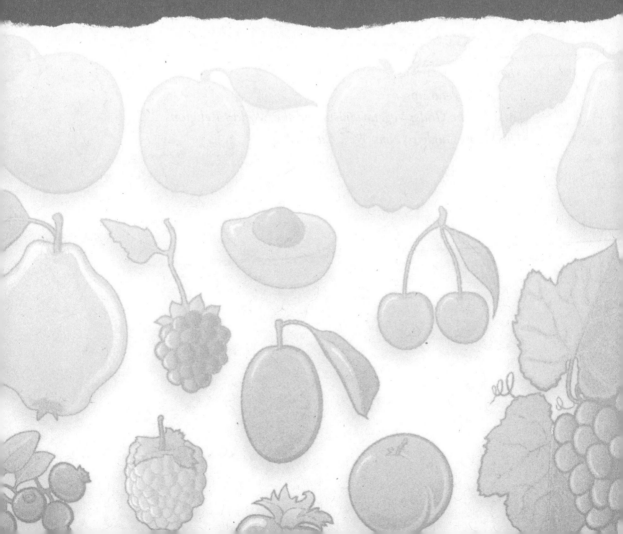

Other books by Brenda Davis and Vesanto Melina:

The New Becoming Vegetarian
Becoming Vegetarian
Becoming Vegan
The Raw Food Revolution Diet (WITH CHERIE SORIA)

Other books by Brenda Davis:

Defeating Diabetes (WITH TOM BARNARD, MD)
Dairy-Free and Delicious (WITH BRYANNA CLARK GROGAN AND JO STEPANIAK)

Other books by Vesanto Melina:

Food Allergy Survival Guide (WITH JO STEPANIAK AND DINA ARONSON)
Raising Vegetarian Children (WITH JO STEPANIAK)
Healthy Eating for Life: To Prevent and Treat Cancer (WITH PHYSICIANS' COMMITTEE FOR RESPONSIBLE MEDICINE)

Other books by Rynn Berry:

The New Vegetarians
Famous Vegetarians
Food for the Gods: Vegetarianism and the World's Religions
The Vegan Guide to New York City

BECOMING RAW

The Essential Guide to
RAW VEGAN DIETS

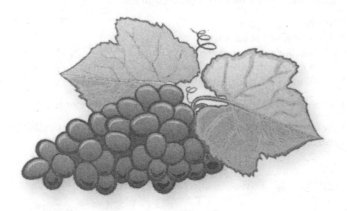

BRENDA DAVIS, RD, and VESANTO MELINA, MS, RD

with Rynn Berry

Book Publishing Company
Summertown, Tennessee

Library of Congress Cataloging-in-Publication Data

Davis, Brenda.
   Becoming raw : The essential guide to raw vegan diets
Brenda Davis, Vesanto Melina; with historical information by Rynn Berry.
    p. cm.
   Includes bibliographical references and index.
   ISBN 978-1-57067-238-5 (alk. paper)
1. Raw food diet. I. Melina, Vesanto, 1942- II. Berry, Rynn. III. Title.
   RM237.5.D38 2009
   613.2'65--dc22

                       2009036367

Cover design: Warren Jefferson, John Wincek
Cover art: Jennifer Blume
Interior design: John Wincek

Book Publishing Co. is a member of Green Press Initiative. We chose to print this title on paper with postconsumer recycled content, processed without chlorine, which saved the following natural resources:

140 trees
5,952 pounds of solid waste
51,040 gallons of wastewater
11,283 pounds of greenhouse gases
98 million BTU of total energy

For more information, visit www.greenpressinitiative.org.

Paper calculations from Environmental Defense Paper Calculator, www.edf.org/papercalculator.

Printed in Canada

Book Publishing Company
P.O. Box 99
Summertown, TN 38483
888-260-8458
www.bookpubco.com

ISBN: 978-1-57067-238-5

17 16 15 14 13 12 11 10   2 3 4 5 6 7 8 9

CONTENTS

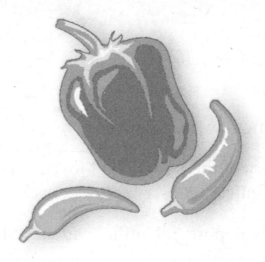

To Brenda's husband, Paul Davis,

for decades of patience, wisdom, support, inspiration, and endless love.

To Vesanto's partner, Cam Doré,

for extraordinary companionship, laughter, joy, and unconditional love.

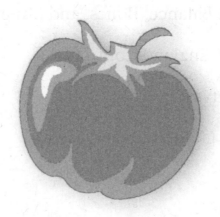

We are grateful for our dear and insightful editors Cynthia Holzapfel and Jo Stepaniak, our wonderful publisher Bob Holzapfel, and Anna Pope, Warren Jefferson, and all the other staff at Book Publishing Company who provide assistance and support whenever we need it. Thank you also to Jennifer Blume for the beautiful cover artwork and the expertise of John Wincek in designing a layout that is both user-friendly and appealing.

We appreciate all those who assisted us with research: dietetics students Angie Dueck and Stacie Andriashyk, Thomas Billings, Claudia Lalita Salas, Patricia Ganswind, the staff at the Ann Wigmore Institute, and Dave Steele.

Sincere gratitude to all those who kindly responded to our queries and requests for information: Dr. Ute Alexy, University of Cologne, Germany; Dr. Paul Appleby, University of Oxford, United Kingdom; Mr. Gilles Arbour, Mont-Saint-Hilaire, Quebec, Canada; Dr. Luciana Baroni, Mestre-Venice, Italy; Dr. Susan Barr, University of British Columbia, Canada; Dr. Steve Blake, author, Maui, Hawaii, United States; Dr. Rick and Karin Dina, Living Light Culinary Art Institute, California, United States; Dr. Michael Donaldson, Hallelujah Acres Foundation, United States; Dr. Scott Doughman, President and Chief Scientist, Source-Omega, North Carolina, United States; Dr. Joel Fuhrman, physician, New Jersey, United States; Dr. Michael Gardner, University of Bradford, United Kingdom; Dr. G. Sarwar Gilani, Health Canada, Ottawa, Canada; Angie McIntosh, Penticton, Canada; Dr. D. Joe Millward, University of Surrey, United Kingdom; Dr. B. Dave Oomah, Agriculture and Agri-Food Canada, Summerland, Canada; Dr. Peter Pellett, University of Massachusetts, United States; Dr. Lawrence Prochaska, Wright State University, Dayton, United States; Dr. Anna-Liisa Rauma Kosonen, University of Kuopio, Finland; Dr. Stephen Rothman, University of California, San Francisco, United States; Dr. Ann-Sofie Sandberg, Chalmers University of Technology, Sweden; Cherie Soria and Dan Laderman, Living Light Culinary Art Institute, California, United States; Dr. Stephen Walsh, Vegan Society, United Kingdom; and Dr. Sascha Rohn, Technical University of Berlin, Germany.

Sincere thanks for outstanding organic foods from Nyjal Brownson of Lady-Bug Organics, and David Nelson and Lisa McIntosh of Urban Harvest; Robert Gaffney and the excellent Omega Nutrition Products; and Margie Roswell, who funded nutritional analysis of the Green Giant Juice and other raw foods.

Love and gratitude to our families and friends: Cam Doré and Paul Davis for continual computer help, recipe tasting, moral support, and patience. Our beloved, nature-loving children, Chris and Kavyo, Leena and Cory, who are among our greatest teachers. Our precious, giving friends—Margie Colclough, Lauren Gaglardi, and Sooze Waldock.

Many thanks to the following chefs and recipe innovators who inspired us and generously allowed us to use or adapt their recipes for this book:

- **Rynn Berry:** Three-Melon Salad (page 291);
- **Jenny Cornbleet:** Mango Pie (page 300);
- **Joseph Forest:** Avocado Dip or Spread (page 269);
- **Chef Patricia Ganswind:** Celeriac Linguine with Bolognese Sauce and Hemp Parmesan (page 280), Pesto and Sundried Tomato Pizza with Veggies (page 284);
- **Francis Janes:** Caesar's Better Salad (page 279);
- **Guylaine Lacerte:** Thai Spring Rolls with Spicy Pecan Sauce (page 292), V-8 Vegetable Soup (page 274);
- **Valerie McIntyre:** Pesto the Best-oh! (page 285);
- **Radha Restaurant** staff (Vancouver): Kale Salad with Orange-Ginger Dressing (page 287);
- **Cathy Carlson Rink, ND:** Elegant Greens with Strawberries, Almonds, and Orange–Poppy Seed Dressing (page 283);
- **Matt Samuelson:** Coconut Crust (page 300);
- **Chef Cherie Soria:** Green Giant Juice (page 259), Garden Blend Soup (page 273);
- **Jo Stepaniak:** Creamy Zucchini Soup (page 272);
- **Ann Wigmore:** Crunchy Sprouts and Veggies (page 282).

We greatly appreciate those who tested and assisted with recipes or menus: Maureen Butler, Tricia Carpenter, Margie Colclough, Josée Fontaine, Lauren Gaglardi, Alice Hooper, Lynn Isted, Echota Keller, Michael Koo, Guylaine Lacerte, and Andrea Welling.

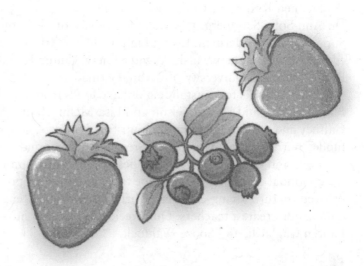

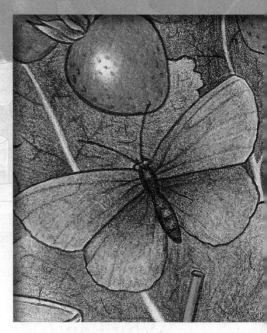

CHAPTER 1

Becoming Raw for Life

Becoming raw is not a new idea. In fact, it may well be the oldest way of eating known to humankind. Although cooking food is now common practice around the world, raw-food practitioners have endured throughout history. Today, raw diets are the latest rage: raw recipe books abound, raw restaurants are thriving, raw-food potlucks and support groups are flourishing, and the Internet is abuzz with raw-food websites, blogs, chat rooms, and newsletters. As the saying goes, everything old is new again, and nowadays, raw is hot.

There is a significant alignment between diet modifications guided by better nutrition and those guided by geophysical prudence; what is good for one's health is often also geophysically and environmentally beneficial and desirable.

GIDON ESHEL AND PAMELA MARTIN[1]

While raw diets may be as old as man, there are doubts about their nutritional viability:

- Can we possibly get enough protein if we eat mainly fruit?
- Won't we end up with osteoporosis if we eliminate dairy products?
- Can we really meet our needs for every single nutrient eating only raw food?
- Don't we require certain fats from fish?
- Where will our vitamin B_{12} come from?
- How will we get enough iron without meat?
- Doesn't cooking help to improve food safety and get rid of the substances in plants that prevent nutrient absorption?

In this book we examine all of these important nutrition issues and many more. We also explore conflicts and controversies that separate raw-food and conventional communities, such as:

1

- Do the enzymes in raw foods really contribute to human digestion, health, and longevity?
- Are cooked foods poisonous?
- Do raw vegan diets cure cancer and other chronic diseases?
- Does cooking destroy nutrients?
- Are most raw diets too high in fat?
- Are sprouted legumes indigestible?
- Are some sprouts toxic?

We've contacted experts who are often quoted but rarely questioned, and we've searched through journals and ancient manuscripts. Our quest has been for answers that stand up to scientific scrutiny and provide a clear, safe path for all those who wish to pursue a raw or high-raw vegan diet.

Why Raw?

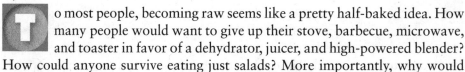 o most people, becoming raw seems like a pretty half-baked idea. How many people would want to give up their stove, barbecue, microwave, and toaster in favor of a dehydrator, juicer, and high-powered blender? How could anyone survive eating just salads? More importantly, why would anyone want to? Becoming raw is unlikely to inspire a celebration within one's social circle; it's more likely to be a source of frustration for friends and family. How are you ever going to be able to enjoy a meal together again? What are they supposed to serve you when you come over?

Despite the less-than-enthusiastic response that commonly comes from others, becoming raw is a choice that is generally embraced with such gusto by practitioners that it is adhered to for years, and often for life. What kind of payoff would inspire such a challenging lifestyle choice? For many individuals, it is the promise of radiant health. For others, the attraction is the ethical and philosophical principles on which the raw vegan diet is based. Some are drawn to its simplicity and ecological rewards. For most, there is a moment of epiphany when something clicks and becoming raw (or simply eating more raw food) is the choice that makes sense. Let's briefly explore the reasons that support such a choice.

HEALTH REASONS

The most popular reason for adopting a raw vegan diet is the belief that it can greatly enhance our physical well-being. Let's consider the three categories of health benefits that win people over to the raw way of eating:

1. General health and well-being

Raw vegan diets are often reported to improve energy and vitality and provide an elevated sense of well-being. With this choice, we eliminate the dietary components that can cause the most damage to our health: harmful fats, chemical contaminants, refined sugars and starches, and excessive animal protein. In their place are whole, raw plant foods, which are packed with vitamins, protective phytochemicals, fiber, and enzymes. Whereas cooking can destroy or damage vital nutrients and phytochemicals in foods, these compounds are preserved and even liberated with common raw-food preparation techniques such as puréeing and juicing.

2. Disease prevention and reversal

Many people increase their intake of raw food because they've been diagnosed with rheumatoid arthritis, fibromyalgia, heart disease, type 2 diabetes, or certain cancers. These conditions inspire a shift away from the standard Western diet, which typically emphasizes meat, dairy products, eggs, and cooked foods containing refined carbohydrates and fats. Along with all the damage from saturated fats and cholesterol, diets centered around animal products and grains can produce a mild metabolic acidosis, or slightly acidic state, which places a burden on the body. (See chapter 9.)

Raw vegetables and fruits, and the antioxidants and other phytochemicals they provide, can reduce our risk of certain diseases or slow their progression. (For specific details, see chapter 3.) Furthermore, a diet that is somewhat low in calories (as most raw vegan diets are) and is nutritionally adequate might also help to slow the aging process!

3. Weight loss and maintenance

Potato chips, donuts, cakes, pies, burgers, and shakes do not qualify as raw foods. In fact, almost all of the foods responsible for our obesity epidemic are automatically eliminated on a raw diet. A well-designed raw vegan diet can be viewed as the ultimate weight-loss regimen. Most raw plant foods are low in calories and high in fiber, making them the perfect choice for those who want to shed a few or many pounds. A visit to a raw-food restaurant will quickly confirm that raw-food adherents tend to be slim. (For more on this topic, also read *The Raw Food Revolution Diet* by C. Soria, B. Davis, and V. Melina, Book Publishing Company, 2008.)

ENVIRONMENTAL REASONS

Although benefits to the environment once were seen as a bonus rather than a primary motivating factor for following a raw vegan diet, environmental reasons have begun to take center stage. The United Nations Food and Agriculture Organization (FAO) report "Livestock's Long Shadow" sent shock waves around the world when it declared that "livestock are responsible for 18 percent of greenhouse gas emissions, a bigger share than that of transport." [2] Our personal contributions to greenhouse gases are significantly reduced when we derive our protein from plants rather than from animal sources.[3] The damage doesn't end with greenhouse gases. According to the FAO report, "The livestock sector may well be the leading player in the reduction of biodiversity, since it is the major driver of deforestation, as well as one of the leading drivers of land degradation, pollution, climate change, overfishing, sedimentation of coastal areas, and facilitation of invasion by alien species."

The environmental effects of vegetarian and nonvegetarian diets have been compared in various parts of the world in terms of their use of natural resources and fertilizers. A California study found that a nonvegetarian diet requires almost three times as much water, two and a half times more energy, and thirteen times more fertilizer than a vegetarian diet. The researchers concluded, "From an environmental perspective, what a person chooses to eat makes a difference." [1-4]

Cooking and processing food also come at great environmental expense. Enormous amounts of natural resources are used to produce power for the industries that bring us these products and to package processed foods. Raw food requires little packaging and no cooking. Compared to the amount of trash produced from a typical diet of cooked and processed foods, the waste from a raw vegan diet is a small fraction—and the majority of it can go straight into the compost bin!

Most raw-food practitioners support organic agriculture, thereby voting with their food dollars against the use of pesticides, herbicides, and chemical fertilizers that would otherwise be dumped into our ecosystem.

PHILOSOPHICAL AND ETHICAL REASONS

Some people are attracted to a raw vegan diet because it is consistent with their deepest philosophical and ethical principles. They recognize the plight of animals in the factory-farming system and are unwilling to fund animal agriculture by purchasing its products. They refuse to support food corporations whose billion-dollar budgets come from refined foods that have been stripped of nutrients. Instead, they want to support organic and sustainable agriculture and the growing of plant foods. Such a choice can strengthen our connection with the natural world and reawaken our spiritual connection to all living beings.

What Is a Raw Vegan Diet?

A raw diet (also called an uncooked diet) is an eating pattern that consists primarily of uncooked, unprocessed foods. Some raw-food advocates suggest that in order for a diet to qualify as "raw," at least 75 percent (by weight) of the diet must be raw food. However, there is no formal consensus on this point, and definitions by raw-food leaders differ according to their unique perceptions of the ideal diet. Foods generally qualify as being raw if they have not been exposed to temperatures in excess of 118 degrees F (48 degrees C), although some raw-food leaders suggest lower maximum temperatures. Freezing food is considered acceptable. Although raw diets are most commonly vegan, raw vegetarian diets (those that include raw dairy products and/or raw eggs) and raw omnivorous diets (those that include raw fish, raw meat, raw eggs, and/or raw dairy products) are not uncommon. For the purpose of this book, we use the term "raw diet" to refer strictly to raw vegan diets.

People who adhere to a raw diet are often referred to as raw-food practitioners, raw foodists, or raw-food adherents. Other commonly used terms are raw-food enthusiasts and raw-food advocates, although these designations may also refer to those who are in the process of shifting toward or are very interested in a raw diet.

The most popular foods enjoyed by raw-food vegans are fresh organic fruits, vegetables, nuts, seeds, sprouts (seeds, legumes, or grains), and sea vegetables. A number of raw foodists include dehydrated foods such as crackers, cereals, sprouted raw breads, and desserts in their diets. Foods are sometimes marinated or warmed in a food dehydrator to create textures and flavors that resemble cooked foods. Food preparation can be simple or gourmet.

Among the fastest growing of all raw-food groups are those who eat a high-raw diet, or a diet that is 50–74 percent raw by weight. These individuals recognize the importance of increasing their intake of raw fruits and vegetables for optimal health. Some are aspiring raw-food practitioners and others are content to eat a high-raw diet that includes a modest amount of cooked foods. If you would rather not take the huge leap to a raw diet of 75 percent or more raw food, you can still enjoy many of the benefits of a raw diet by replacing processed foods, animal products, and some cooked foods with raw, organic plant foods.

There are numerous variations on raw diets, some requiring dietary restrictions or rules that extend beyond the parameters mentioned above. Three of the most well-recognized examples of more restrictive raw vegan diets are fruitarian diets, living-food diets, and natural hygiene diets.

Fruitarian and high-fruit diets. A fruitarian diet is one that is at least 75 percent or more fruit by weight. High-fruit diets are less restrictive, comprising 50–74 percent fruit by weight. Both of these diets include nonsweet fruits that are normally considered vegetables, such as avocados, cucumbers, olives, peppers, squash, and tomatoes. A number of fruitarians also include nuts and seeds in the "fruit" category. The remainder of the diet consists of raw foods that can be gathered without killing the plant. This can include carefully trimmed greens as well as coconut, nuts, and seeds. Some fruitarians believe that it is best to eat just one type of fruit at a time (known as a mono diet) and to wait at least forty-five minutes until another type of food is eaten. Organically grown or biologically cultivated fruits are preferred. Fruitarians may choose this diet based on spiritual and ethical concerns, as they don't wish to end the lives of the plants from which they eat.

Fruitarian and high-fruit diets providing larger amounts of greens, seeds, and nuts can meet nutritional requirements if they include reliable sources of vitamins B_{12} and D and are well planned. (See menus 3 and 4 in chapter 12).

Living-food diets. The terms "raw vegan diet" and "living-food diet" are sometimes used interchangeably, although there is a subtle distinction. While both living foods and raw foods are uncooked and contain enzymes, the enzyme content of living foods is much higher. This is because living-food diets emphasize the soaking and sprouting of raw foods. These processes result in an increase in the activity of enzymes, which are generally dormant in raw foods. The enzymes serve to release storage of carbohydrates, fats, and protein. While unheated nuts and seeds are raw foods, when we soak or sprout the nuts or seeds, they become living foods.

A living-food diet is centered on newly harvested greens, sprouts of all kinds, fresh fruits and vegetables, soaked nuts and seeds, live vegetable krauts, fermented nut and seed cheeses, cultured foods containing acidophilus and other probiotics (friendly bacteria), and some sea vegetables. The consumption of wheatgrass juice, green drinks, and green soups is encouraged, and baby greens, such as sunflower sprouts and pea shoots, are enjoyed in abundance. Foods dehydrated at low temperatures are eaten on occasion. Stimulating and salty foods are limited. A few foods, such as miso and unpasteurized tamari, that are not raw but are alive with friendly bacteria are included in a living-food diet.

Natural hygiene diets. Natural hygiene is a set of principles designed to help a person achieve and maintain optimal health by using fresh clean air, pure water, moderate sunshine, regular exercise, adequate rest, fasting when necessary, and a diet that is consistent with what ancient primitive peoples thrived on. Of all of these factors, diet is considered the most important. The International Natural Hygiene Society (INHS) does not endorse a single diet as being optimal; rather, it promotes a variety of diets that are consistent with what ancient peoples may have eaten. This includes the Paleolithic low-carbohydrate diet, the instincto-omnivorous diet (eating as guided by the senses), the lacto-ovo vegetarian diet, and a modified Herbert Shelton diet (a mainly vegan diet, described in more detail on page 12). All of these diets are predominately raw, most use the rules of food combining (see page 242), and all include a fasting component. The INHS does not recommend vegan or fruitarian diets to the public because "too many hygienists and others have died or become severely damaged using these diets for a long time." While many followers of natural hygiene follow the teachings of Weston A. Price, those on a more vegan natural hygiene diet follow Shelton's teachings, even though Shelton was lacto-vegetarian. The lack of knowledge regarding nutrients such as vitamin B_{12} may explain the early failure of vegan natural hygiene diets. It may also help to explain why proponents were not themselves rigid adherents.

Vegan natural hygiene proponents base their diets on organically grown fresh fruits, vegetables, nuts, and seeds eaten in their raw, natural state. Foods are generally consumed in their simplest form, with very little, if any, preparation, and only in permitted combinations. Dark leafy greens are included in abundance; refined fats (oils) are discouraged; and whole-food fats like avocados, nuts, and seeds are eaten sparingly. Many natural hygienists say no to fermented foods; sprouts; stimulating foods (like chiles, garlic, and onions); condiments (including pungent herbs, salt, and spices); sea vegetables; super-green foods like blue-green algae, spirulina, and wheatgrass; and nutrition supplements.

Are Cooked Foods Harmful?

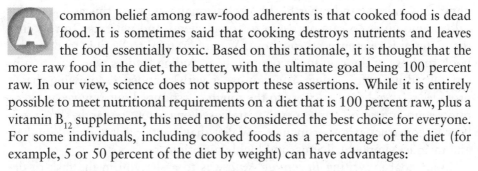 common belief among raw-food adherents is that cooked food is dead food. It is sometimes said that cooking destroys nutrients and leaves the food essentially toxic. Based on this rationale, it is thought that the more raw food in the diet, the better, with the ultimate goal being 100 percent raw. In our view, science does not support these assertions. While it is entirely possible to meet nutritional requirements on a diet that is 100 percent raw, plus a vitamin B_{12} supplement, this need not be considered the best choice for everyone. For some individuals, including cooked foods as a percentage of the diet (for example, 5 or 50 percent of the diet by weight) can have advantages:

- Some methods of cooking are safe and even beneficial in terms of reducing antinutrients and enhancing the availability of nutrients from certain foods. This is especially true for legumes, which provide a rich source of protein, iron, and zinc.
- Whereas this book is designed for adults, at some stages of the life cycle (for example, during childhood), the inclusion of some nutritious cooked foods that are higher in calories can be very beneficial. This can also apply to adults with especially high-calorie needs or when a high-protein diet with a low- or moderate-fat content is needed.
- During cold winter months, cooked foods, such as soups or stews, can be comforting and warming.
- Being rigid in our elimination of cooked foods can be socially isolating.
- In our efforts to move others toward a more compassionate way of eating, adding cooked items to the list of foods to avoid can make such a shift seem daunting. By allowing a greater variety of foods in the vegan diet, the transition becomes more achievable.

Although most of us would be well advised to increase our intake of raw food, the optimal percentage of our diet that should be raw is not clear, and some of the relevant factors extend beyond personal health. While some individuals will thrive on a 100 percent raw diet, others will find they fare better on a diet with some cooked food. No single dietary prescription is ideal for everyone. It is important that your diet be tailored to meet your unique needs.

The Road to Raw

 his book provides a reliable, well-researched guide for those who are moving toward a raw vegan diet (containing 75–100 percent raw food by weight) or a high-raw diet (containing 50–74 percent raw food by weight) and those who want to increase the amount of raw food they are eating. We expect that this book will appeal to people who would like to improve the quality of their diets in an effort to improve their health, though we do not give medical advice. As with our other books (such as *New Becoming Vegetarian, Becoming Vegan,* and *The Raw Food Revolution Diet*), we trust that health professionals—registered dietitians, medical doctors, naturopathic physicians, nurses, and other health professionals—will use this as a scientifically sound guide to raw nutrition for their clients and patients. To this end, the material is referenced throughout. We are grateful to be able to offer this book to those in the raw-food community, including leaders who inspire others toward healthful eating. You can use it with confidence, knowing that it provides science-based answers to the tough questions about raw vegan diets, offers sound nutrition guidelines that are based on current research, shows you how to construct a raw or mainly raw diet that meets recommended intakes, and includes simple, delicious, and highly nutritious recipes.

Our goal in writing *Becoming Raw* was to assist you in the task of designing a raw or mainly raw vegan diet that is not only nutritionally safe and adequate but also optimal. It is our hope that this book will provide the information that you need to construct a diet that will nourish your body and soul. May you move forward with confidence and conviction in your journey toward a gentler, kinder, and healthier world.

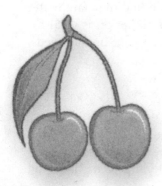

CHAPTER 2

A History of the Raw-Food Movement in the United States

BY RYNN BERRY

Modern raw diets, and even some of the more popular raw recipes, derive from the efforts of health pioneers in Europe and the United States whose work spans almost two hundred years. These early raw foodists run the gamut from religious leaders to showmen, horticulturists, and health professionals. Their motives for adopting and propagating a raw diet were many and various. Some were high-minded health reformers who wanted to protect themselves and others from the spread of infectious diseases and the ill effects of the industrial revolution. Others were utopians who sought to recreate paradise on Earth by reviving humanity's original diet. Still others sought the elixir of longevity, if not immortality, in a raw diet. Not all of them maintained strict raw diets, but many did, and each in his own way propelled the concept of a raw-food lifestyle into the twenty-first century.

The Early Raw-Food Movement

SYLVESTER GRAHAM

The raw-food movement in the United States started in the 1830s with Presbyterian temperance minister and vegetarian food reformer Sylvester Graham (1794–1851). Although best remembered for having given his name to the eponymous graham cracker and graham bread, he is considered to be the founding spirit of the American raw-food movement.

In 1830, a cholera epidemic had emerged from Asia and was cutting a deadly swath through Europe. It was poised to strike the United States when Sylvester Graham dashed to the rescue. Convinced that disease in general, and cholera in particular, could be prevented by drinking pure water and eating fresh fruits, vegetables, and nuts, Graham traveled throughout New England, Pennsylvania, and New York, expounding his dietary principles to overflowing crowds. When the cholera epidemic struck, it was noted that the people who had followed Graham's advice not only survived the epidemic unscathed but also had dramatically improved health. Overnight, Graham boarding houses, serving a vegetarian regimen (with an emphasis on organic whole-grain bread made with unsifted flour, filtered rainwater, and plenty of fresh fruits and vegetables), sprang up in Boston and New York.

Well before the cholera outbreak, however, Graham had argued in his lectures in favor of a vegetarian diet, preferably raw and ideally fruitarian. In his magnum opus, *Lectures on the Science of Human Life*, he writes that the simpler, more natural, and plainer the food of man is, the more health will be in his body, the more perfect may be his senses, and the more powerful may be his intellectual and moral faculties. He concludes: "By simple food, I mean that which is not complicated or compounded by culinary processes."[1]

He quotes ancient thinkers from Moses to Hesiod to Pythagoras, Hippocrates, and Plutarch, suggesting that many ancient peoples who occupy a prominent place in history may have consumed raw, largely vegan diets. Even the American aborigines, Graham contends, "subsisted to a considerable extent on the fruits of the earth."[2] As Graham construed them, all these sages of antiquity concurred in their view that the earliest inhabitants of their respective countries were vegan raw foodists.[3]

Recapturing the bodily perfection and freedom from disease and sexual dysfunction enjoyed by the "first family"—Eve and Adam—bulked large in Graham's program. What Graham meant by "the food of the first family" and "the food of the first generation of mankind" was "fruits, nuts, farinaceous [starchy] seeds and roots, some milk, and maybe honey." (Obviously Graham wasn't a vegan.) As a Presbyterian minister who was steeped in the Holy Scriptures, Graham must have had the image of "the first family," as he quaintly puts it—Eve and Adam and their immediate offspring—constantly in mind. According to Genesis, the first family were near-vegan raw foodists, in fact, fruitarians. Indeed, except for the milk and honey that was on offer, the first family would not have felt wholly out of place in a Grahamite boarding house.

To illustrate further his dietary theory that Eve and Adam were, in effect, "noble savages" who enjoyed heightened sensory powers and robust health while subsisting on fruits, nuts, and vegetables in their uncooked state, Graham cites the contemporary case of Caspar Hauser. Hauser was found living as an *enfant sauvage* (a so-called wild child) in Baden, Germany, confined in a dark dungeon from early childhood. For seventeen years, Hauser was forced to live "on an extremely simple vegetable-and-water diet."[4] At the time of his rescue, it was noted that although he could neither speak nor write, he had acute powers of sight, smell, taste, and touch. He could discern colors in almost total darkness; he could recognize people in a crowd from the distinctive sound of their footsteps; and he could distinguish among apple, pear, and plum trees by smelling their leaves at vast distances. He had an intense aversion to animal flesh and other cooked animal foods but was attracted to fruits, nuts, and vegetables.

Unfortunately, authorities were intent on converting Hauser to a typical German diet of animal flesh and overcooked vegetables. By slow degrees, they succeeded in accustoming him to what Hauser had regarded as "loathsome" fare, with the result that all his supernatural powers of vision, hearing, smell, and touch were diminished.[5] Eventually, he lost them altogether. For Graham, the story of Caspar Hauser recapitulated the fall of humanity through dietary error.

To illustrate the point that humans fare better on a predominantly raw vegetarian diet, Graham cites examples of the laboring classes throughout the world in the eighteenth and early nineteenth centuries, whose members were renowned for their vigor, stamina, and longevity. Unlike the diet of the American worker, which consisted mainly of white bread and overcooked meat and potatoes doused with greasy gravy and washed down with whiskey or beer,[6] the foreign worker's diet consisted mainly of spring water, whole-grain bread, raw fruits, and vegetables, and was just the sort of Edenic diet that Graham was trying to restore in the United States.[7]

BERNARR MACFADDEN

It was Bernarr Macfadden (1868–1955), a proponent of Graham's philosophies, such as temperance, antismoking, and drugless self-healing, who gave vegetarian raw foodism its greatest public exposure in the closing decade of the nineteenth and the first five decades of the twentieth century. During this period he ran a successful publishing empire while living ostentatiously on a raw vegetarian diet. (Later in life he backslid and included some meat in his diet.) As one of America's richest young tycoons, Macfadden could have indulged his appetite on a lavish scale; instead, he ate sparingly. A firm believer that calorie restriction promotes fitness and longevity, he usually limited himself to one meal a day, choosing to live chiefly on raw vegetables and fruit. On rare occasions, when he fell ill, he cured himself through fasting. In fact, a belief of Macfadden's that is similar to Graham's is that modern humans were once a robust species that had been enervated by eating boiled vegetables and the cooked flesh of animals.

In 1902, Macfadden opened one of New York's first vegetarian restaurants, Physical Culture (named after his fitness magazine), which served fresh juices and salads and, for a nickel, entrées like "hamburger steak," made from nuts and vegetables. By 1911, twenty Physical Culture restaurants, all vegetarian, had sprung up in Philadelphia, Chicago, and sundry other locations.

In 1936, Macfadden ran for the presidency of the United States, the first quasi-vegetarian raw foodist to do so. Even as an octogenarian in the mid-1950s, he continued to attract publicity with stunts like parachuting onto the grounds of his health hotel, the Macfadden-Deauville in Miami Beach, in order to exhibit his undiminished physical vigor.

HERBERT SHELTON

One of Macfadden's writers was Herbert Shelton (1895–1985), the moving spirit of modern raw foodism. Shelton felt forever grateful to Macfadden for igniting his interest in unfired food, as raw food was often called at the time. Like his mentors Graham and Macfadden, Shelton preached that cooking food not only robs it of its vital nutrients but also turns it into a toxic mess. Eating cooked food, Shelton contended, actually puts one's health at risk. "Cooking, the most universally employed process of denaturing our foods, is in every way injurious to foods and to man. Whether we cook plant substances or animal products, cooking is ruinous to the properties of the food."

After Shelton had established a health school in Manhattan's Upper West Side in the early 1920s, he moved to San Antonio, Texas, where he founded Dr. Shelton's Health School, supervised fasts, and wrote a spate of books on his new therapeutic system, which he called natural hygiene. An offshoot of naturopathy, natural hygiene is a philosophy of natural living that urges a raw diet of fruits, vegetables, and nuts. The principles of natural hygiene are not really new; they stretch back at least to Hippocrates, who had recognized that there was an innate power in the body to overcome disease and restore itself to health without medical intervention, as long as good health was not undermined by immoderate eating and drinking. In the event of illness, natural hygiene teaches that the body is a self-healing organism, which may be cured through periodic fasting in lieu of the drugs and often unnecessary surgery recommended by practitioners of conventional medicine.

In later years, Shelton failed to follow his own ideal regimen to the letter. According to associates, he often included milk products, such as cheese, clabbered milk, and butter, in his diet.[8] Like so many nineteenth- and early twentieth-century proponents of natural hygiene, Shelton paid lip service to the ideal without always putting it into practice.

However, even as Shelton was being pilloried by doctors who denounced fasting and raw foodism as quackery, he was gaining an international reputation as the ultimate authority on these subjects. His book *The Science and Fine Art of Fasting* had exerted an immense influence on Mahatma Gandhi, who frequently consulted the copy that he kept on his bedside table before making his public fasts.[9] Gandhi's contact with Shelton may have played a role in Gandhi's tendency to eat more raw food later in life. Vegetarian advocate and Nobel Prize–winning author George Bernard Shaw, who had become interested in naturopathy, living nutrition, and fasting as a nonagenarian, corresponded with Shelton shortly before Shaw's death at ninety-four in 1950.

SHELTON'S PROTÉGÉS

Shelton protégé T. C. Fry (1926–1996), author of *The Curse of Cooking*, was an enthusiastic proponent of fruitarian diets. In Texas, Fry founded the Life Science Institute and designed a highly regarded correspondence course in natural hygiene. Among his more illustrious graduates were Harvey and Marilyn Diamond, whose (nonvegetarian) *Fit for Life* books became best-selling popularizations of Fry's teachings. But Fry was less than steadfast in his practice of the fruit diet that he so fervently championed. He could frequently be found cheating massively on his diet with such prosaic dishes as dairy ice cream, macaroni and cheese, and other cooked items.[10] Did cheating on his diet hasten his demise? To be sure, he died an untimely death for a man who benefited from such superior nutrition, passing away at the age of seventy. But what probably hastened his mortality were the contentious bullet fragments that lodged in the back of his head when he was shot with a .22 caliber pistol by a spurned lover in 1982.[11]

Another protégé and colleague of Herbert Shelton was William Esser (1911–2002), a naturopathic physician and author of the book *Dictionary of Natural Foods*. Esser, a pioneering practitioner of natural hygiene and himself an ardent raw foodist, espoused looking to human biology for clues as to the ideal diet: "No less than all other living organisms, man has a need for foods best adapted to his biological needs. Historical evidence, the science of comparative anatomy, as well as comparative studies between meat-eating subjects and fruit-and-vegetable-eating subjects, clearly indicate that humans by nature are frugivores and not constitutionally carnivores."[12]

Esser gained preeminence as a fasting expert at his health retreat, Esser's Health Ranch, in Lake Worth, Florida. By 1983, he had supervised some 35,000 fasts. Unlike T. C. Fry, Esser stuck to his raw vegetarian diet (although he was not averse to eating an occasional piece of cheese). He displayed indefatigable vigor and energy into his nineties. In fact, a year before he passed away at the age of ninety-four, he thrashed his granddaughter at a strenuous game of tennis.

Still another protégé and associate of Herbert Shelton who deserves mention is Vivian Virginia Vetrano (1927–). She supervised innumerable fasts at Shelton's Health School, managed the school upon his retirement, and assisted him in editing his *Hygienic Review*. Like Shelton, Fry, and Esser, she is a practicing fruitarian. In her monograph, *Genuine Fruitarianism: The Ecological Sociable, Satisfying Diet*, she writes: "Superlative health can be maintained on a diet of fruits only, providing nuts and seeds, which are also fruits, are included. However, some individuals do better by the addition of some raw leafy vegetables to the fruit-and-nut diet."[13]

The German Naturalist Influence

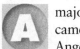

major influence on eating raw fruits and vegetables in the United States came from German émigrés who eventually settled in and around Los Angeles. Gordon Kennedy, in his book *Children of the Sun* (1998), offers two reasons these individuals sought a paradisal existence in Southern California. Germany was heavily industrialized at this time, and the younger generation, born in the 1880s and rebelling against the pollution of the landscape, promoted raw foodism, heliotherapy (the therapeutic use of sunlight), hydrotherapy (the therapeutic use of water), and naturism (nudism). Kennedy also suggests that there had always been a quiescent strain of raw foodism lying just below the surface in Germany, promoted by religious groups that desired to return to the primitive bliss of the Garden of Eden: going unclothed; worshipping nature in a kind of faux, naive pantheism; and feeding on a raw fruitarian diet.

Germany was also popularly perceived to be the seat of carnivorism and warmongering at this time. Despite (or perhaps because of) the bellicose temper of the country in 1896, Adolf Just, a naturopathic doctor, wrote a book called *Return to Nature*. Although Just did not migrate to the United States, his book shaped the thinking of an entire generation of American raw foodists. In *Return to Nature*, Just contends that humans were physiologically designed to live on a diet of raw fruit. Widely acclaimed and widely translated, it had become an international best seller by the turn of the twentieth century, and ads for the book appeared regularly in American papers (such as the *Los Angeles Times*) well into the 1930s.

An ardent admirer of Adolf Just's *Return to Nature* and a midlife convert to fruitarianism was Benedict Lust, born in Germany in 1872. Considered to be the father of naturopathy in the United States, Lust was a graduate of the Kneipp school of hydrotherapy in Germany. In 1896, he traveled to the United States as a representative of the Kneipp water-cure system, and in 1901 he opened the American School of Naturopathy in New York City. There he helped train such illustrious raw foodists as Herbert Shelton and William Esser, cofounders of the American Natural Hygiene Society. Paul Bragg, a noted health pioneer and a sporadic raw foodist, was also trained by Lust. In 1902, Lust founded the Naturopathic Society of America, which later became the American Naturopathic Association.

Shortly after Lust was married, his wife, Louisa, swayed by the writings of Louise Kuhne and Adolf Just, convinced him that he should adopt the fruit, nut, seed, and vegetable diet that Kuhne and Just so fervently touted. So well did Lust thrive on the fruitarian regimen that he started recommending it to his patients.

In 1925, Lust began publishing a best-selling health magazine, *Nature's Path*, and hosted a popular radio show, *The Air Show of Naturopathy*. Many of Lust's medical colleagues dismissed him as a charlatan out for personal gain, but the fact is, the pendulum has swung in Lust's favor—orthodox medicine has begun to incorporate many of the practices that Lust was promoting and his medical confrères were railing against.

Lust also helped Johanna Brandt, famous for her grape cure, to publish her raw-food manifesto. Having cured herself of cancer by living on a raw diet of her own devising (consisting mainly of grapes), the South African housewife was encouraged by Lust to write a newspaper article about it. To help her put it before the public, Lust introduced her to Bernarr Macfadden, the publishing tycoon and fellow raw foodist who had published and written an introduction to Lust's book *Fountain of Youth or Curing by Water* (1923). Macfadden offered to publish a condensed version of *The Grape Cure* on the front page of his newspaper, the *New York Evening Graphic*. When he published the lengthy article in 1928, it caused quite a stir, and when it went on to be published by Lust in book form, it became a raw-food classic.

Another German émigré who played a role in shaping America's raw dietary philosophy was Otto Carque. Born in Alsace in 1867,[14] Carque migrated from Mannheim, Germany, to Chicago in 1893. In 1905, he settled permanently in Los Angeles,[15] where he became a fruit farmer, health-food store owner, horticulturist, and food scientist. Carque was the first to employ the term "natural food" to refer to specific foods that are not refined or adulterated.[16] He was the author of many eloquent books on vegetarian raw foodism, starting with *The Foundation of All Reform* (1904), one of the first two books in the United States to be exclusively devoted to the subject of raw foodism.[17] In his books, Carque argues that a fruitarian diet offers a singular solution to the social and physiological ills that beset "overcivilized" humans.

A lacto-ovo vegetarian, Carque gradually refined his diet, increasing the amount of raw fruit he consumed. (Like most "raw foodists" of this period, however, he continued to eat dairy products and eggs.) The whole notion that a fruitarian diet could be health-sustaining is probably an idea that Carque took over from Just, who had maintained in *Return to Nature* that fruitarianism was a viable lifestyle.

Carque's fruitarian propensities led him to pioneer the use of unsulfured fruits and nuts as staples of the human diet. He is credited with developing the Black Mission fig and other unsulfured dried fruits. He also introduced into the California food landscape a variety of nuts and three different types of unroasted nut butters (almond, filbert, and peanut) that are familiar to us now but were novelties then.

One of Carque's bête noires was the conversion of fruit and grain into spirituous liquors, which he considered to be an enormous waste of nutritious food. Intriguingly enough, he attributes the increase in the thirst for alcohol to the rising consumption of cooked animal flesh and other cooked foods. He writes: "It has been truly said that cooks make more drunks than saloonkeepers." Carque so detested alcoholic beverages that he became a devout teetotaler and set out to popularize the drinking of unfermented wine, or grape juice, as a healthful alternative to wine. In the fall of 1905, using a technique that he had invented, he put up twenty-five thousand gallons of grape juice. Carque's promising life was cut short in 1935 at the age of sixty-eight,[18] when he was struck and killed by a car as he was crossing the street.

Perhaps the most influential of the German naturalists was Arnold Ehret, the author of such raw-food classics as *The Mucusless Diet Healing System* and *Rational Fasting*. Ehret was born in Germany in 1866. At the age of thirty-one, he contracted Bright's disease (an inflammation of the liver); Ehret didn't obtain a lasting cure until he visited an eccentric doctor, who put him on a fruit-and-water diet and told him to take air baths (go nude).

For all its simplicity, the system worked, and Ehret was restored to the vibrant health that he had known only as a youth. After being cured by the fruit-and-water regimen, Ehret was inspired to distill all that he had learned into a series of lectures, which formed the basis of his healing system. Subsequently, Ehret opened a clinic in Switzerland, where he treated thousands of patients by having them fast and follow a fruit diet.

After operating his sanitarium in Switzerland for fifteen years, he moved to Los Angeles in 1914. A popular speaker, he lectured on the health system that he had developed called the "mucusless healing system." Ehret contended that the standard Western diet—which abounds in cooked meats and starches—is mucus forming, and he believed that a diet that is disproportionately high in mucus-creating foods causes ill health and disease. Ehret argued that only through prolonged water fasting and the adoption of the mucusless diet could the body rid itself of accumulated toxins and be restored to its pristine vigor. According to Ehret, our innate desire for sweet-tasting foods after the body has been healed through fasting indicates that humans are physiologically destined to be fruitarians. Echoing the message put forth by Adolf Just in his book *Return to Nature*, Ehret's *Mucusless Diet Healing System* is a clarion call to return to humanity's inborn fruitarian diet.

As fate would have it, Ehret did not live to enjoy the protracted life span that his dietary system would seem to have promised him. After giving a series of lectures in Los Angeles, he fell victim to a freak accident, striking his head on a curbstone and suffering a basal fracture of the skull that killed him almost instantly.

Ehret's writings are more popular and influential today than they have ever been. An example of Ehret's enduring influence in Southern California is furnished by George Fathman, who, with his wife Doris, wrote a widely circulated raw-food recipe book, *Live Foods: Nature's Perfect System of Human Nutrition*. First published in 1967, it was still being advertised in the pages of *Living Nutrition* magazine in the first decade of the twenty-first century. It contains delicious, easy-to-make recipes that bear comparison with the best of today's sophisticated raw-food recipe books. Although Ann Wigmore, a popular raw-food health guru who was born in Lithuania, is commonly credited with creating recipes for nut milks and seed cheeses, the Fathmans' book, which contained similar recipes, appeared a decade before the advent of Wigmore. The Fathmans used nut milks and seed cheeses in place of dairy products, as they did not consider milk products fit for human consumption.[19] After reading Ehret's *Mucusless Healing Diet System*, the Fathmans immediately adopted a fruitarian diet that included soaked-nut milks and fermented nut and seed cheeses, as well as other foods.

The Fathmans were also interested in the writings of another German American apostle of raw foodism, John Martin Beinecke, who throughout the 1950s and '60s wrote a steady stream of articles advocating a raw vegan diet, accompanied by ingenious and delicious raw recipes of his own devising. Beinecke taught the Fathmans in person his techniques of gourmet raw-food preparation.

The first wave of German American naturalists lived off the land as free spirits. The second wave included people like Vera and John Richter (to whom Beinecke gratefully attributed his own dietary conversion to the raw-food program). The Richters started the first raw-food restaurant in the United States in Los Angeles in 1917 called the Eutropheon, which is Greek for "place of good nourishment." Richter became such an authority on the subject of raw foodism in his own right that he gave weekly lectures at the Eutropheon. These lectures were anthologized into the book *Nature: The Healer* (1936), one of the weightier tomes on the raw diet to be published in the United States. Vera Richter wrote one of North America's first raw-food recipe books using dishes from her restaurant's bill of fare; *Mrs. Richter's Cook-Less Book* (1925) became the forerunner of the modern raw-food recipe book.

The German naturalists, along with Carl Schultz (a pioneering naturopathic physician) and Bill Pester (a legendary fruitarian farmer-philosopher), practiced a more authentic strain of raw foodism than did American raw foodists like Herbert Shelton, Bernarr Macfadden, and T. C. Fry. The latter had a tendency to promote raw-food eating in their writings, while being rather fitful in the practice of it in their own lives.

Twentieth-Century Raw-Food Leaders in the United States

That raw foodism is not just a transient fad is further indicated by the fact that books in the United States devoted exclusively to the subject date from the first twelve years of the twentieth century and continue to this day. Eugene and Mallis Christian first attracted the attention of the popular press in 1903 when they threw a gala dinner party at which all the dishes in an elaborate four-course meal were uncooked. Although the Christians enjoyed the distinction of being coauthors of the first book published in the United States devoted exclusively to urging the adoption of a raw diet, *Uncooked Foods and How to Use Them*, their concept was not entirely original. Their book owes a great deal to the works of Adolf Just and other German nature doctors of the nineteenth century, with particular emphasis on Just's *Return to Nature* (1896).

From Just, the Christians borrowed the notion of the emancipation of humanity—especially of women—from enslavement to the tyranny of the cookstove. (This conceit lies at the heart of both *Return to Nature* and *Uncooked Foods and How to Use Them*.) In his *Return to Nature*, Just writes, "Consequently, when men no longer cook, they gain the following advantages: women need no longer ruin their health before the cooking stove, the source of poisonous vapors, where they acquire their many troubles and diseases."[20]

Eugene Christian went on to write several other books on diet, including *Eat and Be Well*, *Wheatless and Meatless Menus*, and *How to Live 100 Years*. The last title was poignantly ironic. During a lecture series he was giving in San Diego, he confidently predicted that he would live to be one hundred, but shortly after making this prophecy, he was taken with the first bad cold, he is quoted as saying, that he had experienced in thirty-seven years. Steadfastly clinging to the raw diet that he had championed since 1900, he died of pneumonia at the age of seventy-two.

In his *Unfired Foods and Tropho-Therapy* (1912), Chicago nutritionist George J. Drews states that "man's natural foods are fruits, the succulent herbs and roots, the nuts and the cereals, which in their natural (unfired) form appeal to his unperverted sense of alimentation." In 1912, influenced by noted raw-food author Benedict Lust, he started a raw-food journal, *The Apyrotrophers' Magazine*, featuring the writings of many of the prominent raw foodists of the 1920s and '30s, as well as a medley of raw-food recipes. A triumvirate of raw-food authors, Carque, Christian, and Drews—albeit largely forgotten today—exerted an immense influence on the nascent raw-food movement that was taking shape in the United States in the early part of the twentieth century and did much to educate Americans about the benefits of a raw vegetarian diet.

In the late 1920s, St. Louis Estes—an even more flamboyant raw foodist than the swashbuckling publisher Macfadden—cut a dash through American society. A wealthy dentist with a thriving practice in Manhattan, Estes converted to a raw diet at the age of forty-eight. In 1928, he wrote a best-selling book on the topic, *Raw Food and Health*.[21]

Although Macfadden may have been the first multimillionaire in the United States to become a raw foodist, Estes was the first health pioneer to become a multimillionaire by virtue of being a professional raw foodist. He lectured to overflow audiences in New York, Chicago, and Los Angeles and successfully marketed a back-to-nature line of food products and cosmetics. His second wife, Esther, authored a raw-food recipe book of her own, *Raw Food Menu and Recipe Book* (1927), which was the second such book penned in the United States after Vera Richter's *Cook-Less Book*.[22]

Today, of course, the raw recipe book, or "uncookbook," has become almost a genre unto itself, starting with Elizabeth Baker's *The UNcook Book*. This new genre includes such evocative titles as *Delights of the Garden*, all seemingly nostalgic for a utopian or Golden Age world.

NORMAN WALKER

Another immigrant to whom the raw-food movement owes much is Norman Wardhaugh Walker. Born in Italy to Scottish missionary parents in 1886, he is described as "the longest-lived, most widely known raw-food faddist of the modern era."[23] Walker moved to the United States at the age of sixteen and, in 1934, he invented what is still regarded as the world's most efficient juicer, the Norwalk Juicer. It subjects fruits and vegetables to the force of a hydraulic press. Not only does this method extract almost twice the yield of any other juicer, but it also produces juice that is said to be higher in enzymes and phytonutrients and lower in oxides.[24] This invention has been a boon to the raw-food movement, along with Walker's numerous books, written in the late 1930s, urging the adoption of a raw vegan diet. His book *Become Younger* (1948) recounts the details of his early life. He was raised on the standard diet of the period, which heavily emphasized animal flesh and starches, and had been a sickly child, suffering from chronic diseases. Alarmed by his enervated condition, his doctor recommended that he should travel to Brittany to convalesce with a peasant family, as he was fluent in French. He found an elderly couple who ate mostly raw vegetables and fruits from their garden and were willing to put him up for two dollars a week. While there, he made his first attempts at juicing. For himself, and for the couple who was fostering him, he manually pressed their soft, peeled carrots through some porous cloth, yielding a zesty juice. He writes: "Since these episodes in my young life, I have advocated a raw fruits and vegetable diet with an abundance of fresh, raw vegetable juices whenever possible."[25]

Walker strongly disapproved of dairy products, which he claimed form excess mucus in the body. But despite his tirades against consuming dairy products, Walker contradicted himself when he recommended relieving the monotony of drinking pure carrot juice by occasionally spiking it with a dash of goat's milk.

Because he died in a small town, Cottonwood, Arizona, to very little fanfare, overzealous raw foodists have exaggerated his age at death (from 109 to as much as 130 years) to give him an aura of superlongevity. Recently, however, reporter Kathryn Friesen decided to find out the truth. After a long search, she was able to determine that Walker died June 6, 1985, at the ripe age of ninety-nine.[26] Not bad for a sickly lad, born in the nineteenth century when life expectancy was about forty.

PAUL BRAGG

With a shock of white hair, bronzed, muscular physique, big toothy grin, and an irresistible sales patter, Paul Chopius Bragg (1895–1976) had all the attributes of a consummate health pitchman. Bragg never missed an opportunity to hawk his health products, which included apple cider vinegar, the supposedly raw Bragg Liquid Aminos (an ersatz soy sauce), and a collection of slickly produced self-help health guides, in addition to a string of health-food stores and expensive lectures. Patricia Bragg, who had been Paul's daughter-in-law,[27] assumed control of Bragg's health empire upon his death.[28]

Bragg was an alumnus of Benedict Lust's School of Naturopathy and doubtless imbibed his early fruitarianism from Lust. In his earlier writings, Bragg extolled the benefits of a fruitarian diet. In his book *Cure Yourself* (1929), Bragg states: "The ideal diet for mankind, undoubtedly, is the exclusive fruit diet, but because the race has lived on cooked and prepared foods for so many centuries, we cannot in one generation become fruit eaters. The most we can do is to change over to a diet of fruit combined with raw, uncooked vegetables, and even this change must be made gradually through what is called 'The Transition Diet System.' The principle of this Diet System is the step-by-step elimination from the diet of concentrated, artificially prepared, and devitalized foods and the gradual substitute of fresh fruits and succulent vegetables."[29]

In 1939, he self-published a raw vegan recipe book titled *Life Food Cookbook and Menus*. The chapter headings say it all: "No Meat," "Poisonous White Sugar," "Salt—The Enemy of Life," "Dairy Products Are Not Human Food," and "No Condiments." But a radically revised edition of Bragg's book was published in 1947 with a new title, *Paul Bragg's Health Cookbook*.[30] Bragg does a complete about-face by recommending that people eat a balanced diet of lean meats and some cooked foods.

Later, in his book *The Miracle of Fasting*, he reverted to an abhorrence of animal slaughter, and in an interview with the *Miami Herald* in 1973, he led a reporter to understand that he was still a vegetarian raw foodist. Unbeknownst to the *Herald* reporter, Bragg, by this time, had strayed far from his raw veg-etarian diet and had become an enthusiastic eater of hamburgers and other fried foods.[31]

That Bragg advocated eating small amounts of cooked meats and cooked vegetables toward the end of his life suggests that he may not have been the superb physical specimen that he made himself out to be. Legend has it that he died in a surfing accident in Hawaii at ninety-six, but as with Norman Walker, Bragg's age at his demise was grossly inflated to make him seem more advanced in years than he actually was. In reality, he died of a heart attack in his hotel room shortly before he was to give a talk at a health, diet, and fitness show in Florida,[32] and according to Bragg's death certificate, he was eighty-one years old—again, a fairly ripe age for a male born in the United States in the nineteenth century, but not exactly in a class with Methuselah. Nor does it inspire confidence in Bragg's ability as a life-extension expert. Yet, throughout his books (and even on their covers), Bragg proclaims himself to be a "Life Extension Specialist!"

Modern Practitioners: Sproutarianism and Living Foods versus Fruitarianism

fter Germany, the country that has contributed the most to the raw-food movement in the United States is Lithuania. (Finland has contributed more in the realm of academic research on raw diets, but Lithuania, through the works of Wigmore and Kulvinskas, has had a greater influence on the dietary practices of American raw foodists.) In fact, the foods that are most closely identified with the sproutarian side of the raw-food movement— sprouted beans, seeds, nuts, and fermented grains, plus the juice of pressed grasses—are the legacy of Ann Wigmore. Born in 1909 in eastern Lithuania, Wigmore learned her potent health secrets at the knee of her grandmother, who had been the village healer.

Remembering how her grandmother had healed her ailing patients by feeding them uncooked gruels and juiced grasses, Wigmore decided to follow the dictum of Hippocrates, "Our food should be our medicine," and start a health institute where she could treat chronically ill patients with food instead of medicine. In 1963, Wigmore founded the first Hippocrates Institute. She achieved miraculous healings there and at the various other Hippocrates heal-ing centers that she founded throughout the United States.

Another Lithuanian native who has contributed much to the American raw-food movement is Viktoras Kulvinskas. As a young man, his health was seriously compromised by his lifestyle proclivities, which included smoking three packs of unfiltered cigarettes and eating hamburgers and other cooked foods, washed down with twenty cups of coffee, every day.[33] Fortuitously, Viktoras found his savior and mentor in Wigmore. He helped her establish a Hippocrates Institute in Boston; then he launched his own successful career as an author and lecturer, promulgating the raw sproutarian diet that he had acquired from her. His book *Survival into the 21st Century* (with a preface by sometime-fruitarian, social activist, and comedian Dick Gregory, who proclaims his fruitarianism in his book *Dick Gregory's Natural Diet for Folks Who Eat*[34]) has become a raw-food classic.

Perhaps because the Wigmore regimen originated in the chillier climes of northeastern Europe where fruit is scarce, fruit composed a small proportion of the diet. For instance, Kulvinskas advocated a mono diet of fruit in his recipe book *Love Your Body: Live Food Recipes*, but, confusingly, he also advocated a diet that included sprouts, green juice, fruit, and steamed vegetables.[35] In Wigmore's book *Dr. Ann Wigmore's Complete Live Food Program*, she devotes almost the entire book to extolling the virtues of mung bean sprouts and alfalfa sprouts; however, fruits, such as melons and apples, are shunted to the back of the book.

Brian Clement, who is carrying on the work of Wigmore at the Hippocrates Institute in Palm Beach, Florida, openly touts sprouts as "a unique superfood with potent medicinal qualities."[36] He has relegated fruit to a tertiary role in his healing program. In his latest book, *Hippocrates Life Force*, he argues that fruit has been hybridized to create produce with a high sugar content, and that most commercially grown fruit is picked unripe.[37]

Two extremes of raw foodism—sproutariansim and fruitarianism—have their passionate adherents. Fruitarian math professor and amateur triathlete Chris Abreu-Suzuki opposes sproutarianism on ethical grounds; she regards germinated seeds as having potential life and believes that eating them is injurious to the unborn tree or plant. Instead, she would prefer to assist in the propagation of the plant by eating its fruit and scattering its seeds. For Abreu-Suzuki, eating sprouted seeds or beans is uncomfortably reminiscent of eating fertilized eggs.

Fruitarian author and food scientist Aris LaTham is an African American native of Panama who moved to the United States as a teenager. He is considered to be one of the founders of gourmet raw vegan cuisine in the United States. He debuted his raw-food creations in 1979, when he started Sunfired Foods, a live-food company in New York City. In the years since, he has trained thousands of raw-food chefs and added innumerable gourmet raw-food recipes to his repertoire, focusing on fruit dishes that require little, if any, preparation. He views sproutarianism as primarily a diet for sick people; while he recognizes its curative powers, he feels it is difficult to sustain as a permanent diet.[38]

David Klein, publisher of *Living Nutrition/Vibrance*, a journal that promotes fruitarianism, was inspired by a disciple of fruitarian advocate T. C. Fry to adopt a fruit-based diet and cure himself of ulcerative colitis. Klein believes that "my experience, studies, and observation of other fruit-eating people confirm that fruit is the ideal food for humans, and a fruit-based diet, including the non-sweet fruits (cucumbers, tomatoes, bell peppers, and avocados) is a key to mastering one's life."[39]

Fruitarian advocate Douglas Graham, author of *Nutrition and Athletic Performance* and *The 80/10/10 Diet*, explicitly recommends a fruitarian diet to competitive athletes and others.

WILD-GROWN RAW FOOD AND DAVID JUBB

Born on a remote island in Tasmania, Australia, in 1953, David Jubb is the author of the *LifeFood Recipe Book* and *Secrets of an Alkaline Body*. He holds that we should be eating only unhybridized, shade-grown fruits and vegetables that either are harvested from the wild or are "wild-grown." Jubb contends that such food is charged with electricity, or stored sunlight. We can recharge the electrical energy that courses between nerves and blood by eating food that is complete and whole and has kept intact its "vital electrics," the strong electrical force in fresh fruit and low-starch vegetables that are whole, organic, unhybridized, uncooked, and preferably in season, sprouted, soaked, and/or fermented. Unfortunately, it is almost prohibitively expensive and time-consuming to seek out unhybridized, shade-grown fruits and vegetables. Such a dietary philosophy, while laudable in theory, seems quixotic and utopian in the real world.

ESSENE AND CHRISTIAN RAW FOODISTS

It is remarkable how many of the leading figures in the contemporary raw-food movement in the United States style themselves as modern Essenes (a Jewish sect that existed in the centuries before and after the time of Jesus, the members of which "lived the same kind of life as that which Pythagoras introduced among the Greeks,"[40] which is to say that they were vegan raw foodists). Many raw foodists of today occupy positions in the modern Essene Church.

One of the most colorful self-styled modern Essenes was Johnny Lovewisdom (1919–2000). Lovewisdom maintained that humans wear out their bodies by subjecting them to a diet that is high in cooked animal protein and starch. According to Lovewisdom, as early as late adolescence the body senses that it is being poisoned and that death is imminent, so it activates the sexual reproductive system in a frantic effort to replicate itself, much as a dying tree puts out more seeds.

He believed that this accounted for the overemphasis on sexual reproduction and the eroticization of the typical Western lifestyle. However, by adopting what Lovewisdom called the Vitarian diet of living water foods, consisting mainly of juicy fruits, he contended that we can fight off the aging process and reverse the unremitting eroticization of our lives.

Although interested in dietary reform for nutritional reasons, Lovewisdom was not insensitive to the cruelty involved in eating foods of animal origin. And he spoke movingly of the heart-hardening effect that such a depraved diet has on those who consume it.[41] Unfortunately, Lovewisdom could not overcome his own addiction to cooked foods, and in later life he became a surreptitious consumer of cooked foods and animal milk—even though he continued to preach Vitarianism. From the start, he had condemned the eating of seeds and nuts, as well as animal flesh, milk, and eggs, and it is likely that his ideal diet was simply too austere for him to maintain. Nevertheless, Lovewisdom served as an inspiration for many young fruitarians.

Other modern Essenes draw their inspiration primarily from the works of Edmund Bordeaux Szekley. His works purport to be translations of original Essene gospels that Szekley is supposed to have discovered in a secret archive of the Vatican Library; they depict Jesus and the Essenes as fruitarians. Patristic scholars have cast doubt on the authenticity of Szekley's writings.[42] Some of the leading lights of the American raw-food movement who have embraced modern Essenism include Viktoras Kulvinskas; Essene minister David Wolfe, author of *Nature's First Law*, *Eating for Beauty*, and *The Sunfood Diet Success System*; and Essene minister Viktoria Boutenko, author of *The Raw Family* and *12 Steps to Raw Foods*.

Essene minister and master raw vegan chef Cherie Soria studied the healing benefits of the raw vegan diet with Ann Wigmore. She was catering the national Essene gatherings at Breitenbush Hot Springs, Oregon, when she met "the father of the raw living-food movement," Viktoras Kulvinskas. Kulvinskas was so impressed with the gourmet raw vegan cuisine that Soria had created utilizing her traditional chef skills that he encouraged her to start teaching chefs. As a result, Soria founded the world's first gourmet raw-food school, Living Light Culinary Arts Institute, which attracts students from all over the world, including top chefs from award-winning traditional restaurants. Soria has written two books (*The Raw Food Revolution Diet* and *Angel Foods*) and is considered the "mother of gourmet raw vegan cuisine."

Gabriel Cousens, author of *Conscious Eating*, *Spiritual Nutrition and the Rainbow Diet*, and *There is a Cure for Diabetes*, runs The Tree of Life rejuvenation center in Arizona, where he conducts Living Essene Way retreats. He offers instruction in Kabbalah as well, and the foods served during workshops at the center are kosher and raw.

HALLELUJAH ACRES

Another modern Christian group that promotes raw foodism is Hallelujah Acres, founded by George H. Malkmus, author of *Why Christians Get Sick*. In his book, he relates how, as a Baptist minister at the age of forty-two, he was diagnosed with colon cancer. He recalled that in Genesis 1:29, God states plainly that humans were destined to eat raw fruits and vegetables. Malkmus writes: "There is not one indication in the Bible that for the first 1,000 years after creation man cooked his food! Today if man wants to experience superior health and avoid sickness and disease, he must consume his food in a state just as close as it can be to the way God created it and intended man to consume it, without processing, additives, or heat, and grown organically."[43]

After healing himself of colon cancer with a raw vegetarian diet, Malkmus decided to dedicate the rest of his life to sharing his healing experience with others. To that end, he purchased a fifty-acre mountain farm in Edison, Tennessee, which he called Hallelujah Acres. Shortly thereafter, he founded the Hallelujah Ministry, envisioning that people could come to Hallelujah Acres and be taught how to make the transition back to the diet that God had given them in the first chapter of Genesis. Since starting his ministry in 1982, Malkmus has trained more than five thousand health ministers to go forth and preach the Christian raw-food lifestyle.

There is a nostalgia in the modern raw-food movement for the pristine diet of the Garden of Eden and the Golden Age. Considering some of the classic titles of books on raw-food preparation—*Delights of the Garden, The Garden of Eden Raw Fruit and Vegetables Recipes, Original Diet, Raw Food Revolution Diet* (which suggests a circling back to the beginning point), and Elizabeth Baker's classic *The UNcook Book*—one might be struck by a longing for a time when humans lived on a diet of unfired fruits and vegetables. Even the title of *The UNcook Book* suggests the idea of undoing, or correcting, the dietary wrongs that humans have wrought, implying that there was an original, right way of eating.

By taking up a raw vegan diet, we seem to be returning to the original diet of humankind. So there is an element of nostalgia in these titles, a hankering for a richer, disease-free mode of living, and a more nutritious way of eating that is popularly associated with the Garden of Eden. The implication is that we have lost our connection with the primordial paradise through cooking and that if we just got rid of our stoves and started eating unfired vegetarian food, we could uncook our way back to the garden of earthly delights.

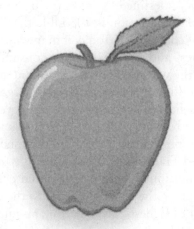

CHAPTER 3

The Raw Report: Scientific Evidence to Date

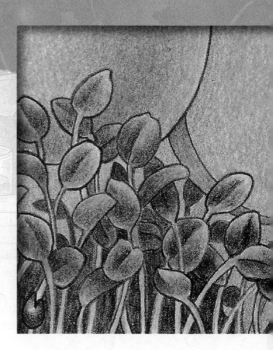

The evidence that vegetarian diets are safe and healthful has been accumulating for many years and is now well accepted within medical and scientific communities. In fact, it's the official position of the American Dietetic Association and Dietitians of Canada that "appropriately planned vegetarian diets—including total vegetarian, or vegan, diets—are healthful, nutritionally adequate, and provide health benefits in the prevention and treatment of certain diseases."[1]

At present, the weight of the evidence rests on lacto-ovo vegetarian diets, and on vegan diets to a somewhat lesser extent. Studies that have examined variations of vegan diets, such as raw- or living-food diets, are few in number. The majority of these studies have looked at only a small number of people for a short period of time. Most have observed raw-food eaters in Europe, although some work has been conducted in the United States. It's worth noting that, in the scientific literature, raw vegan diets and other raw diets and their variations are also described as "living-food diets" and "uncooked vegan diets." While these terms are frequently used interchangeably in scientific studies, distinct definitions exist for each (see chapter 1).

The research published to date on raw vegan and living-food diets in peer-reviewed scientific journals (where submissions are subject to scrutiny by other researchers in that field) is summarized in this chapter. We have excluded studies on raw nonvegan diets (that is, raw diets that include raw milk, raw eggs, or other raw animal products). The findings are divided into two subject areas: (1) raw vegan diets and chronic disease, and (2) the adequacy of raw vegan diets.

our intestines. This change is thought to significantly reduce the symptoms of rheumatoid arthritis. The theory is that living-food diets reduce the harmful by-products of microorganisms that can pass through the intestine into the bloodstream and initiate the formation of antibodies that attack these foreign invaders. In some cases, these antibodies also attack healthy tissue, because the by-products of gut flora found in this tissue are similar to substances that the antibodies were designed to destroy.[3] Five out of the seven above-mentioned studies examined microflora changes in the study participants.[3–6, 8] A significant, favorable diet-induced change in the fecal flora was observed in all the test groups following the living-food diet but not in the control groups.

Another popular theory regarding the success of all types of plant-based diets in reducing the symptoms of rheumatoid arthritis is that such diets generally result in weight loss. This was certainly the case in the above-mentioned studies, with losses averaging 9 percent of total body weight in the studies that reported on weight changes.[5, 7, 8] This theory was tested by pooling the results of three studies that examined the effects of lacto-vegetarian, vegan, or Mediterranean diets on rheumatoid arthritis.[9] The average weight loss was 5.3 pounds (2.4 kilograms) per person over a trial of three to four months. Looking at the change in body weight versus the change in symptoms of rheumatoid arthritis, no significant correlation was observed between weight loss and improvements in rheumatoid arthritis. While this doesn't rule out the possibility that weight reduction is helpful in decreasing the symptoms of rheumatoid arthritis, it suggests that dietary modifications are even more effective.

Some experts argue that the benefits conferred by "extreme" vegan diets are due to the removal of foods that have produced allergies and sensitivities in the patients.[10] Any diet that excludes trigger foods, such as dairy products, gluten-containing grains, or nightshade vegetables, may prove highly effective for those affected. (For more on this topic, see *Food Allergy Survival Guide* by Vesanto Melina, Jo Stepaniak, and Dina Aronson.)

Long-chain omega-3 fatty acids have also been shown to reduce the symptoms of rheumatoid arthritis. In 2003, a research study from Germany noted reductions in tenderness and swelling in participants served a vegetarian diet, while no changes were experienced on an omnivorous diet.[11] When long-chain omega-3 fatty acids (fish oil) were added to both diets, significant reductions in tenderness and swelling were observed, although they were much more pronounced in those consuming the vegetarian diet. Although vegetarians and vegans avoid fish oil, they can use microalgae-based omega-3 fatty acid supplements and take the necessary steps to optimize omega-3 fatty acid status. (See chapter 7 for further information on omega-3 fatty acids).

There are no studies comparing the effectiveness of raw vegan diets relative to cooked vegan diets in the treatment of rheumatoid arthritis. However, one study compared a group of volunteers who consumed a living-food diet for one week with a second group of volunteers who consumed the same items for the same amount of time, but all their food was cooked in a microwave for two minutes prior to consumption. The findings were largely positive for both groups; however, the reductions in toxic compounds and improvements in vitamin status were more pronounced in the participants following the living-food diet.[12] Some of the changes observed in the participants eating the living food have been associated with improvements in the symptoms of arthritis, indicating a potential advantage for living-food diets.

There are numerous studies assessing the use of standard vegan/vegetarian diets (containing greater amounts of cooked foods) for patients with rheumatoid arthritis. The authors of these studies have reported favorable changes in fecal flora, reduced pain and stiffness, and improvements in measurable indicators of rheumatoid arthritis that are comparable to the raw-diet studies.[13-25] In a 1995 Norwegian study, rheumatoid arthritis patients who followed a one-year lacto-ovo vegetarian diet experienced a reduction in the harmful bacteria *Proteus mirabilis*, while healthy omnivores in the study did not. *Proteus mirabilis* promotes urinary tract infections and kidney stones and has been strongly linked to rheumatoid arthritis. The researchers speculated that vegetarian diets may have antimicrobial effects resulting from intakes of compounds known to have antibacterial activity, such as lignans and other estrogen-like compounds. Experts advise that people suffering from rheumatoid arthritis could benefit from antibacterial measures that protect against *Proteus mirabilis*, such as the use of vegetarian diets and a high intake of water and fruit juices, especially cranberry juice.[26]

> **CONCLUSION:** Both living-food and standard vegan diets appear to offer significant benefits in the treatment of rheumatoid arthritis. Limited evidence suggests that living-food diets may provide additional advantages over conventional vegan diets in treating rheumatoid arthritis. However, further studies are necessary before specific recommendations can be made regarding living-food diets in the treatment of rheumatoid arthritis.

FIBROMYALGIA

Based on three studies to date, raw vegan diets appear to offer significant benefits for people with fibromyalgia.[3, 27, 28] Raw and living-food diets have been tested by two groups of investigators, one in the United States and one in Finland. In a U.S. study by Donaldson and associates, twenty patients on a high-raw diet were followed for a total of seven months.[27] Of these participants, fifteen people experienced a significant improvement in health. The severity of symptoms was reduced 46 percent (from 51 points to 28 points) in participants eating the prescribed diet, and their quality of life was rated approximately 20 percent higher after seven months. At the end of the seven-month trial period, the people who improved were no longer statistically different from healthy women of a similar age in scores of general health (with the exception of bodily pain, which was higher), vitality, and emotional and mental health.

A three-month Finnish study using a vegan living-food diet noted improvements in pain scores and significantly less morning stiffness.[28] Symptoms in these patients returned when they resumed a standard diet. These studies suggest that raw and living-food diets can significantly improve the symptoms of fibromyalgia in the majority of patients, at least in the short term. Larger, controlled trials would be needed to confirm these results and to determine whether raw and living-food diets could produce these benefits on a long-term basis.

It's interesting to note that fewer studies have been conducted using standard vegetarian or vegan diets. To date, only two such studies have been published, both of which reported beneficial effects. The first was a small study of ten patients in Norway.[29] In this study, researchers found that a three-week vegetarian diet produced improvement in patients' symptoms and lab-test results. A second study, conducted in India, compared thirty-seven patients treated with a diet free of animal protein and forty-one patients treated with the usual drug therapy, amitriptyline.[30] While the diet treatment resulted in a significant decrease in the patients' pain score, it was a less effective treatment than the pharmaceutical agent.

> **CONCLUSION:** From the available data, raw vegan diets appear to offer a viable treatment option for people suffering with fibromyalgia. Raw vegan diets appear to be even more effective than standard vegetarian and vegan diets, although further research is needed to confirm these findings.

CANCER

There are good grounds for assuming that a raw vegan diet would provide powerful protection against cancer and would be a sensible adjunct to treatment. However, the scientific evidence to date is limited and more research needs to be done.

A 2006 U.S. study by Fontana compared a number of metabolic markers (growth factors and hormones) for cancer. Insulin growth factor, or IGF-1, is known to promote tumor development by increasing cell division and preventing cancer-cell death. High IGF-1 levels have been associated with an increased risk of breast, prostate, and colon cancers. There were three groups of twenty-one participants each, matched for age, sex, and height. One group was composed of sedentary individuals following a low-calorie, low-protein, raw vegan diet for at least two years or longer. The second group was made up of lean endurance runners, averaging forty-eight miles per week, and the third group consisted of slightly overweight, sedentary participants who ate typical Western diets.[31] The body mass index (a measure of body fatness), or BMI, was similar in the raw-food vegans and the endurance runners but significantly higher in the Western-diet group. Growth factors (including IGF-1) were much lower in the raw vegan group than in the Western-diet group and significantly lower than in the endurance runners (even when body fatness was accounted for). Test results for several other metabolic markers of cancer risk were all more favorable for the groups with the raw-food vegans and endurance runners than for the group eating a Western diet. While both the raw-food vegans and the endurance runners have an advantage over the participants on a Western diet, the raw vegan diet appears to afford additional protection because it is associated with significantly lower growth factors such as IGF-1.

A small study out of Finland compared several laboratory markers of cancer prevention in forty women, twenty of whom consumed a living-food diet and twenty of whom consumed an omnivorous diet.[32] Compared to the omnivores, the living-food participants had less damage to DNA and/or better protection against DNA damage. The authors noted that this difference was due to diet and not to antioxidant supplements, as the use of antioxidants did not further improve results in either group. Serum vitamin C and beta-carotene were also higher in the living-food group, although vitamin E levels were lower. Although the results weren't statistically significant (due in part to the small number of participants), a few important differences suggest that living-food diets may confer advantages in cancer risk reduction.

A second Finnish study assessed changes in metabolic markers of cancer in participants who consumed a living-food vegan diet for one month, followed by their usual omnivorous diet for one month. The test participants were compared with a control group that consumed a conventional omnivorous diet for the duration of the study.[33] The researchers measured the activity of four different fecal enzymes, each of which is known to generate toxic compounds that have been associated with increased cancer risk. The activity of all four enzymes declined significantly—from 33–66 percent—within one week of beginning the living-food diet. Two other toxic metabolites declined from 30–60 percent within two weeks of beginning the living-food diet. All these favorable changes quickly disappeared when the participants resumed the omnivorous diet. No changes were observed in the control group. Several other studies have confirmed the positive effects of living-food diets on gut microflora and other factors that may prove beneficial in cancer risk reduction.[5, 6, 8, 34, 35]

There have been over two dozen studies from 1994 to 2008 that have looked at the relationship between raw and cooked vegetables and cancer risk. These studies were not done on people consuming raw or living-food diets; rather, they focused on the possible advantages of specific foods or components of foods. Most studies showed that as vegetable intake increases, cancer risk decreases, but the findings have been more consistent for raw vegetables than cooked vegetables. The 2007 World Cancer Research Fund/American Institute of Cancer Research (WCRF/AICR) diet and cancer report cited twenty-three studies that provided separate risk estimates for raw vegetable consumption.[36] Of these reports, sixteen showed statistically significant risk reductions with raw vegetable intake. None of the studies reported statistically significant increased risk with raw vegetable consumption. The studies also showed that the benefits were greater with higher consumption.

Three literature reviews have shown a more impressive advantage with raw vegetable consumption than with cooked vegetable consumption.[37–39] A 2004 review by Link and Potter from Columbia University in New York and the Fred Hutchinson Cancer Research Center in Seattle looked at studies published from 1994 to 2003 that examined vegetable consumption and the risk of various cancers.[39] A summary of these findings is provided in table 3.1, page 31. The

TABLE 3.1. Studies assessing cancer risk reduction from raw vegetables

Type of cancer	Findings		Comments
	Decreased risk with intake of raw vegetables	No relationship between raw vegetables and risk	
Breast	3 studies	...	Two studies showed raw vegetables but not cooked vegetables provided risk reduction.
Colorectal (colon and rectum)	5 studies	2 studies	One study found an inverse association only for raw vegetables, while 4 other studies found an inverse association for both raw and cooked vegetables.
Esophageal (esophagus)	9 studies	...	Two studies from a low-risk area of China showed very strong risk reduction with raw vegetables but not with total vegetable intake.
Female reproductive organs	2 studies	...	One study found an inverse association only with raw vegetables, not cooked.
Gastric (stomach)	10 studies	...	Three studies found cooked vegetables were unrelated to gastric cancer. One study of a high-risk population in China found raw vegetables to be strongly inversely related to gastric cancer.
Lung	2 studies	1 study	One study showed no association with cooked vegetables.
Oral, pharyngeal (pharynx), laryngeal (larynx)	9 studies	1 study (review article noted that the study was very small)	Two studies showed a much stronger risk reduction with raw vegetables. One study found risk reduction with raw but not cooked vegetables.
Pancreatic (pancreas)	1 study	...	Study found a significant inverse relationship between raw vegetable consumption and pancreatic cancer risk.
Prostate	...	2 studies	No relationship with either raw or cooked vegetables.
Urinary tract	...	2 studies	One study found benefits only with cooked vegetables but not with raw (authors noted that the population in question has a very low intake of vegetables and fruits).

Source: Data from reference 39.

authors suggested several reasons that raw vegetables might be more effective in protecting against cancer than cooked vegetables:

1. Cooking food decreases water-soluble and heat-sensitive nutrients such as vitamin C and numerous phytochemicals.
2. Cooking food disables enzymes that are responsible for converting certain phytochemicals into active compounds with powerful anticancer effects.
3. Cooking food produces changes to the physical structure of the food and alters its physiologic effects. For example, insoluble fiber may decrease, diminishing the food's ability to bind and excrete cancer-causing substances.
4. Certain methods of cooking produce substances that can alter DNA, such as those formed in the Maillard reaction, potentially increasing cancer risk. (See chapter 4, page 68.)

Since the Link and Potter review, three additional studies of interest have been released. One study examining diet and breast cancer risk found a nonsignificant risk reduction with cooked vegetable consumption. However, participants consuming between 67.4 and 101.3 grams of raw vegetables per day had only 63 percent of the breast cancer risk compared to those consuming less than 67.4 grams per day.[40] It is important to note that higher levels of raw vegetable consumption were not associated with breast cancer risk reduction.

Another study assessing the relationship between diet and bladder cancer found no significant associations for fruit, total vegetables, or total cruciferous vegetables.[41] However, when the total amount of raw cruciferous vegetables (or the amount of individual raw cruciferous vegetables) consumed increased, cancer risk decreased. The authors concluded that cruciferous vegetables, when consumed raw, may reduce the risk of bladder cancer. A third study examining the effects of diet on ovarian cancer found no significant association with vegetable or fruit consumption, with the exception of raw endive, which significantly reduced risk.[42]

No scientific studies to date have assessed cancer rates in people on raw diets compared to the general population or evaluated the effectiveness of raw diets in the treatment of cancer. However, with numerous testimonies and anecdotal reports of excellent outcomes, raw vegan diets would seem a reasonable choice for cancer research. Unfortunately, funding for this type of research is scarce, as it's difficult to obtain an exclusive patent (and rights to profits) on natural therapies. The most powerful evidence would be produced by randomizing cancer patients to conventional treatment (such as chemotherapy, radiation, and surgery) or to a vegan raw organic diet, alone or in combination with other natural therapies. However, such a study would be considered unethical because participants receiving the dietary treatment would be denied the established, evidence-based treatment, which is generally accepted as the most effective therapy available.

Another option would be to carefully follow cancer patients who have opted to forgo conventional therapy in favor of an alternative therapy such as a prescribed dietary regimen. Results, including five-year survival rates, could then be compared with those achieved using conventional therapies. An example of this type of study is one that used Gerson therapy to treat melanoma (the deadliest form of skin cancer) at various stages. Gerson therapy is a diet-based program. The daily nutritional regimen includes thirteen eight-ounce glasses of fresh, organic vegetable-and-fruit juice; three organic, largely vegan meals; and several fruit or vegetable snacks, as desired. Supplements of iodine, potassium, and vitamin B_{12} are provided, and coffee enemas are used as a detoxification method. The diet is very low in sodium and fat and excludes concentrated fats and oils, except for flaxseed oil in small amounts. Tobacco, alcohol, fluoride, foods grown with pesticides, and pharmaceuticals are avoided. The study compared five-year melanoma survival rates in 153 patients using Gerson therapy to rates reported in the medical literature with patients using conventional treatments.[43]

The five-year survival rates reported for this predominately raw vegan alternative dietary treatment are considerably higher than those reported using conventional therapy, although the total number of patients studied is too low to provide statistical significance. In addition, seventy-one Gerson patients were lost to follow-up and were excluded from the analysis. This may have biased survival results in favor of the Gerson subjects, as these patients could have died or otherwise responded poorly to the treatment.

Six additional studies have examined Gerson therapy, although they were not as impressive as the aforementioned study. Two studies looked at patients with colon cancer that spread to their liver and patients with breast cancer. Gerson therapy was initiated, and patients were compared to people receiving conventional treatment. In the colon cancer study, the average survival rate was longer for the Gerson subjects, although no significant difference in metastasis (cancer spreading to other parts of the body) or survival rate was

TABLE 3.2 Survival rates of melanoma patients on Gerson therapy and conventional therapy

Number of patients on Gerson therapy*	Stage of melanoma	5-year survival rate of patients on Gerson therapy	5-year survival rate of patients on conventional therapy with similar staging
14	I and II	100%	79%
17	IIIA	82%	39%
33	IIIA + IIIB	70%	41%
18	IVA	39%	6%

Source: Data from reference 43.

Note: Stage I melanoma is the earliest stage of the disease; stage IV is the most advanced.

*The number of patients using Gerson therapy was too small to reach statistical significance. Numbers using conventional therapy were much higher.

reported in the breast cancer subjects.[44] One study involved 108 patients with various late-stage cancers treated at one of three alternative therapy clinics in Tijuana, Mexico: the Gerson regimen clinic, Contreras therapy clinic, or Hoxsey herbal treatment clinic.[45] Of the thirty-eight patients treated with Gerson therapy, twenty did not follow up, seventeen died with an average survival of nine months, and one was still alive at five years. Finally, six patients reported remarkable improvement,[46] and ten noted improvement in overall health and regression of tumor masses.[47]

> **CONCLUSION:** Based on our current knowledge of food and food constituents, raw plant foods and raw vegan diets are very likely beneficial in the prevention of a number of diet-related cancers. Limited research data also suggests potential benefits for raw vegan diets in cancer treatment. However, further research is needed before any firm conclusions about raw diets in the treatment of cancer can be made.

CARDIOVASCULAR DISEASE

It is widely recognized that plant-based diets offer substantial protection against cardiovascular disease.[48, 49] Research has demonstrated significant reversal of the disease using vegan or near-vegan diets,[50-53] although studies of patients on raw vegan diets are limited.

The previously mentioned study by Fontana on metabolic markers for cancer also examined markers for cardiovascular disease (such as cholesterol, triglycerides, and blood pressure) in three groups of twenty-one participants matched for age and gender: low-protein, low-calorie, raw-food vegans; endurance runners consuming Western diets; and sedentary subjects consuming Western diets.[54] Both the raw-food vegans and the endurance runners had lower total and LDL cholesterol and triglycerides than the sedentary Western-diet participants, although the differences were greatest in the raw-food group. Endurance runners had the highest HDL (so-called good cholesterol), although the raw-food vegans had higher levels than those on a Western diet. Blood pressure was lower in the raw-food vegans than the endurance runners and much lower than in the sedentary Western-diet group. This may be explained in part by the raw-food vegans' low sodium intake: they averaged about 1,400 milligrams of sodium per day compared to 3,700 milligrams per day in the other two groups. A marker of inflammation called high-sensitivity C-reactive protein (hsCRP) was lowest in the raw-food vegans; however, both the raw-food vegans and the endurance runners had much lower levels than those in the Western-diet group. The sedentary Western-diet group had significantly thicker artery walls than either the raw-food vegans or the endurance runners. Thicker artery walls are an indication of plaque buildup. This study demonstrates significant cardiovascular advantages in both raw-food vegans and endurance runners; however, the advantages were greater in the raw-food vegans, particularly where blood pressure is concerned.

Another study of sixteen participants from Finland reported that total and LDL cholesterol (indicators of cardiovascular risk) were significantly decreased in two to three months when the participants followed a living-food vegan diet.[2] Other studies have confirmed cholesterol reductions in participants eating living-food diets.[4, 12] A study of 201 participants from Germany examined the effects of a raw vegan diet (70–100 percent raw) on cholesterol, triglycerides, folate, vitamin B_{12}, and total homocysteine.[55] Total and LDL cholesterol (so-called bad cholesterol) and triglyceride concentrations were reduced in the raw-food eaters. At the same time, however, HDL cholesterol was reduced and total homocysteine concentrations were elevated, both of which increase cardiovascular risk.

There is no doubt that whole-food, plant-based diets offer protection against cardiovascular disease. Raw vegan diets may offer additional advantages, as the consumption of antioxidant-rich vegetables and fruits are often increased, while processed foods containing refined carbohydrates and hydrogenated or partially hydrogenated fats tend to be eliminated. However, the protection against cardiovascular disease could potentially be undermined, at least to some extent, if intakes of vitamin B_{12}, vitamin D, and omega-3 fatty acids are too low. A lack of vitamin B_{12} causes a rise in homocysteine levels, possibly increasing the risk of heart disease.[56, 57] (See chapter 8 for more information on achieving excellent vitamin B_{12} status.) Poor vitamin D status is associated with several cardiovascular disease risk factors, including hypertension, obesity, diabetes mellitus, and metabolic syndrome, as well as cardiovascular disease events such as stroke and congestive heart failure.[58] Because raw vegan diets are deficient in vitamin D, warm sunshine and/or supplements become the principle sources. (See chapter 8 for more information on achieving optimal vitamin D status.) Long-chain omega-3 fatty acids (EPA and DHA) can help to reduce a number of markers of cardiovascular disease: high blood pressure, high triglyceride levels, platelet aggregation, inflammation, and cardiac arrhythmias.[59, 60] Long-chain omega-3 fatty acids come mainly from fish; however, raw-food vegans can improve their EPA and DHA status by consuming sufficient quantities of alpha-linolenic acid, the omega-3 fatty acid found in flaxseeds, walnuts, and certain other plant foods. If need be, they can also consume direct sources of EPA and DHA from vegan supplements or fortified foods. (See chapter 7 for more information on improving omega-3 fatty acid status.)

CONCLUSION: Raw vegan diets have considerable potential to prevent and reverse cardiovascular disease, as these diets are typically even richer in antioxidants, phytochemicals, and other protective nutrients than conventional vegan diets, which have proved to be so successful. Raw vegan diets also are lower in harmful compounds, such as trans-fatty acids and pro-oxidants, both of which are formed when foods are cooked. To provide maximum protection against cardiovascular disease, reliable sources of vitamin B_{12}, vitamin D, and omega-3 fatty acids should be included in the diet.

DIABETES

The story for diabetes is remarkably similar to that of cardiovascular disease. Substantial evidence suggests that prevention, treatment, and even reversal of type 2 diabetes are possible using whole-food, plant-based diets.[61, 62] While we would expect results to be at least as good, if not better, with raw vegan diets, to date few research studies have assessed the potential for prevention or treatment of diabetes with raw food.

One research group in the United States reported favorable fasting glucose, fasting insulin, and insulin sensitivity in raw-food vegans compared with people eating standard Western diets.[54] There is also strong evidence that raw vegan diets produce weight loss. (See Overweight and Obesity, page 37.) Studies have demonstrated that weight loss in overweight or obese type 2 diabetic patients is associated with decreased insulin resistance, improved blood glucose control, reduced cholesterol and triglycerides, and decreased blood pressure.[63]

Raw diets naturally have a moderate impact on blood glucose relative to conventional diets. Foods that cause the greatest spikes in blood glucose—such as flour products, starchy vegetables, and sugar-laden foods and beverages—are largely eliminated on raw vegan diets. Grains are limited, and when they are included, they are eaten intact, generally sprouted. In addition, raw vegan diets are rich in antioxidants, phytochemicals, and fiber. They contain few refined carbohydrates and pro-oxidants. While not yet published in a peer-reviewed journal, the work of Gabriel Cousens, a physician and advocate of raw vegan diets, is worth noting and following. Cousens has reported outstanding results with his twenty-one-day living-food program offered at the Tree of Life Rejuvenation Center. In his book *There is a Cure for Diabetes,* he explains his theory on how people can minimize the effects of disease-promoting genes and maximize the potential of protective, disease-preventing genes by making more healthful diet and lifestyle choices.[64] His program begins with a week-long green juice fast, followed by a completely organic living-food diet that is nutrient-dense, vegan, low-glycemic, and high in minerals. Within one to four days after starting Cousens' program, most participants stop taking various medications and insulin, as they no longer need them. In 2006, Cousens tested his clinical outcomes by inviting six people who were eating standard Western diets to participate in his program. He also invited an independent movie producer to film the participants' experiences, including "before and after" medical findings. Four of the participants had a diagnosis of type 2 diabetes, and two had a diagnosis of type 1 diabetes. One person whose blood glucose had fallen from 500 to 200 milligrams per deciliter in two weeks dropped out of the program because he was not willing to follow the diet. Five participants remained. Within four days, all participants, except one with type 1 diabetes, were off insulin and oral antidiabetic medications. By the end of one month, two people had normal fasting blood glucose levels averaging between 70 and 85 milligrams per deciliter. Two had dropped from average blood glucose levels of 250–450 milligrams per deciliter to approximately 120 milligrams per deciliter. One person with type 1 diabetes was able to lower his daily insulin intake from 70 units to 5 units. The other person, with a diagnosis of type 1 diabetes, is no longer on insulin and, according to lab tests, no longer suffers from diabetes. In 2008, the full-length film *Simply Raw: Reversing Diabetes in 30 Days* was released, chronicling the stories of these six individuals.

Less-than-adequate intakes of three nutrients that are consistently low in raw vegan diets—vitamin D, vitamin B_{12}, and omega-3 fatty acids—may accelerate the progression of diabetes. Recent evidence suggests that many people with diabetes or prediabetes have low levels of vitamin D, which may increase the severity of the disease.[65] Popular medications used to treat diabetes, such as metformin, may reduce vitamin B_{12} absorption, further contributing to decreased B_{12} status, increased homocysteine levels, and peripheral neuropathy (nerve damage causing pain and numbness in the hands and feet).[66] There is preliminary evidence suggesting that vitamin B_{12} may be an effective treatment for diabetic peripheral neuropathy.[67] Having low levels of omega-3 fatty acids increases the risk of depression in people with diabetes. There is also some evidence that a low intake of omega-3 fatty acids is associated with an increased risk of type 2 diabetes.[68]

> **CONCLUSION:** There is no doubt that raw vegan diets offer powerful therapeutic potential for the prevention, treatment, and reversal of type 2 diabetes and impressive treatment possibilities for people with type 1 diabetes. It is important, however, that raw-food vegans ensure adequate intakes of vitamin B_{12}, vitamin D, and omega-3 fatty acids.

OVERWEIGHT AND OBESITY

In 2005, approximately two-thirds of American adults were classified as overweight or obese, with about half of them being overweight and the other half being obese. The numbers continue to climb. Raw-food vegans seem to be well protected from unwanted weight gain. The diet and lifestyle habits at the root of the obesity epidemic are far removed from those practiced by raw foodists. When a raw vegan diet is adopted, weight loss almost always follows, especially in those who are overweight.

To date, at least six studies have reported weight loss with the adoption of a raw or living-food diet.[5, 7, 8, 12, 28, 69] Three studies of rheumatoid arthritis patients reported average weight losses of approximately 9 percent total body weight.[5, 7, 8] One study reported weight loss of approximately 22 pounds (10 kilograms) in men and 26 pounds (12 kilograms) in women for those participants who stayed on a raw vegan diet for at least three and a half years.[69] An average of 15 percent of the men and 25 percent of the women fell below the normal BMI range (<18.5 kg/m^2).

One study compared participants following a living-food diet for only one week to those eating the same foods prepared in a microwave oven for two minutes.[12] Interestingly, the living-food vegans lost 3.5 percent of their body weight, while the body weight of the vegans eating the cooked food dropped

4.8 percent. The authors noted that cooking the food in a microwave greatly diminished its palatability, triggering significant complaints from the participants, although they were said to have consumed their food portions as requested.

For further information about raw vegan diets and weight loss, read *The Raw Food Revolution Diet* by Cherie Soria, Brenda Davis, and Vesanto Melina.

> **CONCLUSION:** Raw vegan diets trigger weight loss in people who adhere to the diet. For people who suffer from chronic diseases, weight loss can produce a remarkable reduction in symptoms. Raw vegan diets seem to be a reasonable and effective option for those who struggle with overweight and obesity.

OSTEOPOROSIS AND BONE HEALTH

Only one study to date has examined the bone mass and bone health of raw-food vegans.[70] This study compared bone mass, vitamin D status, and C-reactive protein levels (a marker of inflammation in the body) in eighteen raw-food vegans and eighteen omnivores. The raw-food vegans had a mean body mass index (BMI) of 20.5 (indicating low body fatness but not underweight) relative to the omnivores, who had a BMI of 25.4 (indicating significantly higher body fatness and slight overweight). The bone mineral density at all sites examined (lumbar spine, total hip, and two additional hip sites) were significantly lower in the raw-food group than the omnivorous controls, with overall (total body) bone mineral density only 86 percent that of the controls. Reduced body weight, body mass index, and bone mineral density are strongly associated with increased fracture risk, and these were all lower in the raw-food group than in the control group. However, evidence suggests that bone quality also plays an important role in determining fracture risk. Changes in collagen, as well as oxidation and chronic inflammation, may negatively affect bone quality and increase bone fracture risk independent of bone mass. Circulating levels of C-reactive protein (CRP) were significantly lower in the raw-food group than in the control group. The authors were surprised to find that indicators of bone breakdown and bone formation were not significantly different between the two groups. These findings suggest that bone loss was not increased among the vegans and that their low bone mass may have been due to a temporary increase in bone loss or decrease in bone formation when they initially embarked on a raw diet and lost weight. It is also possible that some of the raw-food vegans had low body weights and low bone mass prior to their adoption of a raw diet.

Although the researchers expected the vegans to have low vitamin D levels because their dietary intake of vitamin D was extremely low, their blood vitamin D levels were significantly higher than those of the omnivores. The favorable vitamin D levels suggested better sun exposure among the vegans, which was verified by questioning the participants.

> **CONCLUSION:** In a single small study, the bone mineral density of raw-food vegans was found to be significantly lower than that of omnivores. However, it is possible that raw-food vegans may not have an increased incidence of fractures because of good bone quality. Clearly, further studies are required to determine the consequences of long-term raw vegan diets for bone health. It would be prudent for raw-food vegans to take the necessary steps to improve and maintain their bone mineral density. (See chapters 8 and 9 for more information.)

The Adequacy of Raw Vegan Diets

aw vegan diets offer tremendous potential for both the prevention and treatment of chronic disease. They can also support excellent health in adults when care is taken to ensure that all nutrient needs are met. However, studies of raw-food vegans suggest that calorie and nutrient shortages are common. It's vital that nutritional inadequacies be averted if these diets are to be embraced as viable alternatives for disease prevention or treatment, or for use by healthy individuals. The following is a brief summary of the research specific to adequacy issues. Further details are provided in the chapters that follow.

NUTRITIONAL ADEQUACY

Vitamin B_{12}

It is well recognized that vegans and other vegetarians who do not regularly consume reliable sources of vitamin B_{12} have poor vitamin B_{12} status.[71–75] Five studies to date have examined the vitamin B_{12} intake and status of raw-food vegans.[55, 76–79] The vast majority of participants in these studies had inadequate vitamin B_{12} status, and many suffered from vitamin B_{12} deficiency. The vitamin B_{12} status of raw-food vegans who do not include a reliable source of this nutrient is consistently poor. (For a complete overview of vitamin B_{12} research on raw-food vegans, see chapter 8, pages 166–172).

Essential Fatty Acids

To date, only one study has assessed the essential fatty acid (EFA) status of raw-food vegans.[80] In blood and other tissues, levels of highly unsaturated omega-3

Nutritional Intake and Nutritional Status

Two terms that are often used when talking about whether a diet is adequate are "nutritional intake" and "nutritional status." These terms are not interchangeable, although good intake often leads to a good status.

"Nutritional intake" or "dietary intake" refers to the amount of a nutrient (or other dietary component) that is consumed in the diet. Supplements may or may not be included in this assessment. "Nutritional status" or "dietary status" refers to a person's state of health as a consequence of both dietary intake and the assimilation of nutrients by the body. Nutritional or dietary status is generally measured by blood, tissue, or urine tests but also includes measurements of height, weight, and body fatness.

fatty acids were only about half that of the omnivores studied. It's very likely that the diet in this study contained high levels of omega-6 fatty acids relative to omega-3 fatty acids, although we don't know this for sure. Raw-food vegans should ensure a healthful intake and balance of essential fatty acids in their daily diets. (For a complete overview of the research on essential fatty acids and raw-food vegans, see chapter 7.)

Other Nutrients and Overall Nutritional Status

The dietary intake and/or nutritional status of raw-food vegans has been assessed in numerous published research studies.[4, 7, 12, 28, 31–33, 35, 54, 55, 70, 76, 78, 81, 82] Most raw vegan diets are rich in vegetables and fruits, moderate in nuts and seeds, low in grains and legumes, and free of meat, eggs, dairy products, and refined foods. As a result, intakes of nutrients that are concentrated in vegetables and fruits are naturally high in these diets. Raw-food vegans consistently have intakes of vitamin A (as provitamin A carotenoids), vitamin C, folate, potassium, magnesium, and phosphorus that are above the Dietary Reference Intakes (DRI). However, raw-food vegans seldom meet the DRIs for calcium, vitamin B_{12}, or vitamin D (although vitamin D is not usually a concern for those receiving adequate sunshine). Intakes of protein, B vitamins (other than B_{12} and folate), vitamin E, calcium, copper, iodine, iron, selenium, zinc, and omega-3 fatty acids can fall in either direction, depending on the specific food choices made. (For more information on each of these nutrients, see chapters 5, 7, 8, and 9).

CALORIE INTAKE AND BODY WEIGHT

The calorie intakes of raw-food adherents are consistently below those of the general population, and below levels commonly recommended for adults. Based on seven studies of raw-food consumers, energy intakes ranged from 1,460 to 1,989 calories per day, averaging approximately 1,700 kcal per person per day.[31, 33, 55, 70, 76, 80, 81, 83] These intakes are significantly lower than those typically considered necessary for healthy adults, although they are suitable for weight-loss diets. (For a more in-depth review, see chapter 5.)

Not surprisingly, these low-energy intakes are reflected in the lower body weights and BMIs of raw-food vegans compared to the general population.[31, 32, 54, 69, 83] While most raw-food vegans fall into the lower end of the healthy weight spectrum, some studies have found that a significant percentage are underweight.[69, 76] In one study, about 30 percent of the women younger than 45 years of age had partial to complete amenorrhea (cessation of menstruation) due to low body weight.[69] The researchers were so concerned about these findings that they advised against the long-term use of a strictly raw diet due to concerns about excessive weight loss.[69] Of course, it is possible to avoid underweight and amenorrhea by carefully planning the diet to include sufficient calories. (See chapter 5, pages 75–85, and chapter 12.)

Body Mass Index (BMI)

The body mass index (BMI) is a measure of body fatness in adults based on an individual's height and weight. Between two people of the same weight, the taller person will have a lower BMI. The formula for calculating BMI is weight in kilograms (kg) divided by height in meters (m) squared. BMI calculators are widely available on the Internet. The standard weight categories associated with various BMI ranges are shown in the table below:

TABLE 3.3 Body mass index (BMI) and standard weight categories

BMI	Weight status
Below 18.5	Underweight
18.5–24.9	Normal weight
25–29.9	Overweight
30 or higher	Obese

While BMI is a relatively good indicator of body fatness, it does have limitations. BMI is considered most accurate for adults aged 20–65 years. Older people generally have more body fat than younger adults. BMI does not factor in muscle mass; consequently, even when men and women have the same BMI, women tend to have more body fat than men. Athletes, particularly male bodybuilders, may have a high BMI due to increased muscle mass rather than increased body fat. Very short people (individuals under 5 feet/1.5 meters tall) may have a higher BMI than would be expected relative to their size.

DENTAL HEALTH

One study has examined the dental health of people whose diets are more than 95 percent raw.[84] This was a relatively large study with 130 subjects and seventy-six individuals in a control group whose age and sex matched the study subjects. Compared to the control group, subjects living on a raw diet had significantly more dental erosions (loss of tooth structure caused mainly by acid from foods such as fruit). Only 2.3 percent of the raw-food group had no erosive defects compared to 13.2 percent of the controls. Over 37 percent of the raw-food vegans had at least one tooth with moderate erosion (versus 55.2 percent of the controls), but 60.5 percent had at least one tooth with severe erosion (versus 31.6 percent of the controls). The results suggest that raw diets bear an increased risk of dental erosion compared to conventional diets. It's important to note that the raw-diet records showed that subjects on this diet ate almost five servings of citrus fruit a day. Total fruit intake was significantly higher than in the control group.

CONCLUSION: While the benefits of adopting a raw vegan diet are often quick and dramatic, the potential shortfalls can take many months or years to realize. The most common nutritional concerns associated with raw vegan diets are insufficient calorie consumption leading to underweight and amenorrhea, and vitamin B_{12} deficiency. Careful planning of raw vegan diets can help prevent nutritional deficits and ensure that all nutritional needs are met.

Well-planned raw vegan diets offer some compelling advantages for human health. The balance of this book is dedicated to assisting you in designing a raw diet that is enjoyable, protective, and nutritionally sound. Let's begin by exploring many of the specific components in foods that give raw vegan diets a unique edge for health.

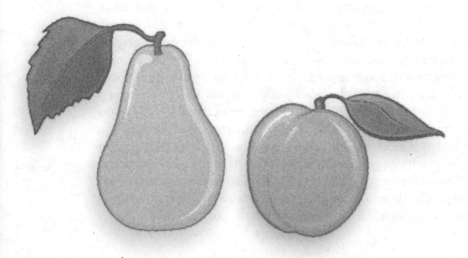

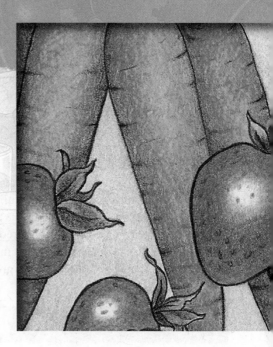

CHAPTER 4

Why Raw Rocks!

aw vegan diets offer impressive advantages, especially when it comes to body weight and to chronic disease. This is no surprise. After all, plant foods deliver nature's most powerful beneficial compounds—phytochemicals, plant sterols, antioxidants, fiber, and healthful fats. Conversely, the most potentially damaging dietary compounds are concentrated in processed foods and animal products. Moreover, cooking, especially at high temperatures, is associated with the formation of a number of compounds that may damage our health (see page 67). Needless to say, the vast majority of harmful foods are eliminated when we shift to a raw vegan diet. In this chapter, we will explore these compounds in some detail so that their relevance to health might be more fully appreciated.

Raw-Food Defenses: How Plants Protect Us

lants provide an army of compounds that defend us in a variety of ways. Let's consider how these little gems work their wonders and how various methods of preparation affect their actions.

PHYTOCHEMICALS

Phytochemicals are, quite simply, chemicals found in plants (*phyto* is the Greek word for "plant"). Whereas vitamin and minerals are essential for human life, phytochemicals are not considered essential for survival, although they appear to offer health benefits. Plants produce phytochemicals primarily for their own survival and protection. Some phytochemicals are responsible for the color, flavor, texture, and odor of plants, and they play a critical role in attracting pollinators and seed dispersers. Others act as an internal defense system that protects plants from pests, pathogens, and potentially hostile environments. Fortunately, when we eat plants, these phytochemicals continue their good deeds on our behalf.

It is estimated that there may be as many as 100,000 different kinds of phytochemicals, and often a hundred or more in a single plant, with thousands of copies of each.[1] Scientists expect many more to be discovered. Phytochemicals support optimal health by reducing the risk of chronic disease and fighting existing disease. With countless mechanisms of action, each phytochemical is a little miracle. The following list gives a tiny glimpse into their amazing activities:

Phytochemical Benefits

- Anticancer activities
  - block tumor formation
  - reduce cell proliferation
  - reduce oxidative damage to DNA
  - repair DNA damage
  - induce enzyme systems that help rid the body of carcinogens (cancer-causing substances)
- Antioxidant activities
  - neutralize free radicals, which damage vital components of cells, including DNA
- Antiestrogenic and weak estrogenic activities
  - antiestrogenic effects may reduce the risk of hormone-related cancers
  - weak estrogenic effects could help maintain bone density and improve blood cholesterol levels
- Anti-inflammatory activities
- Antibacterial, antifungal, and antiviral activities

- Cardiovascular protective activities
  - decrease damage to blood vessel walls
  - decrease oxidation of LDL cholesterol
  - decrease platelet stickiness
  - increase blood flow
  - lower blood pressure
  - reduce blood cholesterol levels
  - reduce blood clot formation
  - slow cholesterol synthesis
- Immune-enhancing activities
  - increase activity of cells that protect the body from microorganisms that cause disease
- Modulation of cell-signaling pathways, which regulate the growth, division, and death of cells
- Prevention of macular degeneration and cataracts
- Prevention of motion sickness
- Prevention of osteoporosis

There are numerous ways of classifying phytochemicals, most of which are based on chemical structure and function. Table 4.1, page 45, provides a detailed list of phytochemicals and their biological activities and food sources. While this is only a partial list, it provides some appreciation for the scope and complexity of this lively new area of research.

TABLE 4.1 Phytochemicals, their sources, and activities

CLASS *Subclass* Type	Food sources	Activities
PHENOLS AND POLYPHENOLS		
Monophenols		
Carnosol	Rosemary	Antioxidant, anti-inflammatory, anticancer
Carvacrol	Oregano, thyme	Antibacterial
Flavonoids (Polyphenols)		
Anthocyanins	Purple/blue foods such as blackberries, black currants, blueberries, cherries, plums	Antioxidant
Flavones (such as apigenin, luteolin, and tangeritin)	Celery, parsley, thyme	Beneficial effects against atherosclerosis, certain cancers, diabetes, osteoporosis
Flavonols (such as kaempferol, myricetin, and quercetin)	Apples, berries, broccoli, cherries, green tea, onions, red wine	Anticancer, antihypertensive, anti-inflammatory, antimutagenic
Flavan-3-ols (such as cathechins, epicatechins, and proanthocyanidins)	Dark chocolate, grapes, green tea, red wine, white tea	Antitumor, anticardiovascular disease activity
Flavanones (such as eriodictyol, hesperetin, and naringenin)	Citrus fruits	Antiallergenic, anticancer, anti-inflammatory, antimicrobial
Isoflavones (such as coumestrol, daidzein, genestein, and glycitein)	Soybeans, soybean products	Exert weak pro- and antiestrogenic effects
Phenolic acids		
Capsaicin	Chiles	Analgesic, anti-inflammatory, possible antitumor
Curcumin	Turmeric	Anticancer, anti-inflammatory, antioxidant, wound healing
Ellagic acid	Berries, grapes, nuts, pomegranates	Anticancer
Salicylic acid	Almonds, certain spices, fruits, peanuts, some vegetables	Anticancer, anticardiovascular disease
Tannic acid or tannins (such as gallic acid)	Tea and red wine	Antioxidant (note: tannins reduce the absorption of trace minerals, particularly non-heme iron)
Vanillin	Vanilla beans, cloves	Antioxidant
Zingerone (metabolized from gingerol)	Ginger	Anti-inflammatory, antioxidant, antinausea
Hydroxycinnamic acids		
Caffeic acid	Coffee, some vegetables and fruits	Antimicrobial
Coumaric acid	Basil, carrots, grapes, green peppers, peanuts, pineapple, strawberries, tomatoes, turmeric, wine	Anticancer, antioxidant
Ferulic acid	Cereal brans, cumin	Antioxidant

CLASS *Subclass* Type	Food sources	Activities
Stilbenes		
Resveratrol	Grapes, peanuts, red wine	Antioxidant, antithrombotic, inhibits carcinogenesis
Lignans		
lariciresinol, matairesinol, pinoresinol, and secoisolariciresinol	Beans, grains, seeds (flax, pumpkin, and sesame), some vegetables and fruits	Antioxidant, phytoestrogenic
TERPENES AND TERPENOIDS		
Carotenoids		
Alpha-carotene	Orange and yellow vegetables	Antioxidant, immune system enhancer
Beta-carotene	Green leafy vegetables, orange and yellow vegetables	Antioxidant, immune system enhancer
Beta-cryptoxanthin	Orange and red fruits and vegetables	Antioxidant, immune system enhancer
Lutein	Dark green leafy vegetables	Filters out harmful light, protects against macular degeneration
Lycopene	Red grapefruit, tomatoes, watermelon	Reduces risk of prostate cancer, may inhibit all cancer cell growth
Zeaxanthin	Corn, dark green leafy vegetables	Filters out harmful light, protects against macular degeneration
Monoterpenes		
Limonoids	Citrus fruits	Cardioprotective, induces enzyme systems required for detoxification of carcinogens
Phytosterols		
Beta-sitosterol, campesterol, stigmasterol	Corn, dark chocolate, legumes, nuts, seeds, soybeans, vegetable oils, whole grains	Reduces cholesterol absorption and total and LDL cholesterol
Saponins		
…	Legumes, especially herbs, soybeans, vegetables	Anticancer, antioxidant, cholesterol lowering, immune-enhancing
THIOLS (ORGANOSULFUR COMPOUNDS)		
Glucosinolates		
Indoles (such as indolyl-3-carbinol)	Cruciferous vegetables	Anticancer, favorably influences estrogen metabolism
Isothiocyanates (such as sulforaphane)	Cruciferous vegetables	Anticancer, potent inducers of Phase II enzymes (see pages 142–144)
Thiosulfinates		
Ajoenes, allicin, allylic sulfides, vinyl dithiins	*Allium* vegetables	Antibacterial, anticancer, antifungal, antiviral, cardioprotective

Source: Data from references 3–7.

In this table, three of the principal phytochemical classes are included: phenols and polyphenols, terpenes and terpenoids, and thiols (organosulfur compounds). Members of each class share some similarity in their chemical structure. Phenols and polyphenols are a huge and impressive class of phytochemicals associated with antioxidant and anti-inflammatory activities. Some also reduce tumor formation and growth, and reduce risk factors associated with heart disease and stroke. Terpenes include many thousands of types of compounds with a variety of beneficial properties associated with a lowered risk of heart disease and cancer. The most important subclass is carotenoids. Thiols are sulfur-containing phytochemicals which often emit a rather conspicuous aroma. Many of these compounds are known to stimulate enzyme systems that may help to reduce DNA damage. They are also recognized as having cardioprotective, antiviral, antibacterial, and antifungal properties. Some thiols serve as phytoestrogens.[2, 3]

Phytochemical Champions

Although colorful vegetables and fruits are the phytochemical champions, legumes, nuts, seeds, grains, herbs, spices, and teas deserve an honorable mention. The benefits of phytochemicals seem much more pronounced when we consume whole foods rather than supplements, as the natural combination of beneficial compounds in a whole food appears to have a synergistic effect. Studies that have examined phytochemicals in supplement form have shown their effects to be generally disappointing. Choosing a wide variety of colorful, whole plant foods is the key to a phytochemical-rich diet. Of course, there are superstars that can help to transform a good eating pattern into a phytochemical feast. Among the most noteworthy are dark greens (such as collards, kale, and spinach), cruciferous vegetables (such as broccoli, brussels sprouts, and cabbage), purple/blue fruits (such as blueberries and blackberries), tomatoes, citrus fruits, garlic, flaxseeds, and soybeans.

ORGANIC FOOD AND PHYTOCHEMICAL ADVANTAGES

Consumers have long speculated that organic produce may have greater concentrations of phytochemicals than conventionally grown produce. This makes perfect sense when we consider that phytochemical production is, at least in part, a function of stress on a plant. If a plant is attacked by microorganisms, it will manufacture greater amounts of phytochemicals in an effort to counter the attack. Organic produce receives more contact with naturally occurring microorganisms and pests than conventionally grown food because synthetic herbicides and pesticides are not used. This would lead us to assume that organic fruits and vegetables grown in rich soil under favorable conditions develop more of the phytochemicals that protect them naturally. The preponderance of research seems to support this theory and suggests that organic production methods lead to increases in phytochemicals, particularly organic acids and polyphenolic compounds.[8, 9] Of nineteen studies comparing the phytochemical content of organic versus conventionally grown foods, thirteen showed greater concentrations in the organic produce.[10–22] Five studies did not find any significant difference.[23–27] One study found that certain phytochemicals were elevated in the organic produce, while other phytochemicals were elevated in the conventional produce.[28] None of these studies showed significantly greater concentrations of phytochemicals in conventionally grown foods.

COOKING AND PHYTOCHEMICAL REDUCTIONS

Many people are aware that refining foods dramatically diminishes their phytochemical content. For example, turning wheat berries into white flour removes over 95 percent of the phytochemicals! However, far fewer people know that cooking can also adversely affect the phytochemical content of food. While the consequences are more variable than with refining, the bulk of the evidence to date suggests that cooking, in general, has a negative effect on total phytochemical content. Table 4.2, page 49, provides a summary of the research findings regarding both the positive and negative effects of cooking on phytochemicals in food.

Some research suggests that cooking increases the antioxidant capacity of certain phytochemicals. When this occurs, it is usually because the plant cell walls soften, making it easier for our bodies to extract these important compounds.[29, 30] These observations are usually associated with carotenoids. For most other phytochemicals, cooking has a negative effect. The cooking method, temperature, and cooking time all factor into the equation. Many phytochemicals are water-soluble, so losses are greater with boiling than with steaming. Losses are accelerated when the cooking time and temperature are increased. Among the most exciting findings, particularly for raw-food adherents, are the discoveries concerning two enzymes in vegetables: myrosinase and alliinase. (For further information about enzymes, see chapter 10.)

THE ENZYME STORY

Most experts in medical and scientific circles dismiss the idea that the enzymes found in raw plant foods survive in the human digestive tract in amounts that are significant enough to positively influence human health. However, there is an enzyme story that is rarely told, yet it is so solidly rooted in science that it sparks no controversy. Within two families of plants there are enzymes that are responsible for converting certain phytochemicals into highly beneficial, bioactive metabolites (breakdown products). The enzymes, myrosinase and alliinase, are physically separated from these phytochemicals in intact foods and are released only when the plant tissue is disrupted (that is, when the food is chopped, mashed, puréed, or chewed). Upon their release, conversion begins. Cooking foods that are rich in myrosinase and alliinase can destroy much or all of these enzymes, potentially wiping out some of the food's most impressive health benefits.

TABLE 4.2 Research summary of the effects of cooking on phytochemicals

Food studied	Findings
NEGATIVE EFFECTS OF COOKING	
Broccoli	Raw broccoli provided about three times more isothiocyanates than cooked broccoli, with myrosinase inactivated.[34]
	Microwave cooking resulted in a 74% loss of glucosinolates and boiling a 55% loss, due to the leaching into cooking water. Steaming had minimal effects.[40]
	Boiling and steaming eliminated the sulforaphane in fresh broccoli, while reduced losses were noted with pressure cooking and microwaving.[41]
	Glucosinolates and phenolic compounds were reduced with microwave cooking, in direct proportion to the cooking time and the amount of water used.[42]
	The estimated sulforaphane in humans was about three times higher after consumption of lightly cooked broccoli than fully cooked broccoli.[43]
Brussels sprouts, kale	19%–57% of the lutein, beta-cryptoxanthin, and zeaxanthin, and 14%–15% of the alpha-carotene, beta-carotene and lycopene were destroyed by microwave cooking.[44]
Cabbage	Glucosinolates were reduced by more than 50% due to leaching into cooking water.[45]
	Lightly cooked cabbage resulted in higher isothiocyanate content than fully cooked cabbage.[46]
	Boiling resulted in a 56% decrease in glucosinolates after 2 minutes, and an over 70% decrease after 8–12 minutes.[47]
Garlic	Raw garlic had significantly greater benefits to several markers of heart health than cooked garlic.[48, 49]
	Microwave heating for 30 seconds destroyed 90% of the alliinase, while 60 seconds virtually eliminated alliinase.[38]
	Cooking for 20 minutes at 212 degrees F (100 degrees C) reduced phytochemicals and antioxidant potential, while shorter cooking times did not.[50]
Greens, rice, wheat	Antioxidant levels were reduced with cooking.[51]
Leafy greens	Antioxidants in 30 different types of leafy greens were higher in raw vegetables compared to cooked vegetables for all samples tested.[52]
Mustard greens and cabbage	Isothiocyanate production was greater in subjects after their consumption of raw mustard greens and cabbage than the cooked vegetables.[53]
Onions	Flavonoid losses were 33% for frying, 21% for sautéing, 14%–20% for boiling, 14% for steaming, 4% for microwaving, and 0% for baking.[54]
Yellow and black soybeans	Boiling and steaming whole black and yellow soybeans resulted in significant decreases in anthocyanins, antioxidants, flavonoids, phenolic content, and tannins.[56]
Zucchini, beans, carrots	Phytochemical losses increased with the quantity of water used in cooking.[57]

Food studied	Findings
POSITIVE EFFECTS OF COOKING	
Carrots	Availability of alpha-carotene and beta-carotene from carrots was highest in cooked, homogenized carrots with oil; lower in cooked, homogenized carrots; lowest still in raw, homogenized carrots; and lowest in raw carrot pieces.[58]
Onions	Roasting onions at 356 degrees F (180 degrees C) led to an increase in bioavailable forms of quercetin, resulting in an overall beneficial effect.[55]
Sweet corn	Cooking at 239 degrees F (115 degrees C) for 25 minutes increased the total antioxidant activity by 44% and raised the phytochemical content (ferulic acid increased 550% and total phenolics by 54%).[59]
Sweet potatoes	Steaming resulted in nonsignificant increases in the concentration of total phenolics and phenolic acids.[60]
Tomatoes	Cooking increased total antioxidant activity and the available lycopene content but produced no significant changes in the total phenolics and total flavonoids.[61]
MIXED FINDINGS	
Artichokes	Cooking decreased flavonoid concentration but increased phenolic acid concentration. The antioxidant capacity of cooked artichokes increased after cooking up to 15-fold with frying and up to 8-fold with boiling.*[29]
Beets and green beans	With typical commercial processing, there was a 32% reduction in phenolic compounds and a 20% reduction in antioxidant activity in green beans, while antioxidant activity remained constant and phenolic content increased 5% in beets.[62]
Broccoli	Steaming increased phytochemical content, while boiling reduced phytochemical content, relative to the raw product. Both steaming and boiling resulted in higher levels of carotenoids and tocopherols compared to uncooked broccoli.[63]
Carrots, broccoli, zucchini	Phenolic compounds were greatest in the raw products, followed by fried, then steamed. Boiled vegetables had no detectable phenolic compounds. Carotenoids were highest in the boiled vegetables, followed by raw, steamed, then fried. Antioxidants were greatest in the fried vegetables, followed by boiled, steamed, then raw.*[30]
Cruciferous (*Brassica*) vegetables	Cooking by steaming, microwaving, and stir-frying did not produce significant loss of glucosinolates, whereas boiling showed significant losses by leaching into cooking water. Most of the glucosinolate losses (approximately 90%) were detected in the cooking water.[64]
Red cabbage	Glucosinolates increased with mild to moderate microwave cooking but were reduced by severe microwave cooking. Plant myrosinase activity was reduced by mild or moderate microwave cooking and destroyed with more severe microwave cooking.[33]

*The increased phytochemical concentrations were attributed to the disruption of the plant cells and increased extractability of the compounds by the chemicals used in the testing. This may not be reflective of what happens in the body.

MYROSINASE IN CRUCIFEROUS VEGETABLES

Myrosinase is necessary for sulfur-containing compounds called glucosinolates to be converted into bioactive metabolites called isothiocyanates. Glucosinolates are concentrated in cruciferous vegetables, giving these foods their distinctive flavor and pungent aroma. Isothiocyanates are highly prized for their ability to induce a group of enzymes in the body that help to inhibit cancer growth and kill cancer cells (for more information, see Phase II enzymes on pages 142–144).[31, 32]

Myrosinase activity increases with temperatures up to about 140 degrees F (60 degrees C), but deactivation occurs with higher temperatures.[33] Unfortunately, most methods of cooking involve temperatures above the critical mark, and further losses occur with increased cooking time.[34] When we eat raw cruciferous vegetables, glucosinolates are quickly broken down into isothiocyanates and absorbed into the bloodstream.[35] Conversely, when we eat these foods cooked, little or no myrosinase remains to initiate this reaction. Some conversion may occur in the intestinal tract through the action of intestinal microflora (friendly bacteria), although this is significantly less than what would be accomplished by active myrosinase.[36] Although unrelated to cooking, it is interesting to note that fresh cabbage juice contains high myrosinase activity, while little activity remains in the cabbage pulp.[33]

Cruciferous Vegetables

Cruciferous, or *Brassica*, vegetables include arugula, bok choy, broccoflower, broccoli, brussels sprouts, cabbage, cauliflower, Chinese cabbage, collard greens, daikon, garden cress, horseradish, kale, kohlrabi, mustard greens, mustard, napa cabbage, radishes, rutabaga, turnip greens, turnips, wasabi, and watercress. These sulfur-containing vegetables are noted for their distinctive anticancer phytochemical content.

ALLIINASE IN *ALLIUM* VEGETABLES

Alliinase is an enzyme found in *Allium* vegetables such as garlic and onions. It converts the organosulfur compound alliin to allicin, its bioactive metabolite. Allicin and its derivatives have been shown to possess anticancer activities (including the induction of Phase II enzymes) as well as antiarthritic, antibacterial, antifungal, antimicrobial, antiparasitic, antithrombotic, antiviral, and lipid-lowering abilities.[37]

Alliinase, like myrosinase, is destroyed by heat.[38] Research has shown that allowing garlic to stand for ten minutes after crushing it allows sufficient conversion of alliin to allicin to blunt some of the effects of heating.[38] However, it is important to note that some of the allicin is still altered or lost during cooking. Allicin in crushed garlic is degraded as cooking temperatures increase. The half-life of allicin (that is, the time it takes for allicin to be reduced by 50 percent) is about one year at 40 degrees F (4 degrees C), thirty-two days at 59 degrees F (15 degrees C), and only one day at 99 degrees F (37 degrees C).[39]

Allium Vegetables

Allium vegetables include chives, garlic, green onions, leeks, onions, and chives. These vegetables contain an extraordinary range of phytochemicals and are the richest sources of organosulfur compounds.

PHYTOCHEMICAL AVAILABILITY

Phytochemicals in raw food appear to have the same or better bioavailability as in cooked food (see sidebar, page 53); however, cooking is generally reported to increase the bioavailability of most carotenoids.[59, 66–71]

Some carotenoids—such as alpha-carotene, beta-carotene, and lutein—appear to be more bioavailable from vegetable juice than from raw or cooked vegetables.[71, 72] Women who consumed vegetable juice had almost three times the alpha-carotene and 50 percent more lutein in their blood than others who consumed the same amount of these carotenoids from raw or cooked vegetables.[73] Adding even a small amount of fat to a meal improves carotenoid absorption from foods, whether the foods are raw or cooked.[73–77] One study found that the addition of fresh avocado was as effective as avocado oil in increasing the lycopene and beta-carotene absorption from salsa, and the alpha-carotene, beta-carotene, and lutein absorption from salad.[78] In addition, consuming 75 grams (about one-half cup/125 ml, sliced) of fresh avocado with the salsa or salad was just as effective as consuming 150 grams.

Juicing, puréeing, or otherwise breaking a food down into smaller particles enhances the bioavailability of phytochemicals.[65, 76, 79] In addition, juicing removes a good portion of the plant's cell walls and membranes, reducing fiber and other compounds that can inhibit the absorption of nutrients and phytochemicals.

Research has shown that the conversion of glucosinolates (phytochemicals found in cruciferous vegetables) to isothiocyanates (the active forms of glucosinolates) is greater when we eat raw cruciferous vegetables than cooked cruciferous vegetables; their subsequent absorption is greater as well.[34, 80–82] One study found substantial differences in the bioavailability and absorption of glucosinolates and isothiocyanates from cooked vegetables, raw vegetables, and raw condiments (arugula, capers, garden cress, horseradish, mustard, and watercress). The amount of isothiocyanates absorbed from cooked vegetables was two to six times lower than from raw vegetables that were thoroughly chewed. This was likely due to the destruction during cooking of the enzyme myrosinase, which is required to convert the glucosinolates into isothiocyanates. The overall average bioavailability of these phytochemicals from raw vegetables was 61 percent compared to only 10 percent for cooked vegetables.[82]

Although cooking may positively affect the bioavailability and absorption of certain phytochemicals from foods, excessive cooking has been shown to

Carotenoids

Over 700 different kinds of carotenoids are found in nature, and nearly 50 are commonly found in our food supply. Six of these account for most (95 percent) of the carotenoids found in blood: alpha-carotene, beta-carotene, beta-cryptoxanthin, lycopene, lutein, and zeaxanthin.[65] Each has been shown to protect cells and tissues from free radical damage, some protecting the retina of the eye, some enhancing immune function, and others defending against heart disease, stroke, or cancer.[65] The carotenoids concentrated in leafy green vegetables (beta-cryptoxanthin, lutein, and zeaxanthin) tend to be more susceptible to destruction by heat than the carotenoids that predominate in yellow, orange, and red vegetables (alpha-carotene, beta-carotene, and lycopene).[44]

Bioavailability

Bioavailability is the fraction of any compound consumed that is absorbed into the bloodstream. If a phytochemical was extracted from a food and administered intravenously, it would be 100 percent bioavailable. However, when a phytochemical comes packaged inside a food and goes through the digestive tract, only a fraction of the phytochemical enters the bloodstream. In other words, only a fraction of the phytochemical is bioavailable. The bioavailability of a nutrient or phytochemical from a food depends on numerous factors:

- How the food is processed or prepared prior to being consumed; some methods—such as juicing, puréeing, mashing, mincing, or cooking—can increase the bioavailability of certain phytochemicals
- The presence of factors in the food that reduce absorption, such as certain types of fiber
- The presence of factors in the food that enhance absorption (for example, fat increases the absorption of fat-soluble phytochemicals)

- The quantity of the compound present in the food—greater concentration improves bioavailability
- The form in which the phytochemical is present; the atoms in a molecule can be arranged in a variety of ways, and some arrangements are more bioavailable than others
- The concentration of the compound already present in the person's bloodstream; high levels in the bloodstream generally reduce further absorption
- The physical state of the person, including the health of the intestinal tract and his or her genetic makeup; if a person has a damaged intestinal tract, bioavailability may be compromised
- Interactions with other compounds in the food and in the colon; some compounds enhance absorption while others reduce it

have an overall negative effect. When food is overcooked, products of oxidation may form, sometimes changing the arrangement of atoms within the food's molecules. This can make the food difficult to break down and be absorbed, resulting in reduced digestibility.[83]

> **CONCLUSION:** Cooking foods (such as blanching, boiling, steaming, frying, and canning) tends to decrease their phytochemical content. At the same time, these processing techniques can help to break down the plant cell walls, liberating certain phytochemicals and making them more easily absorbed.
>
> We can maximize the bioavailability of phytochemicals from raw foods by reducing the particle size of the food (such as by chopping, grating, mashing, milling, processing, puréeing, and chewing well). Juicing, which removes much of the plant cell walls, also can make phytochemicals more available. Including a source of fat when you are eating foods that contain fat-soluble phytochemicals will further boost phytochemical absorption. For example, add avocado or Lemon-Tahini Dressing (page 275) to a salad with carotenoid-rich green, orange, or yellow vegetables.

BOOSTING PHYTOCHEMICALS NATURALLY

Several studies have confirmed remarkable increases in phytochemical content and antioxidant activity when wheat berries were germinated (sprouted).[84–87] In one study, free radical–reducing ability (the ability to quench or stop free radicals) was greater in 1 gram of wheat sprout powder than in 1 milligram of standard, pure reducing compounds (these are agents that are used to stop free radical reactions, such as ascorbic acid, quercetin, reduced glutathione, and rutin).[86] Another study that examined the effects of germination on rye berries found a two- to three-and-a-half-fold increase in certain phenolic compounds.[88] It has been suggested that antioxidants synthesized during germination are essential in protecting new seedlings from the damaging action of free radicals.[89]

Phytochemical increases with sprouting are consistently noted among a variety of plants. Young broccoli sprouts were found to contain up to fifty times more glucoraphanin (a precursor of sulforaphane—both breakdown products of glucosinolates) than mature broccoli. Sulforaphane is the most potent natural inducer of the Phase II enzymes.[81, 90] More recent research has demonstrated that sulforaphane has impressive antimicrobial effects as well.[90, 91] In one study, seven out of nine patients who consumed broccoli sprouts eradicated *Helicobacter pylori* (*H. pylori*) infection within seven days. (*H. pylori* is a major global health problem associated with gastritis, peptic ulcer disease, and stomach cancer.) After thirty-five days, six out of seven patients were still clear of *H. pylori*.[91]

Fenugreek seeds, which are low in phenolic compounds and have poor antioxidant activity, are transformed when sprouted. Phenolic, antioxidant, and antimicrobial properties escalate, with the greatest increases seen during the first few days of sprouting.[92]

Fermentation also appears to boost certain phytochemicals in foods. For example, the levels of phenolic compounds and lignans were increased greatly by fermentation of germinated rye.[93] And the amount of anthocyanins and phenolic compounds were increased, along with antioxidant activity, in fermented black beans compared to nonfermented black beans.[54]

ANTIOXIDANT NUTRIENTS

Antioxidants are compounds that neutralize reactive and highly destructive molecules called free radicals. Free radicals have one or more unpaired electrons, making them extremely unstable. In a desperate attempt to obtain the much-needed electrons and become stabilized, they "steal" them from other molecules. This causes instability in the "victim" molecules, turning them into free radicals and beginning a destructive chain reaction. Some free radicals arise during routine body processes; others are formed by the body's immune system to neutralize viruses and bacteria. External factors, such as pollution, cigarette smoke, radiation, pesticides, chemical contaminants, and food components, can also generate free radicals. Normally, the body can handle free radicals, but if antioxidants are unavailable, or if free radical production becomes excessive, damage and cell death can occur. Free radicals can attack fats, proteins, carbohydrates, DNA, and RNA. Unsaturated fats, which are an essential part of cell membranes, are primary targets, because the more unsaturated the fat, the more vulnerable it is to free radicals. This oxidative damage can accelerate aging, cause degeneration of the brain and eyes, and contribute to numerous chronic diseases such as cancer, diabetes, and heart disease.[94–96]

Antioxidants serve us by donating the necessary electrons to stabilize the free radical; yet they are protected from becoming free radicals themselves because they are stable with or without the electrons they donate. In this way, antioxidants effectively stop the destructive free radical chain reaction. When our bodies are healthy, our internal production and external consumption of antioxidants is sufficient to take care of free radicals before they do too much damage. However, if the body becomes overwhelmed with assaults, free radicals can wreak havoc.

Increasing our dietary intake of antioxidants is one way to boost our defense system. In addition to providing a host of phytochemicals, foods rich in antioxidants offer several nutrients that contribute to our antioxidant army. Antioxidants work as a team, helping to extend one another's lives and improve performance. The nutrients with the most well-recognized antioxidant capacity are the carotenoids, which can be converted to vitamin A (alpha-carotene, beta-carotene, and beta-cryptoxanthin); vitamins C and E; and selenium. Vitamin A from animal meat and milk has no antioxidant activity. For further information on carotenoids, see page 145. In this section, we will focus on vitamins C and E and selenium.

Vitamin C

Vitamin C is a water-soluble compound that is distributed throughout all body fluids. Its storage in the body is very limited, so daily consumption of foods that contain it is important. The best sources of vitamin C are fruits and vegetables, particularly citrus fruits, guava, strawberries, kiwifruit, peppers, broccoli, and brussels sprouts.[97, 98] Vitamin C protects important molecules in the body from damage by free radicals. Vitamin C may also serve to regenerate other antioxidants such as vitamin E.[99]

Vitamin C is easily destroyed by light, heat, and oxygen. Cooking significantly reduces the vitamin C content of foods, often by 50 percent or more.[41, 100–104] However, even with a completely raw diet, significant depletion of vitamin C can be caused when foods are exposed to oxygen (air) and light. To minimize vitamin C losses, practice the following measures:

- Use fresh produce by shopping at least twice a week.
- Store produce in the refrigerator, preferably uncut.
- Eat vitamin C-rich foods as soon as possible after they are prepared.
- Drink freshly squeezed juice immediately.
- Keep food pieces fairly large, if the food must be prepared in advance.
- Slice citrus fruits right before eating them.

Vitamin E

Vitamin E refers to a family of eight antioxidants. The form of vitamin E that has the greatest significance for human health is alpha-tocopherol, which is the only form of the vitamin that counts toward the adult Recommended Dietary Allowance (RDA) of 15 milligrams per day. The form of alpha-tocopherol found in food is the most bioavailable. Although supplements can be made from all-natural sources of vitamin E, many are not. Synthetic vitamin E has only about half the potency of the natural alpha-tocopherol found in food.

Vitamin E is a fat-soluble vitamin and a potent antioxidant. Cell membranes are made of fats, predominantly unsaturated fats, and this makes them very susceptible to attacks by free radicals. Vitamin E is a perfectly designed security force that serves to protect these vital gates to our cells. When vitamin E neutralizes a free radical, it loses its antioxidant status. However, other antioxidants, such as vitamin C, have the ability to restore its activity.

Most people consume about half the recommended intakes for vitamin E, although intakes of those consuming raw vegan diets are significantly higher (see table 8.1, chapter 8). The best sources of vitamin E are nuts, seeds, whole grains, leafy green vegetables, and vegetable oils. Vitamin E is an essential part of the vital, germinating part of a seed, grain, or nut. Almost all methods of cooking result in some reduction of vitamin E as a direct result of oxidation. One study using various heat treatments found declines of vitamin E from less than 20 percent to nearly 70 percent.[105] An unexpected finding was that metal containers may interact with vitamin E to increase its losses. For examples, peas steamed in a metal pot had vitamin-E losses of up to 70 percent compared to no losses when a glass pot was used.[105]

Selenium

Selenium is a trace mineral that is a key component of several antioxidant enzymes. It supports the activity of vitamin E in preventing the oxidation of lipids (a family of fatty compounds that are insoluble in water). The best plant sources of selenium are Brazil nuts, sunflower seeds, whole grains, legumes, and mushrooms. Various cooking methods have not been found to have a significant effect on selenium concentrations in foods.[106] However, one study found that boiling asparagus and mushrooms led to 29 percent and 44 percent reductions respectively, due to losses in the cooking water.[107]

ANTIOXIDANT SUPPLEMENTS

While it may be tempting to take a supplement to boost antioxidant intake, we are a lot better off eating whole foods. Studies that have examined the effects of single-antioxidant supplements have been rather mixed, and several have been unfavorable. A case in point is beta-carotene. Evidence suggests that a diet rich in beta-carotene and other carotenoids protects us against lung cancer.[108, 109] In fact, studies have shown that people with high blood levels of beta-carotene have a reduced risk of several cancers.[110] Yet when beta-carotene was given as a supplement in three large trials, it increased the risk of lung cancer.[111–113] Although the reasons are not yet clear, it may be that carotenoids (and other antioxidants) work synergistically with one another and their collaboration is needed to produce the favorable effect. Loading up on a single carotenoid, such as beta-carotene, in supplement form may saturate the blood and reduce the absorption of the other protective carotenoids.

A second example is vitamin E. Two large studies demonstrated that as vitamin E intake from foods increases, the risk of heart attack decreases.[114, 115] Two additional large studies showed beneficial effects of vitamin E in supplement form.[116, 117] A major clinical intervention, the Cambridge Heart Antioxidant Study (CHAOS), found dramatic reductions in the incidence of nonfatal heart attacks in subjects taking 400–800 IU supplemental vitamin E daily.[118] It seemed that popping a vitamin E pill could be the ideal way to slash heart disease risk. Yet further clinical interventions failed to duplicate these findings—some found no effects from supplemental vitamin E, and others found a negative effect.[119–121] One vitamin E meta-analysis examined the results of nineteen studies with a total of over 135,000 participants receiving either a vitamin E supplement or a placebo (a dummy pill). The researchers found that people who took a high dose (400 IU or more) of vitamin E per day for more than one year had a slightly increased risk of death from a variety of diseases, including heart disease, compared to those taking a placebo.[122] (This "high dose" is the amount of vitamin E in five and one-third cups/one and one-third liters of sunflower seeds.) Another three meta-analyses of randomized controlled trials found no effect on heart disease mortality or deaths from all causes with high doses of vitamin E supplements.[123–125]

> **CONCLUSION:** The mixed results of the research has left both consumers and scientists a little bewildered. Antioxidants tend to work synergistically, and it is possible that when we increase vitamin E, we also need to increase many other antioxidants, such as coenzyme Q_{10} (CoQ_{10}), glutathione, lipoic acid, and vitamin C. Although taking antioxidant supplements in small amounts is likely safe, it is unlikely that taking concentrated extracts will ever provide the same potential for health as eating whole foods.

THE ANTIOXIDANT POWER OF VARIOUS FOODS

There have been many tests developed to measure the free radical scavenging activity of various foods. Each test is slightly different; they all evaluate a food's ability to fight certain free radicals but not necessarily all free radicals. Some foods that have a very high score on one type of test may not score as high on another. The most comprehensive of these tests is called the total antioxidant capacity (TAC). In 2004, a team of researchers measured the TAC in over one hundred foods.[126] The fifty foods with the highest TAC are listed in table 4.3, page 58. Foods that were analyzed in both their raw and cooked states are compared in table 4.4, page 60. You will notice that of the thirteen foods analyzed, eight had higher scores in their raw form, while five had higher scores when they were cooked.

TABLE 4.3 Total antioxidant capacity (TAC) of select foods

Rank	Food	Total antioxidant capacity (TAC)
1	Small red beans, dried (1/2 c/92 g)	13,727
2	Wild blueberries (1 c/144 g)	13,427
3	Red kidney beans, dried (1/2 c/92 g)	13,259
4	Pinto beans, dried (1/2 c/96 g)	11,864
5	Cultivated blueberries (1 c/144 g)	9,019
6	Cranberries, whole (1 c/95 g)	8,983
7	Artichoke hearts, cooked (1 c/84 g)	7,904
8	Blackberries (1 c/144 g)	7,701
9	Prunes (1/2 c/85 g)	7,291
10	Raspberries (1 c/123 g)	6,058
11	Strawberries (1 c/166 g)	5,938
12	Red Delicious apple (1 apple/138 g)	5,900
13	Granny Smith apple (1 apple/138 g)	5,381
14	Pecans (1 oz/28 g)	5,095
15	Russet potato, raw (1 potato/369 g)	4,882
16	Sweet cherries (1 c/145 g)	4,873
17	Black plums (1 plum/66 g)	4,844
18	Russet potato, cooked (1 potato/299 g)	4,649
19	Black beans, dried (1/2 c/52 g)	4,181
20	Red plum (1 plum/66 g)	4,118
21	Gala apple (1 apple/138 g)	3,903
22	Walnuts (1 oz/28.4 g)	3,846
23	Red Delicious apple, peeled (1 apple/128 g)	3,758
24	Golden Delicious apple (1 apple/138 g)	3,685
25	Fuji apple (1 apple/138 g)	3,578

Rank	Food	Total antioxidant capacity (TAC)
26	Deglet noor dates (1/2 c/89 g)	3,467
27	Hass avocado (1 avocado/173 g)	3,344
28	Green pear (1 pear/166 g)	3,172
29	Red Anjou pear (1 pear/166 g)	2,943
30	Golden Delicious apple, peeled (1 apple/128 g)	2,829
31	Hazelnuts (1 oz/28.4 g)	2,739
32	Broccoli rabe, raw (1/5 bunch/85 g)	2,621
33	Navy beans, dried (1/2 c/104 g)	2,573
34	Navel orange (1 orange/140 g)	2,540
35	Figs (1/2 c/75 g)	2,537
36	Raisins (1/2 c/82 g)	2,490
37	Red cabbage, cooked (1/2 c/75 g)	2,359
38	Red potato, raw (1 potato/213 g)	2,339
39	Red potato, cooked (1 potato/173 g)	2,294
40	Pistachios (1 oz/28.4 g)	2,267
41	Black-eyed peas, dried (1/2 c/52 g)	2,258
42	White potato, raw (1 potato/213 g)	2,257
43	Medjool dates (1/2 c/89 g)	2,124
44	Asparagus, raw (1/2 c/67 g)	2,021
45	Red grapes (1 c/160 g)	2,016
46	Yellow sweet pepper, raw (1 pepper/186 g)	1,905
47	Red grapefruit (1/2 grapefruit/123 g)	1,904
48	Beets, raw (1/2 c/68 g)	1,886
49	White potato, cooked (1 potato/173 g)	1,870
50	Orange sweet pepper, raw (1 pepper/186 g)	1,830

Source: Data from reference 126.

TABLE 4.4 TAC (total antioxidant capacity) of selected raw versus cooked foods

Food	TAC raw	TAC cooked
Asparagus	**2,021 (1/2 c/67 g)**	1,480 (1/2 c/90 g)
Broccoli	700 (1/2 c/44 g)	**982 (1/2 c/78 g)**
Broccoli rabe	**2,621 (1/5 bunch/85 g)**	1,322 (1/5 bunch/85 g)
Red cabbage	788 (1/2 c/35 g)	**2,359 (1/2 c/75 g)**
Carrot	**741 (1 carrot/61 g)**	171 (1 carrot/46 g)
Green sweet pepper	**664 (1 pepper/119 g)**	418 (1/2 c/68 g)
Onion, yellow	823 (1/2 c/80 g)	**1,281 (1/2 c/105 g)**
Red potato	**2,339 (1 potato/213 g)**	2,294 (1 potato/173 g)
Red sweet pepper	**1,072 (1 pepper/119 g)**	576 (1/2 c/68 g)
Russet potato	**4,882 (1 potato/369 g)**	4,649 (1 potato/299 g)
White potato	**2,257 (1 potato/213 g)**	1,870 (1 potato/173 g)
Sweet potato	1,173 (1 potato/130 g)	**1,195 (1 potato/156 g)**
Tomato	415 (1 tomato/123 g)	**552 (1/2 c /120 g)**

Source: Data from reference 126.

Note: The numbers in bold indicate the higher TAC.

OTHER PROTECTIVE COMPOUNDS

In addition to phytochemicals and antioxidants, other valuable compounds in plants help to protect our health. We will briefly consider two of these—fiber and healthful fats—and the health implications of consuming them from raw or cooked plant foods. (For more information on fiber, see chapter 6; for more information on healthful fats, see chapter 7.)

Fiber

When it comes to fiber, it seems to matter less whether we eat mainly raw or cooked foods than it does that the bulk of our diet is whole plant foods. Yet cooking changes fiber in a number of ways that could have practical implications for our health.

Although the total fiber content of food can be altered by cooking, the changes are slight. For example, indigestible starches can change into a more digestible form, which slightly decreases the food's total fiber content. Losses of digestible matter (such as sugars and minerals) into cooking water also result in an apparent increase in fiber. In some cases, however, fiber itself is lost in cooking water. Cooking commonly causes some of the insoluble fiber in food to become soluble due to the splitting of cell walls and softening of the plant tissues, although cooking food in salted water may cause cross-linking of some of the soluble pectin molecules, making them insoluble.[127–132]

Changes in plant cell walls also occur with cooking. For example, carrots have dense cell walls with a very clear pectin layer, which cements the cell walls together.[128] Blanching causes the carrot cell walls to swell and split. When more time and heat is used (as with canning), the cell walls swell further and the tissues lose their rigidity and stability. Not surprisingly, raw carrots elicit a lower blood glucose and insulin response than cooked carrots.[131] In addition, cooked carrots have a reduced ability to add bulk to stool. Generally, foods rich in insoluble fiber, such as wheat bran, significantly increase stool bulk;[133] however, cooking diminishes this effect.[134]

Other methods of processing such as blending or grinding alter the size of the fiber particles, changing their physiological effect. Finely ground foods generally do not absorb water when passing through our intestines as well as coarsely ground foods. As a result, coarsely ground food increases fecal volume more than finely ground food because it holds more water. For example, whole flaxseeds increase fecal volume more than finely ground flaxseeds.[135] Larger particles, whether raw or cooked, also slow the emptying of food from the stomach, as more work is required to turn the food into chime (a semifluid state) before it enters the small intestine. This reduces hunger and may help to reduce overweight.

We are still at the early stages of understanding how cooking affects the properties of fiber. While the changes in total fiber content from cooking are relatively small, the physiological benefits of fiber from raw plant foods may turn out to be more significant. It would appear that the maintenance of the cell matrix in raw plant foods positively affects blood glucose, insulin levels, and stool bulk compared with the same foods cooked, although these effects have not been well quantified.

Healthful Fats

Fat used to be considered a dietary villain. Today we recognize that while some fats are harmful to health, others are entirely healthful. There are even fatty acids that are essential (must be consumed) because we cannot make them in our bodies. These essential fatty acids are the most valuable of all fats to human health. Unfortunately, these valuable fats are very susceptible to oxidative damage (damage by free radicals). The more unsaturated the fat, the more susceptible it is to oxidation. The most unsaturated fats of all are polyunsaturated fats, which include the essential fatty acids (for more information on healthful fats and essential fatty acids, see chapter 7).

There are three things that cause free radical damage to fats: light, oxygen, and heat. Whole plant foods are naturally protected by their shells (nuts, for example), their skins (as with avocados), and their remarkable complement of antioxidants. When these foods are refined, these protective elements are often stripped away. When foods are improperly stored, they are subjected to light and oxygen. When foods are cooked, they are subjected to all three destructive factors. The consequences are noteworthy:[136]

1. Fats are damaged and essential fatty acids are destroyed.

2. Products of oxidation are formed that are damaging to human health. These include unstable, fat-based free radicals, such as hydroperoxides, which are responsible for the off-flavors and unpleasant odors of affected foods.

3. Proteins, vitamins, and pigments (phytochemicals such as carotenoids) are degraded.

4. Cross-linkages occur in the fats and other molecules in the food. This can result in molecules that are less digestible and foods that are less appealing and rather rubbery.

Products of oxidation increase in accordance with higher cooking temperatures and longer cooking times. Steaming and boiling produce few products of oxidation, baking produces somewhat more (depending on the oven temperature and length of baking time), and frying considerably more.

It is not difficult to understand why raw plant foods have an advantage over cooked foods where the quality of fat is concerned. One of the three villains (heat) is virtually eliminated on a raw vegan diet. However, the other two (oxygen and light) are still at large, and care must be taken in storing high-fat plant foods to preserve their precious but unstable fats. Once the shells or skins have been removed, fresh plant foods are best covered and refrigerated or frozen.

Damaged Goods: Assaults on Our Health

There is little question that becoming a raw-food vegan is a foolproof way to minimize or eliminate the most damaging dietary components. Transfatty acids, refined carbohydrates, and animal protein are all essentially omitted. Saturated fat, sodium, and pro-oxidants are significantly reduced. Let's briefly consider these dietary components and examine how choosing raw food affects our total intake of these potentially harmful products.

HARMFUL FATS

The fats that have been most consistently linked with chronic degenerative diseases are saturated fats and trans-fatty acids.[137] Saturated fats are found in all fat-containing foods, although they are concentrated in animal products and tropical oils. Saturated fats have consistently been linked to increased blood cholesterol levels, heart disease, several forms of cancer, and insulin resistance. As a result, the World Health Organization (WHO) recommends an upper limit of 10 percent of calories from saturated fat for the healthy population and 7 percent of calories for high-risk populations.[137] Most North Americans take in 20–35 grams of saturated fat every day, or 11–12 percent of calories for adults.[138] Vegetarian intakes are 8–10 percent of calories, and vegan intakes are 4–7 percent. Raw-food vegans fall in a range similar to the general vegan population,[139] although those who consume large amounts of coconut oil and other tropical fats push those numbers a little higher. It is important to recognize that not all saturated fats are created equal, and some appear to be more innocuous than others (for more information on the saturated fats in tropical oils, see chapter 7). Saturated fats are very stable and less prone to oxidation than unsaturated fats; that is why they are often used in cooking and in processed foods.

If we think of poly- and monounsaturated fats as "the good" and saturated fats as "the bad," trans fats are definitely "the ugly." Trans-fatty acids are produced when liquid oils are turned into hard, stable fats by a process called hydrogenation. Approximately 90 percent of the trans-fatty acids in the food supply are produced in this manner. The remaining 10 percent are formed naturally from bacterial fermentation within the intestinal tract of ruminant animals.

Trans-fatty acids raise damaging Lp(a) (a variation of LDL cholesterol and an important risk factor for atherosclerosis), triglyceride levels, and blood pressure, while lowering beneficial HDL cholesterol and raising the ratio of total cholesterol to HDL cholesterol (lower ratios are better).[140, 141] They also increase markers of inflammation.[142] In addition, trans-fatty acids compete against the essential fatty acids for incorporation into cell membranes, negatively affecting the shape, permeability, flexibility, and function of the cells. Not surprisingly, trans-fatty acids have been shown to increase the risk of several chronic diseases, including heart disease and type 2 diabetes. The WHO recommends that trans-fatty acids not exceed 1 percent of calories.[137] The Institute of Medicine did not set an upper limit for trans-fatty acids because any incremental increase in trans-fatty acid intake increases coronary artery risk.[143]

In the Nurse's Health Study, researchers found that the risk of coronary artery disease could be slashed by 53 percent merely by replacing 2 percent of calories from trans fats with unsaturated oils that are free of trans fats. By comparison, replacing 5 percent of calories from saturated fats with unsaturated fats free of trans fats reduces the risk of coronary artery disease by 43 percent.[144] Gram for gram, this makes trans fats more than twice as damaging as saturated fats. One of the tremendous benefits of a raw vegan diet is that trans fats are virtually eliminated. This is not necessarily true of other vegan diets, because processed foods, such as chips and crackers, are often included and can contribute significant amounts of trans-fatty acids.

REFINED CARBOHYDRATES

The majority of calories in typical Western diets come from foods composed of refined carbohydrates—sugars and starches. Heavy reliance on these foods results in disastrous consequences for health. Refined carbohydrates wreak havoc with blood glucose, adversely affect triglyceride levels, and increase the risk of chronic diseases, such as type 2 diabetes and heart disease.[145] In addition, when foods high in refined carbohydrates make up the majority of the diet, there is little room left for foods that nourish and protect us. (For more information on refined carbohydrates, see chapter 6).

Becoming vegetarian or even vegan doesn't guarantee a reduced intake of refined carbohydrates. One of the biggest blunders that vegetarians make when they renounce chicken, steaks, pork chops, and fish is to replace them with pasta, pizza, grilled sandwiches, and veggie burgers. People are attracted to familiar foods, so refined carbohydrates are a popular choice. Raw-food followers never make this mistake. Refined carbohydrates are not in whole, unprocessed plant foods, so intake is minimal in raw vegan diets.

SODIUM

Sodium is a mineral essential to life. It is necessary for maintaining fluid balance, transmitting nerve impulses, and supporting digestive processes. Nonetheless, most North Americans take in far more than is necessary, and in many cases this surplus contributes to health problems. Excessive sodium consumption has been linked to hypertension, increasing the risk of heart attack, stroke, and kidney disease.[146] High sodium intakes may also increase the risk of stomach cancer[147] and induce urinary calcium losses.[148]

The primary source of sodium in the diet is salt (sodium chloride). Salt is 40 percent sodium and 60 percent chloride. Relatively small amounts of sodium occur naturally in foods (other than foods from the sea). Throughout history, salt has been rare and highly prized. Roman soldiers were paid partly in salt; the Latin word *salarium* (meaning "salt money") is the root of the English word "salary." Times have changed! About 77 percent of the salt consumed in North America comes from processed foods, 11 percent from salt added at the table or during cooking, and 12 percent from the sodium naturally present in foods.[146]

The Adequate Intake (AI) for sodium set by the Institute of Medicine[146] is 1,500 milligrams per day for adults nineteen to fifty years of age, and slightly less for older adults (see page 195). These recommendations are for moderately active individuals living in temperate climates; active people living in hotter climates would require higher intakes. The upper limit (UL) for sodium is 2,300 milligrams per day. Over 90 percent of North Americans exceed both the AI and the upper limit for sodium. The UL (2,300 milligrams, or 2.3 grams) of sodium is found in 1 teaspoon (6 grams) of salt (sodium chloride). Vegetarians and vegans don't necessarily consume less sodium than nonvegetarians, although their average intake tends to be somewhat lower. Raw-food vegans do exceptionally well when it comes to optimal sodium intakes. Without processed foods, sodium intakes are naturally low. One study found that men on a raw vegan diet averaged just over 1,500 milligrams of sodium a day and women just over 1,200 milligrams a day.[139] It is possible that some raw-food vegans consume insufficient sodium, especially if they have high requirements due to perspiration losses in hot weather. Reliable sources of sodium, such as sea vegetables, should be included in the daily diet.

ANIMAL PROTEIN

Animal protein has been mistakenly placed on a pedestal in Western society. If people took a good hard look at the science, it would be swiftly knocked down. While eating meat is one way to get protein, it is associated with several negative health consequences:

- **Kidney stones.** Modern diets containing a lot of animal protein, refined carbohydrates, and salt increase the acid load on the body, which raises the risk of kidney stones.[149–151]

- **Cancer.** Animal protein may increase cancer initiation and promotion.[152, 153] The intake of red meat has been positively linked to colorectal cancer[154–157] and possibly prostate cancer.[156, 158, 159]

- **Diabetes.** Animal-protein intake, especially from red meat, and particularly processed meat, is associated with an increased risk of type 2 diabetes.[160–162]

- **Coronary artery disease.** Animal-protein intake may increase the risk of coronary artery disease.[163] Replacing animal protein with plant protein reduces blood cholesterol levels and other markers of coronary artery disease.[164–166]

Meat and other high-protein animal products come packaged with saturated fat, cholesterol, and numerous pro-oxidants. They contain no fiber, no phytochemicals, and very few antioxidants. The best place to get our protein is from plants. Raw-food vegans consume no animal protein, and when protein intakes are adequate, this is likely to work to their advantage.

PRO-OXIDANTS

Pro-oxidants are the antithesis of antioxidants, promoting destructive free radical reactions. When the supply of pro-oxidants exceeds the reserve of antioxidants, cell damage can occur and disease processes escalate. We cannot completely avoid pro-oxidants, as they are all around us. However, we can minimize our exposure to them by making wise lifestyle choices.

Air pollution, tobacco smoke, radiation, sunlight, stress, toxic wastes, and chemical contaminants in the environment can all contribute to oxidative stress. Among the greatest stressors of all are contaminants and other harmful substances found in our foods. The most well-recognized offenders are chemical contaminants, such as PCBs, DDT, dioxins, furans (found mainly in jarred and canned foods), and pesticides (including herbicides and fungicides); rancid fats and fats damaged by high-temperature cooking; metals, including cadmium, chromium, cobalt, copper, iron, mercury, nickel (in specific forms), and vanadium; and finally, alcohol.

Not surprisingly, chemical contaminants, such as PCBs, DDT, dioxins, and furans, move up the food chain, resulting in the greatest concentrations of these compounds in beef, pork, poultry, fish, eggs, dairy products, and other animal products.[167] The highest concentrations of dioxins come from farmed fish, freshwater fish (especially from polluted waters), shellfish, and marine fish.[167, 168] Plant foods contain very low levels of dioxins.

Insecticides, herbicides, and fungicides are found mainly on the surface of the plants that are treated with these chemicals, and in the flesh and milk of animals that consume these plants. A recent study suggested that these chemicals could be an important source of microbial contamination of produce, thereby affecting both the shelf life of these foods and public safety.[169]

While small amounts of a variety of metals are necessary for human health, excessive intakes can be problematic. Iron is a good example. Even though it is an essential nutrient, large amounts of free iron in the blood can act as a pro-oxidant.

There are also some metals that are toxic and should be avoided as much as possible. A case in point is mercury, which is most highly concentrated in fish.[170] A joint statement by the U.S. Food and Drug Administration (FDA) and the Environmental Protection Agency (EPA) recommends against the consumption of king mackerel, shark, swordfish, and tilefish by pregnant and lactating women and young children. Even these somewhat conservative organizations advise a maximum weekly consumption of 12 ounces (340 grams) or less of those fish and shellfish that are lower in mercury.[171]

In 2009, another unexpected source of mercury was discovered. Researchers found that high-fructose corn syrup may contain up to 0.57 micrograms of mercury per gram. (In the samples studied, the content ranged from below the detectable limit of 0.005 to 0.570 micrograms of mercury per gram.)[172] A second study found detectable mercury in one out of every three common food or beverage items tested that included high-fructose corn syrup as a first or second ingredient.[173] The mercury is thought to originate in the chemicals that are added to the syrup, such as caustic soda (used to separate the starch from the corn kernel) and sodium benzoate (a preservative). According to the USDA, the average American consumes 8 teaspoons (about 34 grams) of high-fructose corn syrup per day, almost exclusively from processed foods such as chocolate milk, fruit drinks, granola bars, jam, jelly, soda, yogurt, and other items in which it is used as a sweetener. A 20-ounce (568-milliliter) bottle of Coca-Cola contains 17 teaspoons (about 70 grams) of high-fructose corn syrup. The EPA advises that we should consume no more than 0.1 micrograms of methylmercury per kilogram of body weight per day. (Methylmercury is the form of mercury commonly found in fish and seafood.) There is no reference for total mercury (we don't know what type of mercury is present in high-fructose corn syrup), although all mercury poses a risk.[173] This means that a 120-pound (55-kilogram) woman should consume no more than 5.5 micrograms of methylmercury per day (of course, none would be even better). If this woman eats a standard Western diet, she could, theoretically, ingest as much as 28.5 micrograms of total mercury from high-fructose corn syrup alone.

Diets centered on animal products, processed foods, and deep-fried fast foods promote oxidative damage. Plant-based diets are not only lower in pro-oxidants, they are also higher in antioxidants. Raw vegan diets may offer a significant advantage over other vegan diets, as they avoid the oxidative damage to foods caused by heat and eliminate processed foods, including those containing high-fructose corn syrup. Raw-food adherents can minimize exposure to pro-oxidants in their diets by opting for organic rather than conventionally grown produce and by ensuring that foods are properly stored. All produce should be washed, whether or not it is organic.

COOKING UP CARCINOGENS

When foods are subjected to heat, especially at high temperatures, several by-products can form that are very damaging to human health. Among the most notorious are acrylamide, advanced glycoxidation end products (AGEs), heterocyclic amines (HCAs), and polycyclic aromatic hydrocarbons (PAHs).

ACRYLAMIDE

Acrylamide is a chemical that is used to make polyacrylamide, which is employed in the manufacturing of certain glues, cosmetics, food-packaging materials, grouting agents, plastics, and soil-conditioning agents. It is also used in water treatment. Although polyacrylamide is nontoxic, small quantities of acrylamide residues, which appear to be less benign, remain in finished products.[174]

In April 2002, Swedish researchers discovered the presence of acrylamide in some starchy foods. They noted that acrylamide appears to form spontaneously when certain foods, particularly those that are high in carbohydrates and low in protein, such as potatoes, are subjected to high cooking temperatures. The higher the cooking temperature and the longer the cooking time, the greater the acrylamide concentration becomes.[175] Canadian scientists discovered that most acrylamide in food is formed when the amino acid asparagine reacts with naturally occurring sugars, such as glucose.[176–178] This generally occurs at the later stages of baking, roasting, and frying, when the moisture content of the food diminishes and the surface temperature rises.

The most concentrated food sources of acrylamide are processed foods such as potato chips and other baked or fried salty snacks and french fries, as potatoes are particularly high in asparagine. Other food sources include breads (especially toasted), cold cereals, crackers, crispbreads, pretzels, and other foods processed at high temperatures, such as coffee and cocoa.[179] Acrylamide is also formed during the home preparation of starchy foods, such as frying potatoes or roasting nuts. Any significant formation of acrylamide requires temperatures of 248 degrees F (120 degrees C) or higher.[178] Consequently, it is found only in insignificant amounts in steamed or boiled foods, and is, for all practical purposes, negligible in raw foods.[180]

There are a number of potential health concerns associated with acrylamide consumption. Occupational and accidental exposure to high doses have been shown to cause neurotoxicity in humans. Experimental studies suggest that it could also be toxic to genetic material, increasing the risk of cancer and reproductive problems, although these findings have not been confirmed in humans.[180] Acrylamide was evaluated by the International Agency for Research on Cancer in 1994 and classified as "probably carcinogenic to humans" on the basis of a positive cancer bioassay result.[180] In July 2002, the European Commission's Scientific Committee on Food (SCF) recommended that dietary acrylamide levels be reduced to as low as reasonably achievable.[181]

Vegetarians are not necessarily at an advantage over nonvegetarians in terms of acrylamide intake. If vegetarians consume large amounts of baked or fried starchy foods, they may be at a disadvantage. Once again, raw-food vegans would be expected to have among the lowest intakes of acrylamide of any dietary group.

Advanced Glycation End Products

Advanced glycation end products (AGEs) are harmful end products of the Maillard reaction (see sidebar, below) or of fat oxidation, which occurs when food is heated to high temperatures.[182, 183] AGEs can also be formed within the body when sugar molecules attach to protein, fat, or DNA.[184]

There is evidence that AGEs impair immune-system function, accelerate aging, and contribute to the progression of Alzheimer's disease, cardiovascular disease, diabetes, eye diseases, kidney disease, nerve diseases, and stroke.[185, 186]

Research has shown that about 10 percent of the AGEs in food are absorbed into the system.[187] Restricting foods rich in AGEs has been shown to significantly reduce circulating AGE levels in the body and levels of C-reactive protein, a marker for inflammation (high levels of C-reactive protein indicate greater inflammation in the body).[184]

Foods that have the most concentrations of AGEs are broiled, grilled, and fried meats. (See table 4.5, page 69, for a list of AGEs in common foods.) The average AGE intake (based on food records) for people eating a standard

The Maillard Reaction

The Maillard reaction is a form of nonenzymatic browning that occurs when a sugar, such as glucose or fructose, combines with an amino acid. The chemical reaction, which is called glycation, results in intermediate products of the Maillard reaction. If heating continues, further chemical reactions may result in irreversible bonding of amino acids (protein cross-linking), and the formation of advanced glyation end products (AGEs).[188] The cross-linking of protein may also result in the destruction of essential amino acids or a reduction in their availability.[188] The Maillard reaction occurs when foods are heated to high temperatures. Generally, the reaction begins to escalate at temperatures of 310 degrees F (155 degrees C) or

higher. Products of the Maillard reaction are minimized when foods are boiled or steamed, as temperatures reach only 212 degrees F (100 degrees C). The food industry purposefully uses the Maillard reaction to improve the flavor and color of foods. Good examples of this are breads, cereals, coffee, pastries, and sauces. The potential harmful effects of the end-stage products of the Maillard reaction were not well recognized until the 1970s, when products of nonenzymatically glycated hemoglobin where found in diabetic patients.[189] Glycated hemoglobin is formed when glucose or other sugars react with hemoglobin (in a pathway that does not involve the action of enzymes). This detrimental process increases with poor blood glucose control.

TABLE 4.5 AGE content of common foods

Food group	Amount	AGEs (kU)
ANIMAL PRODUCTS		
Frankfurter, broiled 5 minutes	3 oz/90 g	10,143
Chicken breast, breaded, fried 25 minutes	3 oz/90 g	8,965
Hamburger, fried, fast food	3 oz/90 g	4,876
American processed cheese	1 oz/30 g	2,603
Trout, roasted 25 minutes	3 oz/90 g	1,924
Cottage cheese, 1%	4 oz/120 g	1,744
Egg, fried with margarine	1.5 oz/45 g	1,237
Infant formula	1 c/250 ml	1,212
Chicken breast, boiled 1 hour	3 oz/90 g	1,011
Chicken breast, raw	3 oz/90 g	692
Human milk	1 c/250 ml	16
Whole milk	1 c/250 ml	12
FATS AND OILS		
Butter	1 Tbsp/15 g	3,972
Margarine	1 Tbsp/15 g	2,628
Olive oil	1 Tbsp/15 ml	1,800
PLANT FOODS (INCLUDING PROCESSED FOODS)		
Tofu, broiled	3 oz/90 g	3,696
Nuts, roasted (average)	1 oz/30 g	2,000–3,000
Potatoes, fried, fast food	3.5 oz/100 g	1,522
Waffle, frozen	1 oz/30 g	861
Tofu, raw	3 oz/90 g	709
Rice Krispies cereal	1 oz/30 g	600
Beans, kidney, canned	3.5 oz/100 g	191
Potatoes, boiled 25 minutes	3.5 oz/100 g	117
Beans, kidney, raw	3.5oz/100 g	116
Whole wheat bread, toasted	1 oz/30 g	30
Whole wheat bread	1 oz/30 g	19
Oatmeal, instant, dry	1 oz/30 g	4

Source: Data from reference 185.

Western diet has been estimated at approximately 16,000 kilounits (kU).[185] Vegetarian diets would contain lesser amounts, unless they were very high in processed and fried foods. Raw vegan diets contain minimal AGEs, providing yet another health advantage.

Heterocyclic Amines and Polycyclic Aromatic Hydrocarbons

Heterocyclic amines (HCAs) are chemicals that are created when meat, poultry, fish, or eggs are subjected to high-temperature cooking, such as barbecuing, grilling, or frying. The formation of these compounds increases with higher temperatures and longer cooking times.[190] Cooking methods that use direct heat (such as frying and grilling) produce more HCAs than do methods that use indirect heat (such as poaching, steaming, and stewing).[191]

Many people wonder if cooking vegetables in a similar manner would produce these chemicals as well. The answer is no, because the formation of these compounds involves the condensation of creatinine with amino acids (the building blocks of protein), and creatinine is found exclusively in muscle tissue.[192, 193] In January 2005, HCAs were officially added to the list of cancer-causing agents that is published by the National Institutes of Health.[193]

Polycyclic aromatic hydrocarbons (PAHs) are a group of over one hundred different chemicals that are formed by the incomplete burning of organic substances, such as coal, food, forests, garbage, gas, oil, and tobacco,[194] or the pyrolysis (decomposition) of fat at temperatures in excesses of 392 degrees F (200 degrees C).[195] Food accounts for over 90 percent of PAH exposure. The most concentrated sources of PAHs are grilled or charred meat, poultry and fish, grains, fats and oils, and sweets. Vegetables, fruits, beverages, and dairy products also contribute to overall intake.[195] However, PAHs in vegetables and fruits are due largely to environmental contamination of the air and soil. Where contamination is minimal, produce will also by very low in PAHs.[196]

A host of factors affect PAH formation, apart from environmental contamination. The primary factors include the temperature of cooking, distance from the heat source, duration of cooking, type of fuel used in heating, amount of fat in the food, and whether the fat drips onto the heat source and rises back onto the food.[197] Raw grains tend to be low in PAHs; however, processing techniques, especially those that use direct-combustion gas heating and toasting, can increase levels. For example, a sprouted grain grown in contaminated soil could be a very minor source of PAHs, but a ready-to-eat cereal will contain significantly higher levels. Processed sweets can also contribute to PAH intake. Fats and oils are a significant source, as the foods from which they are extracted are often environmentally contaminated. In addition, direct-combustion gases and solvents used in processing can further increase levels.

Heterocyclic amines and polycyclic aromatic hydrocarbons are known to be mutagenic (that is, they damage DNA). Evidence suggests that HCAs increase our risk of a variety of cancers, including breast, colorectal, pancreatic, and stomach cancers.[193] Cancers thought to be linked to PAH intake include those of the genitourinary tract (related to the genital and urinary organs), lung, and skin.[193] Most of our exposure to these compounds comes through our food, and the vast majority through high-temperature cooking. Vegetarian diets generally contain negligible amounts of HCAs and moderate amounts of PAHs. Although no data exists, it would be reasonable to assume that amounts eaten on a raw vegan diet would be lower than intakes on other diets.

CONCLUSION: Experts consistently agree that we should keep our intake of acrylamides, advanced glycation end products, heterocyclic amines, and polycyclic aromatic hydrocarbons as low as possible. One of the best ways of accomplishing this task is to eat a raw vegan diet. When it comes to maximizing protective dietary compounds and minimizing potentially harmful ones, raw-food vegans rock!

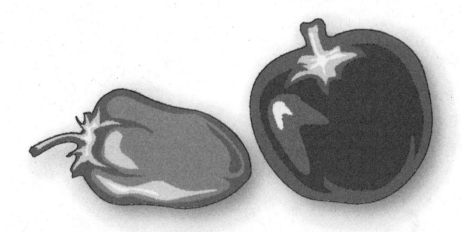

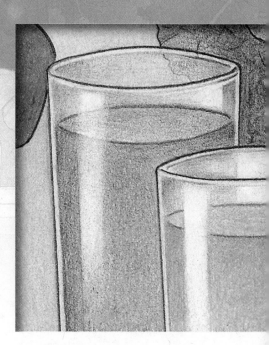

CHAPTER 5

Energy and Power

One of the greatest icons of Western cuisine, the hamburger patty, gets 39–40 percent of its calories from protein. In baby zucchini, 40 percent of the calories comes from protein. In spinach, 39 percent of the calories comes from protein. So instead of fatty, cholesterol-packed burgers, we can just eat raw baby zucchini or a big spinach salad, right?

In practical terms, it is not so simple. A 3-ounce (85-gram) beef-burger patty, the size of a deck of cards, provides 22 grams of protein, which is 40–50 percent of an adult's recommended protein intake for the day. To get 22 grams of protein from the veggies, we need to eat 15 cups (1 pound/450 grams) of spinach *plus* 30 baby zucchini (each the size of the average pinky finger). This substantial serving of spinach plus zucchini gives us just *three-quarters the calories of the burger patty* (see table 5.1, page 74). In other words, the plant foods deliver significantly *more protein per calorie*. The meat and the veggies also differ in terms of their volume, appearance, and mouthfeel, and in the amount of time required to consume them!

The zucchini and spinach combination has advantages over the burger choice in terms of its reduced impact on the environment (and on the cow). The veggies deliver much less fat, and the type of fat in the plant foods is beneficial to our health rather than damaging. For almost every vitamin (except vitamin B_{12}), for minerals (apart from selenium and zinc), and for omega-6 fatty acids, we get a *great* deal more from the big bowl of veggies. In table 5.1 (page 74), the nutrients in these foods are listed, with the amount that is higher shown in **bold** and shaded. Notice that most of the bold numbers are in the column representing the veggies. For zinc and omega-6 fatty acids, the amounts in both columns are close. The ratio of omega-3 to omega-6 fatty acids is ideal in the plant foods but imbalanced in the burger. (For more on the ratio of omega-3 to omega-6 fatty acids, see chapter 7.)

TABLE 5.1 Nutrients in hamburger, spinach, and zucchini*

	Hamburger patty (3 oz/85 g)	Spinach (15 c/450 g) plus 30 baby zucchini (330 g)
Protein, g	**22**	22
Calories	**216**	173
Fat, g	**15**	3
Saturated fat, g	**5**	0.6
Cholesterol, g	**77**	0
Carbohydrate, g	0	**27**
Fiber, g	0	**14**
Water, g	49	**717**
Vitamin A, RAE, mcg	0	**2,191**
Carotenoids, RE	0	**4,383**
Thiamin, mg	0.04	**0.5**
Riboflavin, mg	0.2	**1.0**
Niacin, mg	4	**5.6**
Vitamin B$_6$ (pyridoxine), mg	0.3	**1.4**
Folate, mcg	8	**939**
Pantothenic acid, mg	0.5	**1.5**
Vitamin B$_{12}$, mcg	**2.1**	0
Vitamin C, mg	0	**239**
Vitamin E, mg	0.4	**10**
Vitamin K, mcg	1	**2,173**
Calcium, mg	20	**515****
Copper, mg	0.1	**0.9**
Iron, mg	2.2	**15****
Magnesium, mg	17	**464**
Manganese, mg	0.1	**4.7**
Phosphorus, mg	165	**527**
Potassium, mg	258	**4,026**

	Hamburger patty (3 oz/85 g)	Spinach (15 c/450 g) plus 30 baby zucchini (330 g)
Selenium, mcg	**17.8**	5.5
Zinc, mg	**5.3**	5.1
Omega-3 fatty acids, g	0.05	**1**
Omega-6 fatty acids, g	**0.36**	0.32
Protective phytochemicals	0	**massive amounts**

Source: Data from references 1, 2.

*The nutrients that are the highest are bold and shaded.

**The calcium and iron from spinach are complicated by absorption issues (see chapter 9 for more information about this).

Note: "RE" stands for "Retinol Equivalents"; "RAE" stands for "Retinol Activity Equivalents." These are standard units of measure for carotenoids and vitamin A.

The comparisons in table 5.1 highlight key differences between diets that emphasize meat and dairy products and the beckoning world of raw plant foods. Issues raised here form the basis of this and upcoming chapters.

Energy (Calories) and Body Weight

It is well known that raw diets tend to be low in calories (for typical intakes, see table 5.2, page 77). In fact, this often is a key attraction. Entirely raw and near-raw diets help us to slim down while our cells are supplied with abundant antioxidants, vitamins, and minerals. Vegetables are health superstars because they provide more protective substances per calorie than other foods. With good choices, our raw diet can meet recommended intakes of every nutrient we require. Yet raw food takes time to chew and can take longer to prepare, and over the course of a day, a raw diet tends to contain fewer calories than a nonvegetarian diet. At the same time, it is possible to design raw vegan diets that meet the calorie and protein requirements of those with high activity levels and big appetites, including elite athletes. For sample menus that contain 1,600–2,500 calories, see chapter 12. These menus include examples of how to further increase caloric intakes.

The calories in food are derived from the carbohydrates, fat, and protein they contain. The calories in a wide assortment of raw fruits, vegetables, nuts, seeds, legumes, and grains are shown in table 5.3, page 80. Since many vegetables and fruits contain a lot of water, and water has no calories at all, a heaping plate of plant foods often can be extremely low in calories. For each food, calories are listed per cup (250 milliliters) or per unit (for example, one apple). The percentage of each food that is water is shown in the column at

Caloric Density

Whether you would like to lose weight, gain weight, or simply be healthy, the concept of *caloric density* is of value. A food's caloric density is the number of calories (food energy) per gram of that food. For instance, an avocado has a caloric density of 1.6, which means that it has 1.6 calories in every gram. Most animal products are much higher in caloric density. For example, a broiled hamburger has a caloric density of 2.7, medium cheddar cheese has a caloric density of 3.9, and bacon has a caloric density of 5.6. Small amounts of these foods deliver plenty of calories—and padding for our hips.[1]

Most fruits and vegetables are significantly lower in caloric density. The caloric density of an apricot is 0.5 (meaning that it has only 0.5 calories per gram). Dried apricots, from which the water has been removed, have a caloric density of 2.75. The caloric density of a carrot is 0.4, of broccoli is 0.3, and of romaine lettuce is 0.2. If you want to lose weight, foods with a low caloric density can fill your stomach temporarily without adding to your waistline permanently. Such foods appear in countless research studies and newspaper headlines as the most nutritious choices because their low caloric density is accompanied by abundant vitamins and phytochemicals and respectable amounts of minerals. You can find the caloric density of a food in table 5.3, page 80, by dividing its calories by its weight in grams.

When foods are ground (as when nuts and dried fruit are ground and made into tasty little cookies like Coconut Macaroons, page 298, or are formed into compact energy bars), the end product has a higher caloric density, a feature that is of value for athletes, hikers, and hungry snackers.

the right. As you can see, certain items, such as avocado, coconut, dried fruit, durian, nuts, olives, and seeds, are high in calories. These foods have a high-caloric density compared to other plant foods.

CALORIC REQUIREMENTS FOR ADULTS

The number of calories that adults need varies considerably depending on body size, age, and activity level. Typical requirements are 1,800–2,000 calories for a sedentary or moderately active woman and 2,400–2,600 calories for a moderately active man. The standard used on food labels is 2,000 calories per day.[3–5]

CALORIC INTAKES ON RAW DIETS

If raw-food adherents rely on large quantities of foods that are mostly water, do they get enough to eat? What are typical caloric intakes on raw and near-raw diets? Studies have been done in the United States, Finland, and Germany, and the average daily intakes of the groups studied range from 1,460 to 1,989 calories (see table 5.2, page 77). It seems that some people on raw and mainly raw diets get enough calories (along with most other essential nutrients)—and some don't.

A 2001 U.S. study summarized food records of 141 adults who had been following the high-raw Hallelujah Acres diet (which is 55 percent raw by calories

TABLE 5.2 Average daily calories and protein in raw food studies

Study, country, year, participants, references	Daily calories	Daily protein (or g per kg body weight)	Percentage of calories from protein
Raw vegan diet, USA, 2005, 2006, 11 men, 7 women[11, 12]	1,989	45 g (0.73 g/kg/day)	9.1%
Giessen study, Germany, 2001, 2005, 43 vegans[13]	1,887	39 g	8.2%
Hallelujah Acres diet, USA, 2001, 141 near-vegans and vegans[6]	1,830 (men) 1,460 (women)	47 g (men) 37 g (women) (0.66 g g/kg/day)	10%
Living-food diet, Finland, 1995, 7 vegan women, 1 vegan man[10]	1,674	49.5 g	12%
Living-food diet, Finland, 1995, 20 vegan women, 1 vegan man[15, 18]	1,696	51 g	12%
Living-food diet, Finland, 1992, 7 vegan women, 3 vegan men[16]	1,782	67 g	15%
Average for all participants in the above studies	1,700	43 g	10.1%

and 75 percent raw by weight) for an average of twenty-eight months. Participants typically consumed six to seven servings of fruit, plus eleven to twelve servings of vegetables, with a serving being 1 cup of salad or 1 item—such as an apple, a banana, or a carrot—making a daily total of 3.75 pounds (1.7 kilograms) of fruits and vegetables. This is about three times the typical American intake.[6, 7] Those in the study typically consumed 2 cups of carrot juice, 17 grams of dehydrated barley juice, 2 tablespoons (18 grams) of nuts, and 28 grams of oil per day, on average. Three-quarters of the diet's weight came from raw foods, especially fruits, and one-quarter from cooked grains, vegetables, and legumes.[6]

The survey data showed that the average caloric intakes of the people in this study were well below typical recommendations: the average intake for the women was 1,460 calories per day, and the average intake for the men was 1,830 calories per day. Participants consumed about 73 percent of the recommended caloric intake for each person's specific age, gender, weight, and activity level. Only 11 percent met or exceeded their recommended caloric intake; 89 percent consumed less. One in four people consumed less than 60 percent of his or her recommended caloric intake. For these people, overall nutrient intake became inadequate, with insufficient protein and shortages of most minerals and vitamins. One man and 17 percent of the women were underweight, with a body mass index (BMI) that was below the healthy range of 18.5–24.9.[6, 8]

Nonetheless, the participants' responses to the diet were favorable. They attributed their improved health and quality of life to their near- or entirely raw diets. The main concern was that reduced calorie and protein intakes by those at the low end of the spectrum might result in eventual health problems. As a preventive measure, dietary changes were recommended, such as increasing their intake of nuts and seeds, eating more food, and adding legumes (such as raw peas, sprouted lentils and mung beans, or cooked beans). Including a vitamin B_{12} supplement was also advised.[6, 8, 9]

In table 5.2, page 77, you can see the average daily calories and protein from other studies. Raw-food practitioners in Finland have developed living-food diets centered on sprouted and fermented plant foods. In one study, the eight vegans who had eaten living food for an average of 7.3 years showed caloric intakes that were 8 percent higher than those of eleven control subjects on nonvegetarian diets. Yet the vegans were leaner, with an average BMI that was 82 percent that of the controls and an average weight that was 87 percent that of controls. Researchers speculated that perhaps "nutrients present in this uncooked diet are not utilized as efficiently."[10] Many raw-food adherents believe that raw foods are digested far more efficiently than cooked foods. Yet perhaps we digest at least some raw foods *less* efficiently, making raw diets an excellent way to keep one's weight in check while eating abundant quantities of food.

WEIGHT AND BODY MASS INDEX

Was the Duchess of Windsor right? No! While we can't claim expertise about being too rich, nutrition research gives a clear message about the health risks in being too thin. People on raw vegan diets tend to have lower body weights and lower BMIs compared to those on nonvegetarian diets.[17–19] Though losing weight and keeping it off is a blessing and a health benefit that many adults pray for, losing too much weight can lead to problems, including nutrient deficiencies due to insufficient intakes and loss of bone density.[6, 8, 12, 14] Serious disadvantages at the low end of the caloric spectrum include: (1) too great a reduction in body fat; (2) a change in the body's hormonal balance; (3) amenorrhea and reproduction problems in women of childbearing age; (4) deficiencies of protein, minerals, and vitamins; and (5) low bone density.[6, 8, 14, 20, 21]

You can never be too rich or too thin.

WALLIS SIMPSON, Duchess of Windsor

According to the joint position papers on nutrition and athletic performance by the American Dietetic Association, Dietitians of Canada, and the American College of Sports Medicine, "Low energy intakes can result in loss of muscle mass, menstrual dysfunction, loss or failure to gain bone density, and increased risk of fatigue, injury, and illness." In these documents, the three associations of experts on nutrition and performance also make the point that low caloric intakes can impair performance.[22]

In the Giessen study of 513 Germans who had followed a raw vegan diet for 3.7 years (on average), most had experienced an initial and dramatic weight loss and then their weights had leveled out or increased slightly. The average weight loss for men was 22 pounds (10 kilograms) and for women, 26 pounds

(12 kilograms). For most participants, their BMI ended up within the healthy range, although one woman in four and 15 percent of the men fell below this range. Among the women of childbearing age in this study, one in four had a total absence of menstruation; another 10 percent had irregular menstruation. The low body weights, lack of body fat, and menstrual irregularities were associated with the longest and most rigid adherence to the raw diet.[17]

A study of thirteen men and eight women in the American Midwest who had consumed raw vegan diets for an average of 4.4 years found the average BMI to be 20.5, well within the healthy range, and average daily caloric intakes to be 1,983 calories. In comparison, controls on nonvegetarian cooked diets had average BMIs of 25.4, which is just above the healthy BMI range of 18.5 to 24.9. For those on raw diets, body fat averaged 14 percent in men and 24 percent in women, compared to 21 and 34 percent respectively for the control men and women.[12] A Finnish study of one man and twenty women who had followed a living-food diet for 5.5 years found the average BMI to be 21, and the average daily caloric intake to be 1,672 calories.[18]

Percentage of Weight and Percentage of Calories

Foods, meals, or menus are sometimes described in terms of their percentage of weight that is fat or protein. By weight, 2 percent milk contains 2 grams of fat (and contains 89 grams of, or is 89 percent, water) per 100 grams of milk. By comparison, baby zucchini contains 0.4 percent fat by weight.

When our bodies convert fat, protein, and carbohydrate to calories, we derive approximately 9 calories from each gram of fat and approximately 4 calories from each gram of protein or carbohydrate, but none from water. Accordingly, in 2 percent milk, *35 percent of the calories* comes from fat, 27 percent from protein, and 38 percent from carbohydrate (lactose sugar). In baby zucchini, 13 percent of the calories comes from fat, 40 percent of the calories from protein, and 47 percent of the calories from carbohydrate.

> **CONCLUSION:** Evidence suggests that a well-designed raw vegan diet can be a highly effective choice for weight loss. However, once a healthy weight is achieved, it is important that raw-food practitioners ensure adequate calories to maintain a healthy body weight and adequate nutrient intakes for the long term.

BENEFITS OF LOW-CALORIE DIETS

Research indicates that a diet that is *slightly* low in calories but meets recommended intakes for other nutrients *may* reduce age-related disorders, such as diabetes, cancer, and cardiovascular disorders, and *may* extend the maximum expected lifespan. The exact degree of caloric restriction that is optimal for adults has not been determined.[12, 23–27]

To lengthen thy life, lessen thy meals.

BEN FRANKLIN

Not only might you live longer in good health by reducing caloric intake, you could even improve your memory.[28] Certainly, when we do not overburden our bodies with excess calories and body weight, we lessen our risk of chronic disease. It can be a health benefit to maintain our young-adult weight instead of adding one or more pounds every year past adolescence, as so many people do.

TABLE 5.3 Calories, protein, fat, carbohydrate, and water in raw food

Food	Calories per cup or unit, grams	Protein per cup or unit, grams	% of calories from protein	% of calories from carbo-hydrates	% of calories from fat	% water (by weight)
FRUITS						
Apple, chopped (1 c/125 g)	65	0.3	2	95	3	86
Apples, dried (1 c/160 g)	440	4	4	96	0	26
Apple, medium, each	72	0.4	2	95	3	86
Apricot, medium, each	17	0.5	10	83	7	86
Apricots, sliced, (1 c/165 g)	79	2	10	83	7	86
Apricots, dried (1 c/160 g)	429	6	5	93	2	30
Banana, dried (1 c/100 g)	346	4	4	92	4	3
Banana, medium, each	110	1	4	93	3	75
Banana, sliced (1 c/150 g)	133	2	4	93	3	75
Blackberries (1 c/144 g)	62	2	12	79	9	88
Blueberries (1 c/145 g)	82	1	5	90	5	84
Blueberries, dried (1 c/160 g)	560	4	3	97	0	10
Cantaloupe, diced (1 c/156 g)	53	1	9	87	4	90
Cherimoya, chopped (1 c/225 g)	211	3	5	92	3	74
Coconut, dried (1 c/116 g)	766	8	4	13	83	3
Coconut milk (1 c/240 g)	552	6	4	9	87	68
Crabapple, sliced (1 c/110 g)	84	0.4	2	95	3	79
Currants, red/white (1 c/112 g)	63	2	9	88	3	84
Currants, black (1 c/112 g)	71	2	8	87	5	82
Currants, Zante, dried (1 c/144 g)	407	6	5	94	1	19
Dates, chopped (1 c/178 g)	502	4	3	96	1	21
Durian, chopped (1 c/243 g)	357	4	4	66	30	65
Figs, dried (1 c/199 g)	496	7	5	92	3	30
Fig, medium, fresh, each	37	0.4	4	93	3	79
Gooseberries (1 c/150 g)	66	1	7	82	11	88
Grapefruit, medium, each	103	2	7	90	3	88
Grapefruit, sections (1 c/230 g)	74	2	7	90	3	91
Grapefruit juice (1 c/247 g)	96	1	5	93	2	90
Guava, diced (1 c/165 g)	84	1	6	84	10	86
Honeydew melon, diced (1 c/170 g)	61	0.9	5	92	3	90
Huckleberries (1 c/145 g)	83	1	5	90	5	84
Kiwi fruit, diced (1 c/177 g)	108	2	7	86	7	83
Kiwi fruit, medium, each	46	0.9	7	86	7	83

Food	Calories per cup or unit, grams	Protein per cup or unit, grams	% of calories from protein	% of calories from carbo-hydrates	% of calories from fat	% water (by weight)
Loganberries (1 c/144 g)	62	2	11	80	9	88
Mango, diced (1 c/165 g)	107	0.8	3	94	3	82
Mango, medium, each	135	1	3	94	3	82
Mango, dried (1 c/121 g)	424	0	0	100	0	14
Orange, medium, each	62	1	7	91	2	87
Orange, sections (1 c/180 g)	85	2	7	91	2	87
Orange juice (1 c/248 g)	112	2	6	90	4	88
Papaya, diced (1 c/140 g)	55	0.8	6	91	3	89
Papaya, mashed (1 c/230 g)	89	1	6	91	3	89
Peach, sliced (1 c/170 g)	66	2	8	87	5	89
Peach, dried, each	37	0.7	7	93	0	30
Peach, medium, each	38	0.9	8	87	5	89
Pears, sliced (1 c/165 g)	96	0.6	2	96	2	84
Pear, Bartlett, medium, each	96	0.6	2	96	2	84
Pear halves, dried (1 c/180 g)	472	3	3	95	2	27
Pear, medium, each	100	1	4	88	8	83
Pineapple, diced (1 c/155 g)	74	0.8	4	94	2	86
Plum, sliced (1 c/165 g)	91	1	5	86	9	85
Plum, medium, each	40	0.5	5	86	9	84
Plums, dried (1 c/121 g)	273	3	4	96	0	36
Prunes, dried (1 c/170 g)	408	4	4	95	1	31
Raisins, seeded, packed (1 c/165 g)	488	4	4	95	1	17
Raisins, seedless, packed (1 c/165 g)	493	5	4	95	1	15
Raspberries (1 c/123 g)	64	1	8	82	10	86
Strawberries, dried (1 c/80 g)	300	2	3	97	0	16
Strawberries, halved (1 c/152 g)	49	1	7	86	7	91
Strawberries, whole (1 c/144 g)	46	1	7	86	7	91
Watermelon, diced (1 c/152 g)	46	0.9	7	89	4	91
VEGETABLES						
Asparagus spear, medium, each	5	0.4	35	62	3	93
Asparagus, sliced (1 c/134 g)	26	3	35	62	3	93
Avocado, all types, medium, each	324	4	5	78	17	74
Avocado, all types, puréed (1 c/230 g)	370	5	5	78	17	74
Avocado, all types, sliced (1 c/146 g)	235	3	5	78	17	74
Avocado, California, medium, each	289	3	4	77	19	72
Avocado, California, puréed (1 c/230 g)	384	5	4	77	19	72

Food	Calories per cup or unit, grams	Protein per cup or unit, grams	% of calories from protein	% of calories from carbo-hydrates	% of calories from fat	% water (by weight)
Avocado, Florida, medium, each	365	7	7	24	69	79
Avocado, Florida, puréed (1 c/230 g)	276	5	7	24	69	79
Basil, fresh, chopped (1 c/42 g)	11	1	31	52	17	91
Beans, snap, green/yellow (1 c/110 g)	34	2	20	77	3	90
Beets, sliced (1 c/136 g)	58	2	14	83	3	88
Beet juice (1 c/236 g)	83	3	12	88	0	88
Beet greens (1 c/38 g)	7	0.7	31	67	2	92
Bok choy, shredded (1 c/70 g)	9	1	36	53	11	95
Broccoli, chopped (1 c/70 g)	20	2	33	58	9	91
Brussels sprouts, cup (88 g)	38	3	26	69	5	86
Cabbage, green, chopped (1 c/89 g)	21	1	20	76	4	92
Cabbage, napa, chopped (1 c/85 g)	15	1	29	71	0	92
Cabbage, pe-tsai, chopped (1 c/76 g)	12	0.9	25	66	9	94
Cabbage, red, chopped (1 c/89 g)	28	1	16	80	4	90
Cabbage, red, shredded (1 c/70 g)	22	1	16	80	4	90
Carrot, chopped (1 c/128 g)	52	1	8	87	5	88
Carrot, medium, each	30	0.7	8	87	5	88
Carrot juice (1 c/236 g)	50	1	11	83	6	93
Cauliflower, chopped (1 c/100 g)	25	2	26	71	3	92
Celery, diced (1 c/120 g)	17	0.8	17	74	9	95
Celery, rib, large, each	9	0.4	17	74	9	95
Celery root, chopped (1 c/156 g)	66	2	13	81	6	88
Chile, hot green (1 c/150 g)	60	3	17	79	4	88
Chile, hot red (1 c/150 g)	64	3	15	65	20	88
Cilantro (1 c/46 g)	11	0.9	27	58	15	92
Collard greens, chopped (1 c/36 g)	11	0.9	27	63	10	91
Corn, yellow/white (1 c/154 g)	132	5	13	76	11	76
Cucumber, peeled, each	24	1	19	69	12	97
Cucumber, peeled, sliced (1 c/119 g)	14	0.7	19	69	12	97
Cucumber, with peel, sliced (1 c/104 g)	14	0.7	18	74	8	96
Daikon radish, chopped (1 c/88 g)	16	0.5	12	83	5	95
Dandelion greens (1 c/55 g)	24	1	20	68	12	86
Eggplant, cubed (1 c/82 g)	20	0.8	14	80	6	92
Garlic cloves (1 c/136 g)	203	9	16	81	3	59
Garlic cloves, medium, each	5	0.2	16	81	3	59
Green Giant Juice, page 259 (1 c/250 ml)74	36	3	35	58	7	96

Food	Calories per cup or unit, grams	Protein per cup or unit, grams	% of calories from protein	% of calories from carbo-hydrates	% of calories from fat	% water (by weight)
Horseradish, grated (1 c/240 g)	144	7	18	78	4	77
Jerusalem artichokes, sliced (1 c/150 g)	114	3	10	90	0	78
Kale, chopped (1 c/67 g)	34	2	22	67	11	84
Kale juice (1 c/250 ml)[74]	70	7	39	50	11	92
Kelp, Japanese, chopped (1 c/80 g)	34	1	14	76	10	82
Leeks, chopped (1 c/89 g)	54	1	9	87	4	83
Lettuce, butterhead, chopped (1 c/55 g)	7	0.7	33	55	12	96
Lettuce, iceberg, chopped (1 c/55 g)	6	0.4	26	66	8	96
Lettuce, leaf, chopped (1 c/56 g)	8	0.8	30	62	8	95
Lettuce, red leaf, chopped (1 c/28 g)	4	0.4	33	55	12	96
Lettuce, romaine, chopped (1 c/56 g)	10	0.7	24	63	13	95
Mushrooms, shiitake, dried (1 c/145 g)	483	38	31	62	7	12
Mustard greens, chopped (1 c/56 g)	15	2	34	60	6	91
Okra, sliced (1 c/100 g)	31	2	22	76	2	90
Olives, ripe (1 c/160 g)	206	2	4	7	90	80
Onion, green, each	5	0.3	19	77	4	90
Onions, green, chopped (1 c/100 g)	32	2	19	77	4	90
Onions, red/yellow/white (1 c/160 g)	67	1	8	90	2	89
Parsley, chopped (1 c/60 g)	22	2	27	57	16	88
Parsnips, sliced (1 c/133 g)	100	2	6	91	3	80
Peas (1 c/145 g)	117	8	26	70	4	79
Pea pods, snow (1 c/63 g)	26	2	26	70	4	89
Peppers, bell, green, chopped (1 c/149 g)	30	1	14	79	7	94
Pepper, bell, green, medium, each	24	1	14	79	7	94
Peppers, bell, red, chopped (1 c/149 g)	39	1	13	78	9	92
Pepper, bell, red, medium, each	31	1	13	78	9	92
Radish, medium, each	4	0	16	79	5	95
Radishes, daikon, dried (1 c/116 g)	314	9	11	87	2	20
Radish, daikon, medium, each	61	2	12	83	5	95
Radish, sliced (1 c/116 g)	19	0.8	16	79	5	95
Radish sprouts (1 c/38 g)	16	1	29	28	43	90
Rutabaga, chopped (1 c/140 g)	50	2	12	83	5	90
Spinach, chopped (1 c/30 g)	7	0.9	39	49	12	91
Spirulina, dried (1 c/80 g)	345	68	58	24	18	5
Squash, acorn, cubed (1 c/140 g)	56	1	7	91	2	88
Squash, butternut, cubed (1 c/240 g)	108	2	8	90	2	86

Food	Calories per cup or unit, grams	Protein per cup or unit, grams	% of calories from protein	% of calories from carbo-hydrates	% of calories from fat	% water (by weight)
Squash, crookneck, cubed (1 c/130 g)	25	1	17	73	10	94
Squash, hubbard, cubed (1 c/116 g)	46	2	17	73	10	88
Sweet potato, cubed (1 c/133 g)	101	2	8	91	1	80
Tomato, medium, each	27	1	17	74	9	95
Tomato, cherry, each	3	0.2	17	74	9	95
Tomatoes, chopped (1 c/180 g)	32	2	17	74	9	95
Tomatoes, green, chopped (1 c/180 g)	41	1	18	75	7	93
Tomato, plum, each	11	0.6	17	74	9	95
Tomatoes, yellow, chopped (1 c/139 g)	20	1	21	66	13	95
Tomatoes, sun-dried (1 c/54 g)	139	8	18	73	9	15
Turnip, cubed (1 c/130 g)	36	1	12	85	3	92
Turnip greens, chopped (1 c/55 g)	36	1	12	85	3	90
Yam, cubed (1 c/150 g)	177	0.8	5	94	1	70
Zucchini, baby, each	2	0.3	40	47	13	93
Zucchini, cubed (1 c/124 g)	20	2	25	67	8	95
NUTS AND SEEDS						
Almonds (1 c/142 g)	850	29	13	13	74	5
Almond butter, cup (256 g)	1,620	39	9	13	78	1
Brazil nut, large, each	31	0.7	8	6	86	3
Brazil nuts (1 c/140 g)	965	21	8	6	86	3
Cashew nuts (1 c/130 g)	736	24	12	18	70	5
Cashew butter (1 c/256 g)	1,503	45	11	18	71	3
Chia seeds, dried (1 c/160 g)	784	25	12	34	54	5
Flaxseeds, ground (1 c/128 g)	576	27	14	23	63	7
Flaxseeds, whole (1 c/176 g)	792	40	14	23	63	7
Hazelnuts (1 c/135 g)	848	20	9	10	81	5
Pecans (1 c/108 g)	768	10	5	8	87	4
Pine nuts (1 c/136 g)	915	19	8	7	85	2
Pistachio nuts (1 c/128 g)	713	26	14	19	67	4
Poppy seeds (1 c/134 g)	716	24	13	17	70	7
Psyllium seeds (1 c/156 g)	367	2	2	8	90	0
Pumpkin seeds (1 c/138 g)	747	34	17	12	71	7
Sesame seeds, hulled (1 c/150 g)	888	30	13	10	77	5
Sesame seeds, unhulled (1 c/144 g)	825	25	12	15	73	5
Sesame tahini (1 c/240 g)	1,421	42	11	14	75	3
Sunflower seeds, hulled (1 c/144 g)	821	33	15	12	73	5

Food	Calories per cup or unit, grams	Protein per cup or unit, grams	% of calories from protein	% of calories from carbo-hydrates	% of calories from fat	% water (by weight)
Sunflower seed butter (1 c/256 g)	1482	50	13	18	69	1
Walnuts, black (1 c/125 g)	759	30	15	7	78	4
Walnuts, English (1 c/120 g)	785	18	9	8	83	4
Water chestnuts, Chinese, sliced (1 c/124 g)	120	2	5	94	1	73
LEGUMES						
Adzuki beans, dried (1 c/197 g)	648	39	24	75	1	13
Lentils, dried (1 c/192 g)	649	54	32	66	2	11
Lentil sprouts (1 c/77 g)	81	7	28	68	4	67
Mung beans, dried (1 c/188 g)	640	44	27	70	3	9
Mung bean sprouts (1 c/104 g)	31	3	32	64	4	90
Pea sprouts (1 c/120 g)	154	11	23	73	4	62
GRAINS						
Amaranth, dry (1 c/195 g)	729	28	15	70	15	10
Barley groats, unhulled, dry (1 c/164 g)	500	13	9	87	4	13
Buckwheat groats, dry (1 c/164 g)	560	20	14	80	6	8
Buckwheat sprouts (1 c/33 g)	65	2	14	80	6	48
Kamut, dry (1 c/188 g)	692	24	14	82	4	9
Millet, dry (1 c/200 g)	756	22	12	78	10	9
Oat groats, dry (1 c/164 g)	610	21	13	73	14	10
Oat groats, organic, dry (1 c/164 g)	750	25	14	71	15	3
Quinoa, dry (1 c/170 g)	636	22	14	72	14	9
Rye berries, dry (1 c/169 g)	566	25	16	78	6	11
Spelt berries, dry (1 c/174 g)	588	25	17	77	6	11
Wheat berries, hard, red, dry (1 c/192 g)	631	30	18	78	4	13
Wheat berries, hard, white, dry (1 c/192 g)	656	22	13	83	4	10
Wheat sprouts (1 c/108 g)	213	8	15	80	5	48
Wild rice, dry (1 c/160 g)	571	24	16	81	3	8
REFINED OR EXTRACTED FOODS (NOT NECESSARILY RAW)						
Agave syrup (1 c/336 g)	960	0	0	100	0	not available
Cane sugar, organic, granulated (1 c/192 g)	764	0	0	100	0	1
Flaxseed oil (1 c/218 g)	1,923	0	0	0	100	0
Maple syrup (1 c/320 g)	835	0	0	99	1	32
Olive oil (1 c/216 g)	1,909	0	0	0	100	0

Source: Data from references 1, 2, 74.

Note: "Vegetables" include sea vegetables, fruits (such as tomatoes), and grains (such as corn) that are commonly used as vegetables. Grains include seeds that are often used as grains. Data for nuts and seeds is before soaking unless indicated. Foods are fresh (raw) unless otherwise indicated. Grams of protein are rounded off above 1.0.

Digestion

hough tables may list the nutrients in various foods, such as mangoes or sunflower seeds, all foods must be "changed" before the body can use them as nourishment. Digestion is our body's ingenious way of breaking down foods into smaller particles so that the nutrients can be absorbed. "Digestibility" means the proportion of calories, protein, or other nutrients that is absorbed over the entire length of our gastrointestinal tract.[29] After being absorbed, the products of digestion (amino acids from protein or breakdown products from fat or carbohydrate) are transported to cells, where they can be used as building blocks, transformed into useable energy, or stored. Vitamins, minerals, essential fats, and protective phytochemicals are used for a multitude of bodily functions.[30]

DIGESTIVE ENZYMES

The key "workers" in the digestive process are proteins known as digestive enzymes, which can break down food into small particles without the worker enzymes themselves being changed. For example, one enzyme's role may be to unravel a long, coiled protein molecule; another's may be to split the protein at certain junctions into shorter chains of amino acids. Further along in the digestion process, other enzymes break these chains into individual amino acids, which are absorbed and become the building blocks for the protein made in our body. Specific enzymes are released in the mouth, stomach, and small intestine and get mixed into the food at various stages.[30] (For more information on enzymes and digestion, see chapter 10.)

THE DIGESTIVE PROCESS

Stage 1

Before food reaches the stomach, the process of digestion has already begun. Chopping, blending, or juicing food greatly increases the surface area and breaks down cells, releasing or activating the enzymes that are present in many plant foods. When we bite and chew the food, the cells are broken down further. The salivary glands in the mouth release a fluid rich in enzymes, which begin the digestion of starch. In order to act, the enzymes need the food to be in small particles, allowing them access to the maximum surface area; they also need food particles to be suspended in water.[30, 31]

Stage 2

After passing down the esophagus, the wet mixture of food and saliva reaches the top part of the stomach, where it may be held for about forty minutes, like a plane on standby for takeoff. Enzymes from food and saliva continue to act during this holding phase. Then, cells lining the lower part of the stomach secrete strongly acidic juices, which can uncoil the long, convoluted protein molecules, exposing the bonds between amino acids so they can be broken down in the small intestine. Stomach juices also contain unique enzymes known as pepsins, which are activated rather than destroyed in this acidic environment. This acid-enzyme team terminates the activity of enzymes from food and saliva that has been continuing in the stomach until now. The powerful, thick muscles of the stomach wall churn and grind the mixture; larger pieces of food have by now become tiny particles. The stomach lining is covered in thick mucus; otherwise, this acid, in partnership with the protein-attacking stomach enzymes, would digest the stomach muscle itself.[30-33] If food hasn't been chewed thoroughly, it is possible that larger particles might pass through the stomach and reach the intestines before being thoroughly broken down.

Stage 3

As the wet mixture passes into the small intestine, its acidity is neutralized by alkaline juice from the pancreas. From this point on, the body adds digestive enzymes, which work best within the slightly alkaline pH mixture in the small intestine. Digestive action began in the mouth, but along this twenty-foot tube coiled within the abdomen, it really gets going. The small intestine consists of a series of specialized sections where disassembly of various food components takes place. (Picture a car-wrecking yard where car radios are removed at one spot, bumpers at another spot, and tires at another location along the line.) Specific digestive enzymes are secreted that break very long protein molecules into shorter segments at specific junctions, until the fragments are just one, two, or three amino acids long, at which point the fragments can be absorbed for our use. Various spots along the small intestine are designed as the entry points for particular vitamins or minerals. A spot near the end of the small intestine is the location for the absorption of vitamin B_{12}.[30]

Our intestine is home to about four hundred different types of bacteria; this population is known as our intestinal flora. The exact mix of bacteria depends on what sustenance is available to them, and it is markedly affected by a change to a vegetarian or raw vegan diet. Some of these bacteria assist our cells with the digestive process, keep the growth of unwanted and harmful microorganisms in check, and may protect us from inflammatory conditions and cancer.[34-37]

Stage 4

Our large intestine is so named due to its diameter rather than its length. Here, unwanted materials are prepared for disposal. Fiber, which assists with moving food through the intestines, has not been absorbed and remains. The body disposes of waste materials by adding them to the fibrous mix that is passing through. Insoluble fiber, which is preserved to a greater extent in raw rather than cooked plant foods, is effective in ridding the body of carcinogens. (For more on fiber, see chapter 6.) Water and salts are removed from the wet mixture and, finally, the waste is allowed to exit through the anus.

Protein

There are two ways to ascertain how much protein we require for the maintenance of our muscles, blood, bone, and cells. One method is to determine the grams of protein per day that are recommended for our body weight. Another approach is to consider the percentage of our total daily caloric intake that should be derived from protein (see Percentage of Calories from Protein, page 93).

RECOMMENDED PROTEIN INTAKE IN GRAMS

The Recommended Dietary Allowance (RDA) for protein is the amount that scientists determine will meet the needs of practically all healthy people based on human research using mixed rather than raw vegan diets.

> *Although it is frequently pointed out that plants can provide all human protein needs, the misconception persists that they are nutritionally inferior to animal proteins.*[38]
>
> **D. JOE MILLWARD,**
> Centre for Nutrition and Food Safety,
> School of Biological Sciences,
> University of Surrey, Guilford, UK

Protein needs of adults are proportional to body weight because larger people have more protein maintenance to do. For adults, the daily protein RDA is 0.8 grams (0.028 ounces) per kilogram (2.2 pounds) of body weight. This figure includes a safety margin to cover differences in the digestibility of foods and variations from one individual to another. It is designed to meet the needs of 97 percent of the population.[39]

There can be substantial differences in protein requirements from one individual to another, but they seem to defy classification. An elderly vegetarian man living in the tropics (whose protein losses through perspiration are slightly greater) *may* need a little more protein per kilogram of body weight than a young female meat eater in a temperate climate.[40] Yet the research on age, diet, gender, and climate differences is too limited to make sound recommendations. Certainly, because our metabolic rates and therefore caloric requirements drop a little with age, we need to get a little more of our calories from protein as we get older.[40, 41]

PROTEIN QUALITY

When we take into account protein requirements, we must consider not just the total amount of protein but also the balance of indispensable amino acids (those required in our diet) that make up the protein.[39] This is particularly true when protein intakes fall very close to the protein RDA, which is the case for the protein intakes on raw diets that are shown in table 5.2, page 77. We require the full complement of indispensable amino acids as building blocks, and a shortage of any amino acid halts the body's ability to manufacture proteins. With vegetarian and near-vegetarian diets, the amino acid that tends to be in short supply is lysine. This fact draws our attention when we explore the topic of protein and amino acid balance in raw diets.[6, 8, 20, 21, 43, 44]

Note that while raw-food practitioners sometimes use the very low proportion of protein in human breast milk as a standard for adult protein needs on raw vegan diets, the comparison doesn't bear scrutiny due to the high digestibility of protein in human breast milk and the highly favorable balance of indispensable amino acids it contains.

PROTEIN REQUIREMENTS FOR RAW-FOOD VEGANS

Some people assume that the recommended protein intake for individuals on a raw vegan diet would be the same as for those on any other diet. Others believe that raw-food vegans need less protein because digestion is superior with this way of eating. Some believe that any cooking severely damages protein, resulting in amino acid deficiencies, which can cause all sorts of health problems, and that for this reason raw protein is superior and better utilized. Another camp suggests that raw-food vegans need more protein because protein from plant foods is less digestible than protein from animal products, and that plant protein provides a less desirable balance of amino acids. While the protein requirements of raw-food vegans have not been well defined, there appear to be reasonable arguments for the various positions.

Why Raw-Food Vegans Might Have Protein Requirements that Are Higher than the RDAs

1. **Some experts have recommended that protein intakes for vegetarians should be higher than those for nonvegetarians**. These experts have advised that the protein intakes for vegetarians should be 10–20 percent higher than that of nonvegetarians because research has shown the protein in many plant foods, such as cooked beans and grains, is significantly harder to digest compared to animal protein.[20, 44, 45]

2. **The amino acid lysine can be low in vegetarian diets.** The amino acid scoring pattern that is used as the standard for all people over the age of one sets the optimal proportion of lysine at 51 milligrams per gram of protein. However, lysine is typically low in grains, averaging 31 milligrams per gram of protein. Grains feature prominently in most vegetarian and near-vegetarian diets. (In fact, it may come as a surprise that grains provide approximately half of the protein for human diets worldwide.) Insufficient lysine limits the body's ability to manufacture proteins that require lysine as a building block.[6, 20, 21, 42–44] Legumes, with 60–70 milligrams of lysine per gram of protein, can help the situation by contributing more than their share. This amount is comparable to the 85 milligrams of lysine per gram of protein in animal products.[1, 2, 39, 47–50]

3. **Cooking at moderate temperatures improves protein digestibility.** The protein digestibility of some raw plant foods is lower than the digestibility of that same protein when the food is boiled or steamed.[51–53]

4. **Raw foods contain enzyme inhibitors.** Enzyme inhibitors protect plants from being digested by the enzymes of outside organisms; enzyme inhibitors do their job by binding to enzymes. They also can inactivate the enzymes that we use to digest protein. These enzyme inhibitors are destroyed by cooking, allowing the digestive process to proceed.[44, 52, 54–57]

Why Raw-Food Vegans Might Have Protein Requirements that Are Lower or Equivalent to RDAs

1. **Research supporting higher protein requirements was on cooked beans and grains, not on typical foods eaten in raw diets.** Research on the digestion of protein in plant foods is centered on beans and grains.[20, 44, 58] Apart from a small amount of research on the effects of sprouting, little research has been done on digestion of the protein in fruits, vegetables, nuts, and seeds that make up raw vegan diets.

2. **Sprouting makes plant protein more digestible.** For example, when peas are soaked for twelve hours and then sprouted for two days, protein digestibility increases by about 25 percent.[59] Sprouting buckwheat improves the digestibility of its protein.[52]

3. **Sprouting can improve protein quality.** Though raw oats, millet, and wheat are low in lysine, the process of sprouting increases their lysine content significantly. When seeds, grains, and legumes are sprouted, the reserve protein that is in storage for just this occasion is broken down into amino acids, and some conversion to lysine occurs.[54, 56, 57, 60, 61]

4. **Cooking lowers the lysine content of foods.** Lysine is lost even at mild cooking temperatures, and fried foods and browned foods show even greater lysine losses and lower protein digestibility than foods that are boiled or steamed.[64–67]

5. **High-temperature cooking lowers protein digestibility.** Whereas boiling can increase the protein digestibility of some foods, higher temperatures decrease digestibility.[43, 44, 64]

6. **Sprouting, soaking, or fermenting foods destroys enzyme inhibitors.**[54, 56, 57, 59, 62, 68–70]

7. **The optimal proportion of lysine for adults may be lower than 51 milligrams per gram of protein.** Whereas the optimal proportion of lysine in the amino acid scoring pattern for anyone above the age of one year is 51 milligrams per gram of protein, expert opinion is far from unanimous in supporting this number, which may be more appropriate for young children. The Food and Nutrition Board of the Institute of Medicine proposes a lower lysine requirement for adults of 47 milligrams per gram

How to Calculate Your Specific Protein Requirements

1. Divide your weight in pounds by 2.2 to give your weight in kilograms (1 kilogram = 2.2 pounds).

2. Multiply your weight in kilograms by 0.8 to find your recommended protein intake (0.8 grams of protein are needed for each kilogram of body weight).

For examples, see the column on the right in table 5.4 (page 91).

TABLE 5.4 Recommended daily protein for various body weights

Body weight, pounds	Body weight, kilograms	Recommended protein (0.8 g protein/kg)
105 lb	48 kg	38 g
120 lb	54 kg	43 g
135 lb	61 kg	49 g
150 lb	68 kg	54 g
165 lb	75 kg	60 g

of protein, while recognizing the possible validity of British protein expert D. J. Millward's suggestion for adults of a level of 31 milligrams of lysine per gram of protein.[38, 39, 71]

8. **Seeds, vegetables, nuts, and fruits contain more lysine per gram of protein than grains.** Whereas lysine is typically low in cereal grains (barley, oats, rye, and wheat), some seeds that we may use in a similar way (such as amaranth, buckwheat, and quinoa) are botanically not grains, do not contain the protein gluten, and have quite different patterns of indispensable amino acids, including more than the 31 milligrams of lysine per gram of protein in cereal grains. Amaranth contains 55 milligrams of lysine per gram of protein, quinoa has 54 milligrams, and buckwheat has 50 milligrams. Vegetables contain an average of 47 milligrams of lysine per gram of protein, and fruits and nuts contain an average of 45 milligrams.[1, 2, 47, 48, 50] These can provide adequate amounts of lysine, even when the recommended protein intakes are just met.[1, 39, 46]

CONCLUSION: While there are arguments for both reduced and elevated protein intakes in raw vegan diets, current data is simply not strong enough to establish a separate RDA. The American Dietetic Association states that an overview (meta-analysis) of the research found no significant difference in protein needs due to the source (plant, animal, or mixed) of dietary protein.[42, 73] Therefore, until we have further evidence, we will use the current RDA of 0.8 grams (0.028 ounces) per kilogram (2.2 pounds) of body weight as a guideline for raw-food vegans, the same as it is for the general population. This recommendation is based on a mixed diet that includes raw vegetables, fruit, nuts, and seeds, with optional grains and legumes, in order to ensure an assortment of the indispensable amino acids.

PROTEIN INTAKES ON RAW VEGAN DIETS

Meeting Recommended Protein Intakes on a Raw Vegan Diet

The average daily protein intake in various studies of raw vegan diets are shown in table 5.2, page 77. At the high-protein end of the spectrum, the 1992 Finnish living-food diet that is listed included plenty of sprouted foods: mung beans, lentils, buckwheat, seeds, nuts, and other sprouts, as well as a fermented oat "yogurt." Raw soups included avocado and many vegetables. At the other end of the spectrum, diets in the Giessen Study were centered around 3 1/3 pounds (1.5 kilograms) of fruit along with just over a pound (519 grams) of vegetables and an average of 2 ounces (56 grams) of nuts and seeds daily. The average caloric intake of participants was 1,887 calories. Yet from this diet, which was about three-quarters fruit by weight, the average protein intake was low at 39 grams; protein provided just 8.2 percent of calories.[13, 14]

To meet recommended intakes, it is important to increase reliance on some of the higher-protein foods listed in table 5.3, pages 80 to 85, such as vegetables, nuts, and seeds, with optional grains and legumes. It may also be necessary to avoid the oils and sweeteners listed at the end of the table. Select nuts, seeds, avocados, and olives as fat sources and fresh and dried fruits as sweet treats instead.

Table 5.5, page 93, shows a day's food intake providing 54 grams of protein. Here, 20 percent of the calories and 41 percent of the protein come from greens (peas in the pod, kale, and romaine lettuce). This is over ten cups of greens! The day's food plan meets recommended intakes for protein, calcium, and other minerals, while it is low or moderate in calories and fat, having less than 30 percent of calories from fat. A diet high in greens is one good way to get abundant protein and calcium along with low or moderate amounts of fat and calories; 1.32 pounds (600 grams) of greens per day has been suggested.[72] Kale can be used in a smoothie (see page 258), soup (see page 273), and/or as part of a salad (see pages 278 and 287). Pea pods make a delicious snack and are easy to include in meals. Seeds are important protein providers. Sunflower seeds can be eaten as a snack, used in a soup (see page 273), or made into a cookie along with dried fruit. Ground flaxseeds can be added to a smoothie (see page 258) or salad dressing (see page 276) or made into crackers (see page 265). Note that the five pieces of fruit, four figs, and one cup of berries contribute 40 percent of the calories (689 calories) in this menu, yet only 17 percent of the protein. For protein intakes in other menus, see chapter 12.

Do you think horses and elephants worry about not having any animal protein in their diet? Elephants are bigger and stronger than you.

RUTH HEIDRICH,
six-time winner of the Ironman Triathlon

ATHLETIC PERFORMANCE ON A RAW VEGAN DIET

Elite athletes meet their energy needs with somewhat larger quantities of food, and higher protein intakes also can be achieved on raw diets. Here are a few examples of athletes who

TABLE 5.5 A sample day's food intake with calories and protein

Food	Quantity	Calories	Protein in Grams
Sunflower seeds	1/2 c (72 g)	410	16
Snow peas	2.75 c (400 g)	168	11
Kale	4 c (268 g)	134	9
Flaxseeds	2 Tbsp (19 g)	103	4
Oranges	3 (393 g)	185	4
Bananas	2 (236 g)	210	3
Walnuts	2 (16 g)	105	2
Romaine lettuce	4 cups (188 g)	32	2
Raw vegetable strips (carrot, celery, zucchini)	1 c (123 g)	29	1
Blueberries	1 c (148 g)	84	1
Figs	4 (34 g)	84	1
Apple	1 (242 g)	126	0
Total	...	1,670	54

Note: The distribution of calories for the day's food intake equals 12% of calories from protein, 59% of calories from carbohydrate, and 29% of calories from fat.

have fueled themselves with raw vegan and mostly raw vegan diets: triathletes Brendan Brazier, Ruth Heidrich, and Tim VanOrden; body builders Storm Talifero, Charlie Abel, and Robert Cheeke; yogi Rainbeau Mars; dancer Tonya Kay; cyclist Bradley Saul; cyclist and runner Harley Johnstone; distance hiker Doug Walsh; and tennis player Martina Navratilova.

PERCENTAGE OF CALORIES FROM PROTEIN

It is recommended that a minimum of 10 percent or more of our calories comes from protein (when caloric intake is adequate). A glance at tables 5.3 (page 80) and 5.5 (above) show that this proportion can be achieved using a wide assortment of raw food. However, some raw diets fall below this level, and the situation is worsened because total calories are low. Every whole plant food supplies us with small or moderate amounts of protein. Insufficient protein intake can result in hair loss, skin problems, and poor wound healing and can be detrimental to bone health. Other symptoms of protein deficiency are muscle wasting, weakness, and fatigue. The calories from protein in most green vegetables and legumes range from 20 to 40 percent and in nuts and seeds from 9 to 17 percent. At the low end of the spectrum is fruit, with just 2–10 percent of the calories from protein.

Note that when people consume insufficient calories, as they intentionally do when a raw diet is part of a weight-loss plan, the percentage of their total calories from protein must be significantly higher (more like 15–20 percent of calories); otherwise, they will lose not only weight but also body protein. Raw diets centered on fruit can fall short of protein requirements. This can be remedied by including plenty of vegetables, moderate amounts of nuts and seeds, and optional sprouted or cooked legumes and grains. (For more on protein, see our books *The New Becoming Vegetarian* and *Becoming Vegan*.)

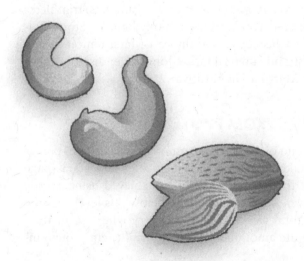

CHAPTER 6

Carbohydrates in the Raw

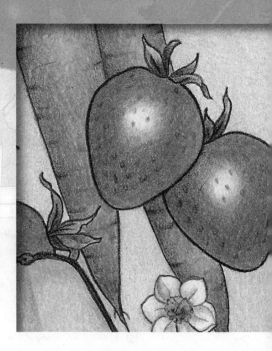

When we make a giant leap from the standard Western diet to a raw vegan diet, our carbohydrate intake undergoes a rather remarkable transformation. In most Western diets, approximately 80 percent of the carbohydrates comes from the white flour and sugars in highly processed foods and beverages. Smaller amounts of carbohydrates come from starchy vegetables, whole-grain breads and cereals, legumes, vegetables, fruits, and other plant foods. In raw vegan diets, white flour is avoided and added sugars are usually a very minor part of the diet. In contrast to conventional vegan diets, bread, cookies, crackers, pasta, and other products made with whole wheat flour are greatly reduced or eliminated. Cooked legumes, whole grains (such as cooked brown rice and barley), and starchy vegetables are also dramatically reduced or eliminated.

You may be wondering what carbohydrate sources remain. All plant foods contain carbohydrate, so it can be found in everything raw-food vegans consume, except oil. Some raw diets are centered on carbohydrates because of high fruit intake. Yet, apart from fruit, the foods that form the foundation of many raw diets are not considered high-carbohydrate foods. This is because these foods are either low in calories (as with nonstarchy vegetables and sprouts), resulting in a low total-carbohydrate content, or most of their calories come from fat, as with nuts and seeds. In this chapter, we will explore the world of carbohydrates and the practical implications of the changes that occur in both quality and quantity of carbohydrates consumed when a raw vegan diet is adopted.

Types of Carbohydrates

Carbohydrates are packages of the sun's energy that are used to support all life on earth. They are created through photosynthesis, a process in which carbon dioxide, water, and the green pigment chlorophyll join forces to trap the sun's energy. (*Carbo* means "carbon" and *hydrate* means "water.") Carbohydrates are categorized according to the number of sugars that are bound together in the carbohydrate molecule.

Monosaccharides. The molecule that results from photosynthesis is glucose—a simple carbohydrate, or sugar. Plants make other sugars, such as fructose and galactose, by rearranging this glucose molecule. These single-sugar units are called monosaccharides (*mono* means "one"). Monosaccharides cannot be broken down into smaller units by digestion, and they are the only carbohydrates that can be absorbed directly into the bloodstream. Other carbohydrates require the help of enzymes to break the bonds between the sugar molecules before they can be absorbed and used for energy.

Disaccharides. Two units of sugar are linked together by bonds to make disaccharides (*di* means "two"), such as sucrose (common table sugar), maltose (malt sugar, which forms when grains are sprouted), and lactose (milk sugar). Both monosaccharides and disaccharides are simple sugars, and they make foods taste sweet. Plants store energy for later use by stringing these sugars together to make larger carbohydrates called starches. When young plants start to grow, as we see in sprouting, they convert these starches back into simple sugars to be used for energy.

Oligosaccharides. When three to nine molecules of sugar are bound together, these relatively small carbohydrates are called oligosaccharides (*oligo* means "few"). Many oligosaccharides are not digested in the small intestine, so they pass through it and serve as fuel for beneficial bacteria in the large intestine. These compounds are also known as prebiotics.

Polysaccharides. When tens, hundreds, or thousands of sugar molecules are linked together, these carbohydrates are called polysaccharides (*poly* means "many"). Polysaccharides are further divided into two groups called starch and nonstarch polysaccharides (NSP). These groups are based on whether the plant uses the polysaccharide for storage or structure. Starch polysaccharides are the plant's energy stores, while nonstarch polysaccharides provide structure to the plant. Nonstarch polysaccharides are more commonly known as fiber. They contain bonds that cannot be completely broken down by the body's enzymes, which is why they are also called nondigestible carbohydrates. (Table 6.1, page 97, provides a summary of the different types of starches.)

How Carbohydrates Are Digested

Carbohydrates begin their journey toward digestion before food even enters our mouths. As plants ripen, carbohydrates are converted into simpler sugars. Processing, juicing, or blending food breaks down cell walls and liberates starch-digesting enzymes in the plant. Once food enters the mouth, amylase (a starch-digesting enzyme in saliva) begins to split some of the

TABLE 6.1 Carbohydrate classifications

Carbohydrate class (number of sugar molecules)	Type of carbohydrate	Examples	Notes
Sugars (1–2)	Monosaccharide	Galactose Glucose Fructose	Absorbed as is; not further broken down by digestion
	Disaccharide	Lactose Maltose Sucrose	Broken down by enzymes—sucrase, lactase, and maltase
Oligosaccharides (3–9)	Malto-oligosaccharide	Maltodextrin	Made from the breakdown of starch; used to thicken or bind processed foods
	Other oligosaccharides	Fructans (inulin and fructo-oligosaccharides) Raffinose Starchyose	Most are not broken down in the small intestine; provide food for friendly bacteria in the large intestine; contribute to flatulence
Polysaccharides (≥10)	Starches	Amylase Amylopectin Modified starches	Digestible starches that are broken down into sugars during digestion
	Nonstarch polysaccharides (fiber)	Cellulose Hemicellulose Mucilages Pectin Plant gums	Components of plant cell walls; gums and other indigestible parts of plants

Sources: Data from references 1–4.

bonds in starch. However, the greater part of starch digestion occurs in the small intestine, where the breakdown into simple sugars is completed. These sugars are converted to glucose in the liver, and from there they are distributed to body cells where they are used as energy or stored for later use. The body is not able to store much of these sugars (only enough for a few hours or perhaps a day), so if your stores are overloaded and you have all the calories you need for immediate energy, excess sugar will be converted into fat for long-term storage.

Some carbohydrates, such as fiber and certain oligosaccharides, are not broken down in the small intestine. They move on to the large intestine undigested, where they either add bulk to the stool or are used as food by intestinal bacteria.

Why We Need Carbohydrates

Carbohydrates are the main source of energy for the body and the preferred fuel for the brain, red blood cells, and nervous system. The only other sources of energy are protein, fat, and alcohol. Protein can be used as a fuel, but it is far from ideal, as it must be processed by the liver and kidneys first, requiring extra work by the body. Protein is used primarily to build new body tissue; make enzymes, hormones, and antibodies; regulate fluids and electrolytes; and act as an acid-base buffer. To ensure that protein is used for these important tasks instead of as a source of energy, it is important that we eat sufficient carbohydrates. This is called the protein-sparing effect of carbohydrates. Fat is used as a fuel, but it is not an ideal energy source. If the body uses fat for energy on an ongoing basis, by-products called ketones can accumulate. In extreme cases, this can cause ketoacidosis, dropping the body's pH to dangerously low levels. Alcohol is not a desirable fuel source, as it is highly toxic to the body, especially the brain, liver, and pancreas. That leaves us with carbohydrates, which are used efficiently and safely by the entire body for energy.

Carbohydrates supply approximately four calories per gram. When nutritional analyses are done on a particular food, all carbohydrates are counted, regardless of the degree to which they are digested. Consequently, the usable calories in many high-carbohydrate foods, particularly whole foods containing fiber and other nondigestible carbohydrates, may be overestimated. Some experts suggest that for carbohydrates (such as fiber) that reach the large intestine, the caloric count should only be two calories per gram.[1] This means that high-fiber foods may provide somewhat fewer calories than what is listed in nutrient databases and on food labels. Bacterial fermentation of fiber and other nondigestible carbohydrates do result in a small amount of available energy (calories) in the form of short-chain fatty acids.

In addition to serving as our major energy source, carbohydrate-rich whole foods can help to reduce hunger, control blood glucose and insulin metabolism, and keep cholesterol and triglyceride levels in check. These foods are also essential to the healthy functioning of the gastrointestinal tract, keeping waste products moving along rapidly, thereby protecting against constipation and intestinal disorders. Most of these beneficial effects are the result of nondigestible carbohydrates (fiber).

The Most Concentrated Sources of Carbohydrates

Plants provide the majority of carbohydrates in the human diet. Animal products (with the exception of milk) contain little or no carbohydrates. The form of carbohydrate in dairy products is lactose, or milk sugar. About 90 percent of the calories in fruits and starchy vegetables comes from carbohydrates. In grains, around 75 percent of the calories comes from carbohydrates, and in legumes, about 70 percent. In nonstarchy vegetables, close to 60 percent of the calories comes from carbohydrates. Only about 12.5 percent of the calories in most nuts and seeds comes from carbohydrates, as these foods are more concentrated in fat. (See table 5.3, page 80, and figure 6.1, page 97, for the percentage of calories from carbohydrates in common foods.)

It is interesting to note that when seeds are germinated, or sprouted, their carbohydrate composition changes. The storage carbohydrates (starches and oligosaccharides) are broken down into sugars so they can provide energy to the germinating embryo as necessary.[5] This change has some important consequences from a practical perspective. One of the reasons some people avoid legumes is because they cause flatulence. Humans do not make the enzymes that are necessary to break the bonds between the sugars in oligosaccharides. When you germinate legumes, this unpleasant side effect is largely eliminated, as the offending carbohydrates have been converted into sugars.[6]

FIGURE 6.1 Percentage of calories from carbohydrates in common foods

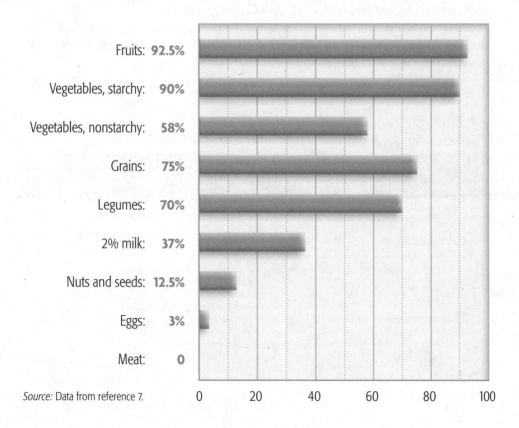

Source: Data from reference 7.

Recommended Carbohydrate Intakes

T he World Health Organization (WHO) recommends that 55–75 percent of our calories comes from carbohydrates, while the Institute of Medicine (IOM), the body that determines Dietary Reference Intakes in North America, recommends that 45–65 percent of our calories comes from carbohydrates.[3, 8] (The IOM recommends higher levels of fat and protein than the WHO; more calories would be provided from these sources.) Both organizations agree that the bulk of our carbohydrates should come from whole plant foods, such as vegetables, fruits, whole grains, legumes, nuts, and seeds.

Average carbohydrate intake in the United States is approximately 50 percent of calories, which falls within the IOM recommendations but below the WHO recommendations.[9] Most of the carbohydrates in standard Western diets come from refined and processed foods. Vegetarian and vegan diets tend to average closer to 50–65 percent of calories from carbohydrates, although people following popular low-fat vegan diets consume closer to 75 percent of their calories from carbohydrates.[10, 11] When you consider the percentage of calories from carbohydrates in plant foods, it is easy to understand why people eating plant-based diets tend to have relatively high carbohydrate intakes. It may be a bit surprising, however, to learn that many raw-food eaters have carbohydrate intakes that are lower than those seen in standard vegan diets, and in many cases, even lower than those of nonvegetarians.

The carbohydrate intakes of raw-food eaters are variable, with published reports ranging from 47 to 67 percent. The findings of research to date are provided in table 6.2, below.

TABLE 6.2 Carbohydrate, fat and protein intakes of raw-food adherents

Researchers, country, date	CHO intakes (% of calories)	Fat intakes (% of calories)	Protein intakes (% of calories)	Diet description
Giessen study, Germany, 2008[12]	Women: 58% Men: 57%	Women: 34% Men: 34%	Women: 8% Men: 9%	High-fruit diet; often one type of food per meal
Raw vegan diet, USA, 2006[13]	48%	43%	9%	Mixed raw diet, including vegetables, fruits, grain and legume sprouts, nuts and seeds, plus olive oil
Giessen study, Germany, 2005[14]	61%	30%	9%	High-fruit diet; often one type of food per meal

Researchers, country, date	CHO intakes (% of calories)	Fat intakes (% of calories)	Protein intakes (% of calories)	Diet description
Hallelujah Acres diet, USA, 2001[15]	Women: 67% Men: 66%	Women: 24% Men: 23%	Women: 10% Men: 10%	55% raw by calories; more grains and cooked starchy vegetables than most raw diets
Living-food diet, Finland, 1995[16]	50%	38%	12%	Raw diet, high in sprouts, fermented foods, nuts, and seeds
Living-food diet, Finland, 1995[17]	46%	42%	12%	Raw diet, high in sprouts, fermented foods, nuts, and seeds
Living-food diet, Finland, 1993[18]	47%	38%	15%	Raw diet, high in sprouts, fermented foods, nuts, and seeds
Living-food diet, Finland, 1992[19]	53%	32%	15%	Raw diet, high in sprouts, fermented foods, nuts, and seeds
Living-food diet, Finland, 1992[20]	55%	30%	15%	Raw diet, high in sprouts, fermented foods, nuts, and seeds
FOR COMPARISON				
WHO[8]	55–75%	15–30%	10–15%	Population Dietary Intake Goals*
IOM[3]	45–65%	20–35%	10–35%	Dietary Reference Intakes: Acceptable Macronutrient Distribution Range (AMDR)**

Note: In the Hallelujah Acres study of people consuming high-raw diets, intakes of carbohydrates were higher and intakes of fat were lower than in other studies.[15] This is because the Hallelujah Acres diet included greater amounts of high-carbohydrate, low-fat foods, such as cooked grains, starchy vegetables, and legumes. Generally, in raw vegan diets, starchy vegetables and legumes are eaten more sparingly.

The German raw-food eaters tended toward high-fruit, raw mono diets, eating only one food per meal.[11, 13] The Finnish living-food followers consumed diets rich in sprouts (including grain and legume sprouts), fermented foods, vegetables, nuts, and seeds. Rejuvelac (a drink made from sprouted and fermented wheat) and wheatgrass juice were often consumed as part of the daily fare.[16–20]

*Population nutrient intake goals are suggested for the prevention of diet-related chronic diseases.

**Acceptable Macronutrient Distribution Range (AMDR). The range of intakes for protein, carbohydrates, and fat that is associated with an adequate intake of essential nutrients and a reduced risk of chronic disease is known as the AMDR. This is expressed as a percentage of total energy intake.

Average Carbohydrate Intakes for Raw Foodists

While data has not been published on carbohydrate intakes in the wider raw vegan community in North America, intakes can be expected to vary considerably depending on the type of raw diet adopted. At one extreme are high-fruit diets, which tend to be very concentrated in carbohydrates (often as much as 70–80 percent of calories comes from carbohydrates, with 10–20 percent of calories coming from fat and about 10 percent from protein). At the other end of the spectrum are high-fat raw diets, which rely heavily on avocados, coconut, concentrated oils, nuts, and seeds. One raw-food leader contends that such diets may contain up to 65–70 percent of their calories from fat, although this view is not based on peer-reviewed research.[21] If we estimate protein intake at 10 percent of calories, this leaves only 20–25 percent of calories from carbohydrates. On a 2,000-calorie diet, total carbohydrate intake would be 100–125 grams (assuming 4 kcal per gram in carbohydrate). The Recommended Dietary Allowance (RDA) for carbohydrate, based on the minimal amount required for adequate brain function, is set at 130 grams per day. If calories from fat become excessive, carbohydrates may drop below intakes that are considered safe.

While high-fruit and high-fat diets demonstrate extremes in carbohydrate intakes, most raw-food eaters land somewhere in between. (See chapter 12 for a variety of menus with nutritional analyses to explore common ranges of carbohydrate intakes in different types of raw-food eating patterns.) One of the main reasons for the relatively high WHO and IOM recommendations for carbohydrates is that when carbohydrate intakes fall below these levels, fat is pushed up beyond the recommended upper limit of 30–35 percent. Some experts question the relevance of this upper limit for fat for people following a raw vegan diet. The upper limits set for large populations are based on mixed diets containing a variety of potentially harmful fats, including those from processed foods, deep-fried foods, and animal products. The evidence concerning the health consequences of consuming high-fat plant foods such as avocados, nuts, and seeds is overwhelmingly positive. However, when fat comes from concentrated fats and oils, nutritional concerns increase. (See chapter 7, pages 118–121, for further information.)

Raw-food adherents who wish to reduce fat intake often do so by shifting toward a high-fruit diet. Meeting recommended dietary allowances with this type of eating pattern can be challenging, as fruit tends to be low in essential fatty acids, B vitamins, protein, iron, and zinc, and lacks vitamins D and B_{12}. Another option for boosting carbohydrates and reducing fat would be to consume more sprouted grains and sproutable legumes (such as lentils and mung beans), and starchy vegetables such as raw corn and squash. These foods are high in carbohydrates but very low in fat. Of course, those who wish to consume a 70–80 percent raw diet or a high-raw diet could select cooked foods that are very low in fat, such as lentil soup and steamed yams. This type of dietary pattern would more readily provide a balance of energy-giving nutrients that are within the limits set by the WHO and the IOM (see page 100).

Comparing the Dietary Needs of Humans to Great Apes

Some advocates of high-fruit diets believe that the diets of wild, nonhuman primates provide a good rationale for a similar eating pattern in humans. Wild primates consume high-fruit diets, with lesser amounts of young leaves, flowers, bark, seeds, and other parts of plants. Animal products (generally insects) make up less than 5 percent of their total diet, and often less than 1 percent. It is important to recognize that there are significant differences in the nutritional profile of wild and cultivated fruits. Cultivated fruits, such as those available in our local supermarkets, have been selectively bred for appearance, sweet taste, succulent pulp, and few seeds. Wild fruits, which were featured in the diets of early humans, are less sweet and more concentrated in protein, vitamins, and minerals.

The intestinal tract of human and nonhuman primates differs both in physiology and function. Relative to body size, human intestines take up less volume than the intestines of great apes. In humans, the small intestine predominates, while in great apes, the large intestine is the more predominant organ. Unlike modern humans, the gut of nonhuman primates is adapted to an extremely high-fiber diet. The bacterial fermentation of indigestible carbohydrates in this diet provides an estimated 57 percent of the calories in the great ape's diet. This is because the bacteria that reside in the ape's large intestine use the indigestible carbohydrates as a food source. Among the by-products that result from the breakdown of these indigestible carbohydrates are short-chain fatty acids. The short-chain fatty acids are absorbed by the primate and become their largest source of calories (energy). The average 15.4-pound (7-kilogram) howler monkey is said to consume an average of 88 grams of fiber a day. This would be comparable to a 154-pound (70-kilogram) person eating 880 grams of fiber, or about 73 pounds (33 kg) of fruit!

Consequently, humans require more highly digestible foods, while great apes can manage with greater amounts of plant fiber and woody seeds. While most people would be wise to move closer to the diet of nonhuman primates—eating more plants, fewer processed foods, and little to no animal products—trying to emulate wild apes may be taking things a step too far.[22-25]

Fiber: The Whole Story

The term "dietary fiber" was adopted in 1953, and one might assume that its definition has been pretty much set in stone since that time. Nothing could be further from the truth. It may come as a surprise that the definition of dietary fiber has been a major source of controversy in the nutrition field for over a decade. In fact, various national and international bodies have proposed their own unique definitions, but a consensus has been extremely difficult to reach. Some believe that fiber should include only the intrinsic, intact components of plants that are neither digested nor absorbed in the small intestine. Others argue that it doesn't matter whether the substance comes naturally from a plant or is manufactured—anything that is not digested in the small intestine should count.

In 2002, the Institute of Medicine (IOM) updated its definition of fiber to include oligosaccharides and functional fiber, which have been traditionally excluded from the definition. Oligosaccharides include raffinose and starchyose, which are concentrated in legumes, and fructans, found mainly in Jerusalem artichokes and onions. Functional fiber is fiber that is not part of a whole plant; rather, it is isolated, or extracted, from plants or synthetically produced. The IOM definition of "total fiber" is not universally accepted. It has been internationally criticized because it creates an artificial, analytically impossible distinction between fiber found in plants and those extracted from plants or synthetically produced.[2]

In 2008, an FAO/WHO Codex Committee agreed on a definition for fiber that includes only carbohydrates with at least ten or more sugar units bound together (such as polysaccharides) that are not broken down by enzymes in the small intestine. Of course, this excludes oligosaccharides, which have only three to nine sugar units bound together.[25]

The major difference between the IOM definition and the WHO/FAO Codex Committee definition is the acceptance of indigestible oligosaccharides as fiber. The Codex Committee opposes the inclusion of indigestible oligosaccharides, as they believe that including oligosaccharides as fiber could lead to consumer confusion.[26] For example, oligosaccharides could be added to bottled water and sold as a rich source of fiber. Consumers may then think that getting fiber from this water would provide the same benefits as getting fiber from beans, fruits, vegetables, and whole grains. Although these isolated or synthetic carbohydrates have demonstrated beneficial effects, most authorities believe that the benefits of getting fiber from whole plant foods outweighs the benefits of getting fiber from isolated compounds.[2] While health organizations around the world have had difficulty reaching consensus about the definition of fiber, there is one thing that is universally agreed upon: fiber brings with it a host of health benefits.

Soluble and Insoluble Fiber

The terms "soluble fiber" and "insoluble fiber" have long been used as a way of dividing high-fiber foods according to their physiological effects. Soluble fiber has been said to reduce cholesterol and help control blood glucose, while insoluble fiber has been noted for its benefits to the gastro-intestinal system. Soluble fiber dissolves in water, but insoluble fiber does not.

Although these terms are still commonly used, they are being phased out, particularly in scientific circles. This is because the physiological benefits observed in scientific studies have been highly inconsistent. For example, some types of soluble fiber have little influence on blood glucose or cholesterol but do improve gut health and regularity. Likewise, some insoluble fiber is rapidly and completely fermented in the large intestine, and therefore would not contribute to stool bulk as expected. Many of the studies on which this terminology was based were done using isolated fibers, even though in plants these fibers exist together. These terms work well when referring to specific, isolated fibers. However, they do not work as well when it comes to whole foods. An effort is under way to replace these outmoded terms with others, such as "viscous" and "fermentable," which are more specific to physiological effects. Table 6.3, page 105, provides a list of the major types of fiber, their health effects, and their common sources.

TABLE 6.3 Types of plant fiber, health effects, and common sources

Type of fiber	Description	Health effects	Common sources
Beta-glucans	Glucose chains that are smaller in size and more branched than cellulose; become viscous in water	▪ Little effect on stool bulk or laxation ▪ Beneficial effect on blood glucose and cholesterol levels	Oats, barley, and mushrooms
Celluloses*	Large polysaccharides that contain only glucose in straight chains; insoluble and resistant to digestion; principle woody components of plant cell walls	▪ Increase stool bulk ▪ No significant effect on blood glucose or blood cholesterol levels	Grains, fruits, legumes, nuts, seeds, and vegetables
Gums and mucilages	Mixed polysaccharides that hold plant cell walls together; viscous and sticky	▪ No effect on stool bulk or laxation ▪ Beneficial effect on blood glucose and cholesterol levels	Seeds such as psyllium and guar seeds, sea vegetable extracts (carageenans and alginates); used in food manufacturing to thicken, stabilize, and add texture to foods
Hemicelluloses**	Large polysaccharides that contain a wide variety of sugars; associated with cellulose in plants; usually insoluble, but may be soluble	▪ Increase stool bulk ▪ May have a beneficial effect on blood glucose or blood cholesterol levels (depending on whether they are the soluble type)	Fruits, grains (especially outer husks), legumes, nuts, seeds, and vegetables
Lignins	Woody components of plants; not carbohydrates, but are bound to fibrous polysaccharides in plant cell walls and included as fiber	▪ Increase stool bulk ▪ No significant effect on blood glucose or blood cholesterol levels	Stringy vegetables and outer layer of cereal grains
Nondigestible oligosaccharides	Oligosaccharides that are not broken down in the small intestine; includes natural and synthesized compounds, such as inulin and fructans (for example, fructo-oligosaccharides)	▪ Some act as prebiotics, stimulating the growth and/or activity of friendly bacteria in the colon ▪ Increase stool bulk ▪ Improve intestinal health	Fruits, grains, legumes, and vegetables
Pectins	Polysaccharides that dissolve in hot water and form gels when cooling; present in cell walls, helping to give structure to fruits; when fruits are overripe, pectin breaks down and the fruits become mushy	▪ Little effect on stool bulk or laxation ▪ Beneficial effect on blood glucose and cholesterol levels	Berries and fruits (especially apples and citrus fruits)
Resistant starches	Starches that are not absorbed in the small intestine	▪ Beneficial effect on blood glucose, insulin sensitivity, and cholesterol levels	Legumes, raw potatoes, underripe bananas

Source: Data from references 2, 3, 4, 27.

*Cellulose accounts for about 25% of the fiber in grains and fruits and 33% in vegetables and nuts.

**Hemicellulose accounts for about 33% of the fiber in plants.

RESPECT YOUR ROUGHAGE

Fiber has been hailed as being "nature's broom" for our intestinal tract. While this analogy is quite reasonable, the benefits of fiber go beyond the broom. The more research that unfolds, the more powerful our understanding and respect for fiber becomes.

The most obvious benefits of fiber are to our gastrointestinal system. Fiber is important for preventing constipation, diverticulosis (small sacs in the wall of the intestines pressing outward), and hemorrhoids (painful, swollen tissues in the anus and rectum). It may also protect us against intestinal cancers (especially colorectal cancers), gallstones, and inflammatory bowel diseases, such as ulcerative colitis. A high-fiber diet makes stools softer and heavier, helping them pass more easily and rapidly out of the colon. While the insoluble, nonviscous, nonfermentable fibers, such as cellulose and lignin, are particularly helpful in this regard, fiber that is fermented in the colon also contributes to stool bulk. Much of this added weight comes from bacteria, as about 1 ounce (30 grams) of bacteria is produced for every 3.5 ounces (100 grams) of carbohydrate that is fermented.[2]

Many fermentable carbohydrates serve as prebiotics, stimulating the growth of friendly bacteria. During the fermentation process, by-products such as carbon dioxide, hydrogen, methane, and short-chain fatty acids are formed. The friendly bacteria and their products of fermentation provide a host of health benefits:

- The pH of both the colon and feces is reduced, inhibiting the growth of harmful yeast and bacteria.
- Carcinogens are reduced and cancer cells are attacked.
- Mineral absorption is improved.
- Food intolerances and allergies are reduced.
- Favorable changes in glucose and lipid metabolism occur (due to the absorption of short-chain fatty acids produced).[2]

Fiber has also been shown to reduce the risk of coronary artery disease, diabetes, gallstones, and kidney stones. Soluble, viscous fibers appear to have a significant cholesterol- and triglyceride-lowering effect. These fibers also delay the absorption of fat and carbohydrates from the small intestine, favorably influencing insulin levels and blood glucose response. Fiber also helps increase feelings of fullness after a meal, preventing overeating and weight gain. As absorption of carbohydrates and fat is delayed, satiety is prolonged.

FIBER RECOMMENDATIONS AND RAW-FOOD VEGANS

The World Health Organization recommends at least 25 grams of dietary fiber per day.[8] The Institute of Medicine recommends 14 grams of fiber per 1,000 calories for everyone over one year of age.[3] While Recommended Dietary Allowances have not been set for fiber, Adequate Intakes (AIs) were set in accordance with this 14-gram figure. Based on average energy intakes for various ages and genders, the AI is 38 grams per day for men (nineteen to fifty years of age) and 25 grams per day for women (nineteen to fifty years of age), and 30 and 21 grams respectively for older men and women.

The average fiber intake in the United States is approximately 15 grams per day.[9] Intakes of those eating vegan diets, raw or otherwise, consistently exceed Adequate Intakes. Raw-food eaters average intakes close to 50 grams per day. Table 6.4, below, provides a brief summary of studies that have assessed the fiber intakes of raw-food adherents. In the six different menus in chapter 12, fiber ranges from 56 to 84 grams.

EXCESSIVE FIBER

While it is possible to get too much fiber, it is unlikely if you are consuming whole foods and drinking sufficient fluids. Excessive fiber is more of an issue when people use concentrated fiber sources, such as wheat bran, in large amounts.

Very high fiber intakes can make the diet too bulky, thereby jeopardizing energy (caloric) intake and potentially leading to failure to thrive in children. This is seldom a concern in healthy adults. Fiber can also reduce the absorption of certain minerals. However, when fiber binds with minerals (such as calcium, magnesium, and iron), the minerals can at least be partially liberated during fermentation in the large bowel. Short-chain fatty acids can then help to facilitate their absorption.[2]

TYPES OF FIBER IN RAW VEGAN DIETS

Grains and legumes are concentrated sources of a number of different types of fiber. You might wonder, then, if intakes of these fibers, and perhaps intakes of total fiber, would be reduced in raw diets relative to conventional vegan diets.

TABLE 6.4 Fiber intakes of raw-food adherents

Study, country, year, reference	Fiber intakes in grams	
	MALES	FEMALES
Giessen study, Germany, 2008[12]	59	48
Hallelujah Acres diet, USA, 2001[15]	47	38
Raw vegan diet, USA, 2006[13]	60	37
Living-food diet, Finland, 1993[18]	47*	...
Living-food diet, Finland, 1992[19]	45	...

*The authors noted that incomplete analysis tables were used and estimated actual intakes at 79 g.

While total fiber intake appears to be similar in raw vegan diets and conventional vegan diets, resistant starch and beta-glucans would likely be lower in raw diets, as these types of fiber are concentrated in grains and starchy vegetables. The benefits associated with these types of fiber relate to the fermentation of carbohydrates in the colon and improved microflora.[2, 28] Evidence suggests that raw diets favorably affect microflora, although the raw diets used in the studies showing such improvements generally relied on a high percentage of fermented foods, which are not always included in raw diets.[19, 29–32] While there are no studies comparing the microflora of raw-food vegans with those eating conventional vegan diets, there is evidence that conventional vegan diets also favorably affect fecal flora.[33–35]

TABLE 6.5 Fiber content of whole plant foods

Amount of fiber per cup or serving*	Food and serving size
Very high-fiber foods 10 to 19.9 grams	Beans (all varieties), cooked, 1 c/250 ml
	Split peas, cooked, 1 c/250 ml
	Avocado (1 medium), 6.7 oz/200 g
High-fiber foods 5 to 9.9 grams	Berries (raspberries, blackberries), fresh, 1 c/250 ml
	Fruit (Asian pear, papayas, pear), 1 medium
	Coconut, fresh, shredded, 1/2 c/125 ml
	Flaxseeds, 2 Tbsp/30 ml
	Grains (most whole grains), cooked, 1 c/250 ml
	Potatoes, regular or sweet, baked, 1 medium
Moderate-fiber foods 2 to 4.9 grams	Berries (blueberries, strawberries), fresh, 1 c/250 ml
	Fruit (most varieties), 1 medium/2 small, or 1 c/250 ml
	Vegetables (most), raw, 2 cups/500 ml
	Nuts and seeds (most varieties), 1/4 c/60 ml
	Grains (brown rice, millet, oats), cooked, 1 c/250 ml
Lower-fiber foods 1.9 grams or less	Sprouts** (grain, legume, or vegetable), 1 c/250 ml
	Melon, 1 c/250 ml
	Fruit or vegetable juice (all varieties), 1 c/250 ml

Source: Data from reference 7.

*Rounded to the nearest gram.

**The fiber in sprouts is far lower than the fiber in an equal volume of the unsprouted food. This is because it takes only a few tablespoons of the unsprouted food to produce a cup of sprouts (which are largely water), and some of the fiber in the seeds or legumes gets converted to simple sugars during the sprouting process.

Carbohydrates: Unrefined or Refined, Simple or Complex

If you were to ask the average person on the street which is a more healthful choice, simple or complex carbohydrates, chances are that he would choose complex carbohydrates. That's because most people think of simple carbohydrates as refined sugars (such as white sugar or brown sugar), and they think of complex carbohydrates as starches like whole-grain breads and cereals. Of course, they are partly correct, as refined sugars are less healthful than starches from whole grains. However, they are not completely correct, as some complex carbohydrates are far less nutritious than some simple carbohydrates.

UNREFINED AND REFINED CARBOHYDRATES

Think about the carbohydrate sources most commonly consumed by raw-food eaters—fruits and nonstarchy vegetables top the list. In both of these nutritious types of foods, the majority of carbohydrates are in the form of simple sugars rather than more complex carbohydrates. On the other hand, some complex carbohydrates have very poor nutritional value. White flour and the multitude of products made from it are good examples. Whether a carbohydrate is simple or complex is not the important issue. What really matters is whether the food has been refined and stripped of nutrients important to human health before it is eaten. If the antioxidants, phytochemicals, fiber, vitamins and minerals in a food remain intact prior to its consumption, that food is a healthful source of carbohydrates; otherwise, it is not. Unrefined, carbohydrate-rich foods include fruits, legumes, vegetables, and whole grains. Refined, carbohydrate-rich foods include white-flour products and other refined grains, soda and other sweet beverages, and candy. Fortunately, raw and high-raw vegan diets include few refined foods. So although raw-food vegans eat their fair share of simple carbohydrates, these carbohydrates are health-promoting.

THE NEW JUDGES: GLYCEMIC INDEX AND GLYCEMIC LOAD

One of the practical failings of the terms "complex carbohydrates" and "simple carbohydrates" is that they were based on the assumption that consuming foods high in complex carbohydrates would lead to small, gradual increases in blood glucose, while foods high in simple carbohydrates would cause blood glucose to spike and then fall rapidly. This assumption turned out to be overly simplistic and technically false.

There are other, far more accurate ways of judging the effects of carbohydrates on our blood glucose: the glycemic index and the glycemic load. The glycemic index (GI) is a measure of how quickly carbohydrates are digested and absorbed into the bloodstream. Foods with a high glycemic index are those that are quickly digested and absorbed, causing a rapid rise in blood glucose. These foods may increase insulin response (negatively affecting long-term blood glucose control), increase triglycerides, and reduce protective HDL cholesterol. Foods with a low glycemic index are those that are slowly digested and absorbed, releasing sugars gradually into the bloodstream (see figure 6.2, below). These foods may positively affect insulin response, triglycerides, and HDL cholesterol levels.[36-38]

In order for researchers to determine the glycemic index of a food, several different people must consume sufficient amounts of the test food to provide 50 grams of carbohydrate. For each study participant, changes in blood glucose are monitored over time and compared to changes in blood glucose after the consumption of a control food (usually pure glucose). The values from all of the participants are averaged to obtain the glycemic index of the food. For example, white bread has a glycemic index of 73 relative to glucose, which means that the blood glucose response to the carbohydrate in white bread is 73 percent of the blood glucose response to the pure glucose. By comparison, barley has a glycemic index of 28 relative to glucose.[37]

Sometimes these comparisons lead to interesting and surprising results. For example, white sugar has a glycemic index of 68—slightly lower than that of white bread. How can it be that white bread, a complex carbohydrate, has a glycemic index that is higher than table sugar, a simple carbohydrate? After all, white sugar is a disaccharide, which is more rapidly converted to monosaccharides than the starches in bread. The main reason that bread has a higher glycemic index than white sugar is that all sugars do not affect blood glucose in the same way. The monosaccharides glucose and galactose have a much greater effect on blood glucose than fructose. Most of the sugars from the white bread are glucose, while white sugar is half glucose, half fructose. Therefore, while bread may be more slowly digested

FIGURE 6.2 High versus low glycemic index

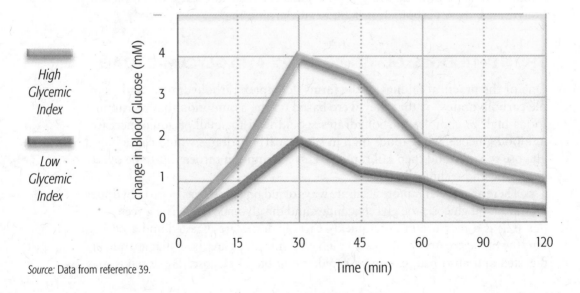

Source: Data from reference 39.

and absorbed than white sugar, the eventual effect of the sugars it contains will be greater. The end result is that the glycemic index of white sugar and bread are only a few points apart.

To throw in another twist, apples have a glycemic index of 36. In the old system, which pitted complex carbohydrates against simple carbohydrates, white bread and barley would have been viewed as complex carbohydrates, and white sugar and apples would have been viewed as simple carbohydrates. As you can see, the classification as a simple or complex carbohydrate has little bearing on how a particular food affects blood glucose and health.

The glycemic index tells us how a serving of food containing 50 grams of carbohydrates will affect our blood glucose. However, it does not tell us how much carbohydrate is in a typical serving of the food. For example, watermelon has a glycemic index of 72, which is very high (higher than white bread or white sugar). However, a 3.5-ounce (100-gram) serving of watermelon provides only 8 grams of carbohydrate. In order to get the blood glucose results predicted by the glycemic index, a person would need to eat about 6.25 servings, or 22 ounces (625 grams), of watermelon. A second useful tool, the glycemic load (GL), was created to provide a better indication of a food's effects. The glycemic load factors in the amount of carbohydrate a typical serving of the food contains. It is calculated by multiplying the glycemic index by the grams of carbohydrate provided in a serving of the food and dividing the total by 100. A 3.5-ounce (100-gram) serving of watermelon has a very low glycemic load; it therefore can be expected to have a relatively minor effect on blood glucose.

Factors that Affect Glycemic Index (GI)

- Type of monosaccharide in the food (glucose and galactose increase GI more than fructose)
- The kind of starch the food provides (amylopectin increases GI more than amylose)
- The amount and type of fiber present (viscous fibers reduce GI more than nonviscous fibers)
- The ripeness of the food (ripeness increases simple sugars and GI)
- Whether the food is raw or cooked and how much it is cooked (cooking increases GI because it breaks down the food, causing more rapid absorption)
- Particle size (whenever particle size is reduced, as with wheat berries ground into flour or foods that are blended, GI is increased)
- The degree of food processing (light and fluffy foods, such as rice cakes and white bread, have a much higher GI than heavy, dense foods)
- The presence of dietary components that slow digestion, such as fats, phytates, and tannins

Source: Data from references 37, 38, 40, 41, 42.

It is important to recognize that glycemic index and glycemic load should never be used in isolation to determine the nutritional value of a food. These tools help us to ascertain the effect of a food on blood glucose. Foods that contain little, if any, carbohydrate have a very low glycemic index, whether or not they are healthful. Deep-fried pork rinds have a low glycemic index; watermelon has a high glycemic index. That does not mean you should start eating deep-fried pork rinds; nor does it mean you should scratch watermelon off your menu. In order to assess a food's nutritional worth, we need to consider its antioxidant, fiber, mineral, phytochemical, and vitamin content. We must also look at the potentially harmful dietary components the food contains, such as pro-oxidants and trans-fatty acids. However, since eating substantial amounts of foods with a high glycemic load can lead to weight gain and diabetes, it's helpful to see how a raw vegan diet can protect against these.

The Glycemic Load of Raw Vegan Diets Compared to Other Diets

Raw vegan diets tend to have a very low glycemic load compared to almost any other diet, although high-fruit or fruitarian diets often have a higher GI than other types of raw diets. The glycemic index of most nonstarchy vegetables is not available. This is because most nonstarchy vegetables are so low in carbohydrates that eating 50 grams of carbohydrates from these foods would require participants to consume more food than would be considered reasonable (except possibly by raw-food eaters!). For example, to get 50 grams of carbohydrates, you would have to eat one of the following: two and one-half heads of romaine lettuce, one and one-quarter heads of broccoli, one and one-half heads of cauliflower, five medium cucumbers, or nine medium carrots. To obtain 50 grams of carbohydrates from most sprouts, you would need to eat three to forty cups, depending on the type of sprout.

Nuts have a glycemic index ranging from 21 to 27. Fruits also have a relatively low glycemic index. The fresh fruit that provides the highest glycemic load is bananas, and the glycemic index of bananas varies depending on the ripeness of the fruit (a less-ripe banana has a lower GI). Dried fruits generally have a comparable glycemic index to fresh fruit, although they have a higher glycemic load because they contain more carbohydrates per serving. Of the dried fruits, prunes have the lowest GI (29) and raisins have the highest (64). Raw vegan diets are generally completely lacking in foods with the highest glycemic index, such as puffed foods and products made with white flour and white sugar.[37]

A popular sweetener among raw-food advocates has been raw agave syrup. Agave syrup consists of varying amounts of fructose and glucose, but it is predominately fructose. Its glycemic index ranges from 10 to 19, depending on the percentage of fructose present (a higher percentage of fructose means a lower GI). While it would seem that agave syrup is the ideal sweetener, there are concerns about consuming too much concentrated fructose (that is, fructose that is not part of a whole food like fruit). When fructose is concentrated and consumed in large quantities, it may interfere with our appetite-control hormones and have negative consequences for health, including weight gain, elevated triglycerides, and increased risk of metabolic syndrome.[43, 44, 45] For more detailed information on glycemic index and glycemic load, and for a comprehensive list of these values in various foods, see www.mendosa.com.

CONCLUSION: The carbohydrates in raw vegan diets come almost exclusively from whole plant foods. Whenever carbohydrates come from these sources, they have been shown to be beneficial to human health. The types of carbohydrates that have been most strongly associated with negative health consequences are largely removed from raw vegan diets.

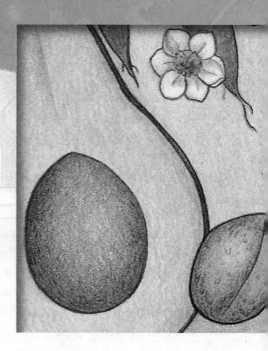

Fat: Friends and Foes

ost people believe that eating too much fat is bad for our health. Fat is viewed as a villain that is instantly deposited on our thighs and belly and in our arteries. You might imagine that fat intake would plummet when a raw vegan diet is adopted. Often, quite the contrary happens—the percentage of calories from fat escalates. Of course, the fat in raw vegan diets differs from that in conventional diets in a number of important ways. Most of it comes from high-fat whole foods, such as avocados, nuts, and seeds. If concentrated fats and oils are used, they are usually unrefined, meaning that they are not subjected to the high temperatures that cause the formation of those nasty products of oxidation. The saturated fat in raw vegan diets doesn't come from meat and dairy products; rather, it primarily comes from coconut and, in smaller amounts, from nuts, seeds, avocados, and oils.

What does all this mean from a practical perspective? Does the high quality of fat in raw food compensate for the relatively high percentage of fat in many raw vegan diets? Are raw diets that contain a lot of olive oil and coconut oil less healthful than those that derive most of their fat from whole foods? In this chapter we will explore the current issues and controversies concerning fat in the raw vegan diet and provide practical recommendations for fine-tuning both the quantity and quality of fat consumed.

Optimal Fat Intake

etermining optimal fat intake is among the most hotly debated issues in nutrition, and the deliberations are no less steamy in the raw-food community. Some high-fruit, low-fat eating plans promote intakes of less than 10 percent of calories from fat.[10] Gabriel Cousens, author of *There Is*

A Primer on Fats

Lipids. Lipids are a family of fatty compounds that do not dissolve in water. They include fats and oils (made up of fatty acids), sterols (such as cholesterol), and phospholipids (such as lecithin). While fats are only one type of lipid, the words "fat" and "lipid" are commonly used interchangeably. The main feature that distinguishes fats from oils is their consistency: fats are solid at room temperature and oils are liquid. Fats are generally found in animal products, such as meat, poultry, and dairy, while oils are commonly derived from plant seeds like olives, rapeseed, corn, and sunflower seeds. Lipids are a source of energy for the body and are our major vehicle for energy storage. They assist in the absorption of fat-soluble vitamins and phytochemicals. Lipids are an essential part of cell membranes. They also are used to make hormones and hormonelike substances that help to control many body systems.

Fatty acids. Fatty acids are basic components of fats and oils. Foods contain three types of fatty acids in varying amounts: saturated, monounsaturated, and polyunsaturated. Fatty acids are built from a chain of carbon atoms with hydrogen and oxygen molecules attached. The degree of saturation of a fatty acid depends on the amount of hydrogen attached to the carbon atoms.

Saturated fat. Saturated fat refers to fatty acids that are completely packed, or saturated, with hydrogen. Fats containing primarily saturated fatty acids are generally hard at room temperature. High intakes of saturated fat have been linked to an increased risk of chronic disease, particularly coronary artery disease.[1] Animal products are the main sources of saturated fats in Western diets. In fish, 20–30 percent of the fat is saturated; in poultry, 33 percent; in red meat,

40–44 percent; and in dairy products, 62 percent. Most high-fat plant foods contain much less fat, with 5–20 percent of it being saturated; the exceptions are tropical oils. Coconut fat is over 90 percent saturated, palm kernel oil over 85 percent, and palm oil about 50 percent.

Monounsaturated fat. Monounsaturated fat refers to fatty acids that have one spot in the carbon chain where hydrogen is missing (one point of unsaturation). Monounsaturated fat has been shown to have neutral or slightly beneficial effects on health, with modest effects on blood cholesterol levels. Replacing saturated fat, trans-fatty acids, and refined carbohydrates with monounsaturated fat reduces total and LDL cholesterol and slightly increases beneficial HDL cholesterol.[2, 3] Oils rich in monounsaturated fat are generally liquid at room temperature but become cloudy and thick when refrigerated, as with olive oil. The richest dietary sources of monounsaturated fat are avocados, canola oil, nuts (except for butternuts, pine nuts, and walnuts), olives, and olive oil.

Polyunsaturated fat. Polyunsaturated fat refers to fatty acids that have more than one spot in the carbon chain where hydrogen is missing (more than one point of unsaturation). Oils that are high in polyunsaturated fat are liquid at room temperature and when refrigerated. There are two distinct families of polyunsaturated fats: the omega-6 and omega-3 families. Polyunsaturated fats generally have favorable effects on health. When they replace saturated fats, trans-fatty acids, or refined carbohydrates in the diet, total and LDL cholesterol levels decrease, and HDL levels may slightly increase.[4] The main dietary sources of polyunsaturated fats are legumes, nuts, seeds, vegetable oils, whole grains, and other plant foods.

Essential fatty acids (EFAs). Most of the fatty acids that we need for survival can be produced in the body, but there are two that we cannot make and must obtain from food. These are called essential fatty acids. One is a parent in the omega-6 family called linoleic acid (LA). The other is a parent in the omega-3 family called alpha-linolenic acid (ALA). LA and ALA are called "parent" fatty acids because it is from them that the body can produce all the other family members, the highly unsaturated fatty acids (HUFA). From LA the body can make other omega-6 family members, and from ALA the body can make other omega-3 family members.

Highly unsaturated fatty acids (HUFAs). Larger polyunsaturated fatty acid molecules are called highly unsaturated fatty acids; they are also known as long-chain fatty acids. Our bodies can convert essential fatty acids into these more complex fatty acids, or we can consume them directly from food. In the omega-6 family, linoleic acid (LA) can be converted to gamma-linolenic acid (GLA), dihomo-gamma-linolenic acid (DGLA), and arachidonic acid (AA), or we can consume GLA directly from black currant, borage, or primrose oil, and AA directly from animal-based foods, such as meat and dairy products. In the omega-3 family, alpha-linolenic acid (ALA) can be converted to eicosapentaenoic acid (EPA) and docosahexaenoic acid (DHA), or we can consume EPA and DHA directly from fish (which contains both EPA and DHA), eggs (which contain only DHA), sea vegetables (which have small amounts of EPA), or microalgae (which are single-celled organisms that provide both EPA and DHA).

Trans-fatty acids. Trans-fatty acids are unsaturated fatty acids in which the position of one hydrogen atom changes the curved, flexible molecule to a straight, rigid molecule. Most trans-fatty acids are formed during hydrogenation, a process that turns liquid oils into solid, stable fats, though some are naturally present in dairy products. Fats in processed foods are hydrogenated to improve their shelf life. Other fats, such as shortening, are hydrogenated to increase their melting point (which is better for deep-frying) and permit high-temperature cooking. Trans-fatty acids have been found to be more damaging to health than any other fats. Trans-fatty acids strongly increase the risk of cardiovascular disease by adversely affecting a multitude of risk factors.[5–8] The trans-fatty acids found naturally in animal products do not appear to be as damaging as those that are commercially produced during hydrogenation.[7] However, evidence does suggest that these natural trans-fatty acids can impair insulin sensitivity in insulin-resistant individuals to a greater extent than manufactured trans-fatty acids.[9] Efforts are currently under way in North America to remove artificially produced trans-fatty acids from the food supply.

Cholesterol. Cholesterol is a sterol that is necessary to the structure of every cell. Because the human body makes 800–1,000 milligrams of cholesterol a day, there is no need for any cholesterol in the diet. Cholesterol comes from animal products and is concentrated in eggs and organ meats. High intakes increase the risk of chronic diseases, especially those of the heart and blood vessels.

Phytosterols. Phytosterols are sterols naturally present in plants. Plant sterols help to block cholesterol absorption from the gut. All whole plant foods contain small amounts of these compounds, although avocados, legumes, nuts, seeds, sprouts, vegetable oils, and wheat germ are the most concentrated sources. Plant-based diets are naturally higher in phytosterols than omnivorous diets.

a Cure for Diabetes, recommends a fat intake of 10–20 percent of calories.[11] The greater majority of raw-food authorities suggest more liberal fat intakes. Let's explore the ups and downs of fat intake and their practical implications.

ULTRA-LOW-FAT DIETS

Some of the most highly respected vegetarian and vegan proponents in the medical community advocate diets providing no more than 10 percent of calories from fat.[12-15] Promoters of high-fruit diets in the raw-food community concur, at least as far as total fat goes. The primary argument used by very low-fat advocates is that fat increases the risk of disease, particularly chronic diseases, such as heart disease, type 2 diabetes, and certain cancers. Researchers have clearly demonstrated that by reducing fat calories to no more than 10 percent and dramatically reducing harmful fats, heart disease can not only be prevented, but it can be very successfully treated and reversed in the majority of patients.[12, 14, 16] No drug therapy or surgery can claim as much. Such diets have also been shown to provide more effective therapy for people with type 2 diabetes than the conventional diet advocated by the American Diabetes Association.[15] While there is not yet peer-reviewed research examining the effects of very low-fat raw vegan diets on patients with coronary artery disease and diabetes, there are compelling anecdotal reports (see pages 34–37). It appears as though these diets produce results that are even more powerful than those reported with conventional vegan diets. This is not surprising when one considers that raw vegan diets go a step further and eliminate most processed foods.

Both the raw-food and conventional low-fat proponents advise against the use of concentrated fats and oils. These foods are not necessary in a healthful diet, and their elimination increases the nutrient density (amount of nutrients per calorie) of the diet. However, many also advise against the use of higher-fat plant foods, such as avocados, olives, nuts, and seeds. Studies that have examined the health effects of consuming these and other higher-fat whole plant foods are overwhelmingly positive (see pages 135–137 for more details). Eliminating or severely restricting high-fat plant foods, particularly when following a raw vegan diet, may prove a disadvantage. The most important justifications for the inclusion of higher-fat plant foods are outlined below:

1. Low-fat raw diets consist predominately of fruit, with the addition of smaller amounts of greens. These are highly nutritious foods; however, when they are consumed exclusively, the diet may fall short in a number of nutrients, including protein and a variety of trace minerals. Higher-fat plant foods, such as nuts and seeds, can help to bring nutrient intakes closer to recommended levels. This is less of an issue in conventional low-fat vegan diets, where legumes and grains are regularly consumed.

2. The absorption of fat-soluble vitamins and phytochemicals can be reduced in very low-fat diets compared to diets containing moderate amounts of dietary fat.[1, 17, 18] The absorption of certain nutrients (iron and zinc in particular) is already lower in plant-based diets; consequently, further

reductions could potentially compromise nutritional status, especially for vulnerable individuals. Although studies suggest that relatively small amounts of fat are required for the absorption of carotenoids, there is some evidence that more may be required when raw rather than cooked foods are eaten, as food processing and heating break down the plant cell walls and promote the release of these nutrients.[19] Fat-soluble nutrients and phytochemicals play vital roles in protecting health and reducing the risk of disease, so consumers are generally well advised to consume enough fat to ensure the optimal absorption of these nutrients.

3. Very low-fat diets may not provide sufficient essential fatty acids. In conventional low-fat vegan diets, grains provide adequate omega-6 fatty acids; however, intakes of omega-3 fatty acids average only about one-quarter of recommended intakes (unless omega-3–rich nuts or seeds are permitted). In raw vegan diets, fruits and greens tend to predominate. When these foods are used exclusively, omega-6 and omega-3 fatty acids are consumed in almost equal amounts (depending on the selection of fruits). While this provides an optimal balance of essential fatty acids, the quantities of essential fatty acids may not be sufficient. In a 2,000-calorie diet, the intakes of the two essential fatty acids average approximately one gram each (intakes are even lower in reduced-calorie diets). This is below both recommended and adequate intakes. In order to boost total essential fatty acid intakes, seeds and/or walnuts would need to be added to the diet. To maintain fat intake at less than 10 percent of calories, not more than one ounce of seeds and walnuts could be consumed in a 2,000-calorie diet. A combination of seeds high in omega-3 and omega-6 seeds could be selected (such as flaxseeds and pumpkin seeds) or seeds and nuts containing a healthful balance of the two essential fatty acids (such as hempseeds and walnuts). This would bring total intakes to a healthful range.

4. Very low-fat diets tend to be bulky (that is, there are few calories in a large amount of food), providing insufficient calories for some people, particularly children. Individuals with high energy needs, such as pregnant and lactating women or competitive athletes, may also have difficulty meeting energy requirements on very low-fat diets.

HIGH-FAT DIETS AND HEALTH

The greater majority of nutrition and health experts, including those who advocate raw diets, suggest more liberal fat intakes. Many believe that determining an acceptable quantity of fat depends on the quality of the fat consumed. Some promote high-fat intakes using Mediterranean-style diets as evidence of the benefits of diets rich in fat, especially olive oil.[20] In the raw-food community, higher-fat diets are common.

In 1980, Ancel Keys' classic Seven Countries Study demonstrated a strong connection between total fat, saturated fat, and coronary artery disease.[21, 22] The link was unmistakable: as fat intake increased, so did rates of coronary artery disease. However, there was one important exception—residents of the Greek island of Crete. In Crete, people averaged 37 percent of calories from fat, yet they had the lowest coronary artery disease rates of all countries studied—even lower than Japan, with an average fat intake of only 11 percent. What seemed to separate the people of Crete and other populations eating high-fat diets were their sources of fat. In Crete, the diet was rich in plant foods and olive oil; intakes of meat, poultry, and fish totaled less than two ounces per person per day. It should also be noted that an estimated 60 percent of the study participants fasted during the forty days of Lent, and an unknown number also followed the Greek Orthodox Church dietary doctrines that prescribe almost 180 days of fasting per year.[23] These doctrines define "fasting" as abstaining from meat, fish, dairy products, eggs, cheese, and olive oil on certain Wednesdays and Fridays. While these practices were not mentioned or factored into the results of Keys' study, leading experts from the University of Crete Faculty of Medicine believe that the regular restriction of certain foods, notably those of animal origin, had significant, positive health effects.[23]

Mediterranean-style diets provide a compelling argument that the quality of fat trumps the quantity of fat as a predictor of health outcomes. However, even when the fat is predominately "good" monounsaturated and polyunsaturated fat, high intakes of concentrated fats and oils may increase health risks. Some of the primary concerns are outlined below:

1. Concentrated fats and oils are high in calories (approximately 120 calories per tablespoon) and low in nutrients. When raw diets contain liberal quantities of fats and oils, more nutrient-dense foods (that is, foods with more nutrients per calorie) may be crowded out. This can make it difficult to meet recommended intakes for nutrients, especially for those that are already marginal in raw diets (for example, trace minerals, such as iron and zinc). The typically low-caloric intakes of raw-food vegans add to the challenge, as nutrients per calorie become even more significant. Concentrated fats and oils generally contribute little more than calories, essential fatty acids, and vitamin E. It makes more sense to obtain these nutrients from nutrient-dense whole foods that offer protein, unrefined carbohydrates, fiber, and a host of vitamins, minerals, and phytochemicals.

2. High-fat diets have been linked to chronic medical conditions, such as cardiovascular disease, diabetes, gallbladder disease, and some cancers. The bulk of the evidence against high-fat diets is specific to diets rich in saturated fats and/or trans-fatty acids.[1, 24, 25] Trans-fatty acids are not consumed in raw vegan diets, and saturated fat intakes are generally low. However, there is some evidence that diets very high in fat (42–50 percent of calories from fat) may increase several markers of blood coagulation and thrombosis, potentially elevating the risk of heart disease.[26, 27]

3. High-fat diets may result in increased oxidative damage to body tissues. Free radicals are more likely to react with polyunsaturated fats (unstable molecules),[28] so people who consume greater amounts of these fats, especially from concentrated oils, could be more susceptible to oxidative damage. Oxidative damage has been linked to numerous disease processes, including arthritis, age-related diseases, cancer, diabetes, heart disease, and neurological disorders.[28, 29] (For more information about this, see pages 66–67.)

4. There is some evidence suggesting that when high-fat diets are consumed, fewer essential fatty acids are converted to the more biologically active highly unsaturated fatty acids compared to lower-fat diets.[30] Adequate conversion of essential fatty acids is important in many aspects of health and disease (see page 126 for more information).

THE BIG FAT MYSTERY SOLVED

It's somewhat mystifying to see such positive results stemming from what appear to be such diametrically opposed eating patterns. In fact, the eating patterns described are less divergent than they might appear. In most cases, both lower- and higher-fat plant-based diets are centered around foods that are loaded with fiber, phytochemicals, vitamins, and minerals. Neither eating pattern provides excessive amounts of saturated fat, trans-fatty acids, cholesterol, animal protein, or refined carbohydrates—the dietary components most strongly linked to chronic disease.

The lesson learned from the low-fat advocates is that low-fat plant-based diets provide powerful therapeutic treatment for chronic diseases, particularly heart disease and type 2 diabetes. However, we cannot assume that these diets set the gold standard for all raw-food vegans, regardless of age or state of health. There are many factors that must be considered when establishing recommended fat intakes for any given population.

The lesson learned from the Mediterranean diet is that high-fat diets can be healthful, if the quality of fat is good. It is not high-fat whole foods, such as avocados, nuts, olives, and seeds, that are responsible for the epidemic of chronic disease that plagues us.

CURRENT RECOMMENDED INTAKES FOR FAT

Most major health organizations concur that fat intake for most people should range from 15 to 35 percent of calories.[1, 24, 31] They also agree that saturated fats, trans-fatty acids, and cholesterol should be restricted.

While experts recognize the potential adverse health consequences of fat intakes that are too high or too low, optimal fat intake depends on your age, your state of health, and the quality and balance of the fats you consume. If you're very physically active or have a fast metabolism (that is, you require a lot of calories to maintain your body weight), you may find it preferable to aim for total fat intakes at the higher end of the suggested range. If you're overweight, have a slow metabolism, or have a chronic disease, such as heart disease, you will likely find intakes near the lower end of the range to be more health-supportive. Fat intakes below 15 percent of calories from fat have proved to be safe and effective in the treatment and reversal of chronic disease; however, they are not generally advised for healthy individuals. Fat intakes above 35 percent of calories are not normally suggested, as they may lead to excessive intakes of saturated fat and trans-fatty acids, and insufficient intakes of carbohydrates and fiber.

Leading health organizations offer varying advice when it comes to the amounts of fat to consume. The World Health Organization has set "population dietary intake goals" for macronutrients. A total fat intake between 15 and 30 percent of calories is suggested, although it adds that highly active people with diets rich in fruits, legumes, vegetables, and whole-grain cereals may sustain a fat intake of up to 35 percent of calories without risk of unhealthy weight gain.[24] It also recommends that saturated-fat intakes be less than 10 percent of calories (7 percent for high-risk populations) and trans-fat intakes be less than 1 percent of calories.

In North America, the Institute of Medicine's new Dietary Reference Intakes for Energy, Carbohydrates, Fiber, Fat, Protein, and Amino Acids has not set a Recommended Dietary Allowance (RDA), Adequate Intake (AI), or Upper Limit (UL) for total fat (except during the first year of life). However, it has set a criterion known as the Acceptable Macronutrient Distribution Range (AMDR).[1] The AMDR for fat is 20–35 percent of calories for adults, 25–35 percent for children age four to eighteen, and 30–40 percent of calories for children age one to three. A gradual transition from the high-fat diet of infancy (55 percent of calories during the first six months of life, and 40 percent of calories from six to twelve months) to childhood is recommended. The report doesn't set maximum levels for saturated fat, cholesterol, or trans-fatty acids, as risk increases no matter how much is consumed. However, it recommends eating as little as possible of these and consuming a diet adequate in important essential nutrients.

The American Heart Association strongly advises that all Americans over the age of two limit fat to less than 25–35 percent of daily calories, saturated fat to less than 7 percent of daily calories, trans fat to less than 1 percent of daily calories, and cholesterol to less than 300 milligrams per day for most people and less than 200 milligrams per day for people with coronary artery disease.[31]

Although the American Diabetes Association does not suggest a range for total fat intake, it does recommend that saturated fat be less than 7 percent of calories, trans-fatty acids be minimized, and cholesterol be kept under 200 milligrams per day for people with diabetes.[32]

FAT INTAKES OF VEGANS AND RAW-FOOD VEGANS

In conventional vegan diets, average fat intakes range from 28 to 33 percent of calories.[33] This compares to 36 percent of calories in the average Western diet.[34] From research reported to date, fat intakes of raw-food vegans average 36 percent of calories (see table 6.2, page 100), with the exception of Hallelujah Acres followers, who consume an average of only 23–24 percent of calories from fat. However, the Hallelujah Acres diet, with 55 percent of calories derived from raw foods, differs significantly from standard raw-food eating patterns, as intakes of cooked foods (particularly grains and starchy vegetables) are higher.

TOTAL FAT RECOMMENDATIONS
FOR RAW-FOOD ADHERENTS

At the present time there is insufficient data to set a definitive recommendation for total fat intake for raw vegan diets. While the upper limits suggested by the

World Health Organization and the Institute of Medicine are certainly reasonable, they may be less relevant to raw-food eaters than the general population. This is because these figures are based on omnivorous eating patterns, which are more concentrated in potentially damaging fats such as saturated fat, trans-fatty acids, and oxidized fats produced by frying and other high-temperature heating methods.

There is very little data to suggest that increased health risks are associated with generous intakes of avocados, nuts, seeds, and other high-fat plant foods. A handful of small raw-food studies have reported favorable health outcomes with fat intakes exceeding 35 percent of calories.[35–37] A 2006 U.S. study of raw-food adherents consuming almost 43 percent of calories from fat in a moderately low-calorie diet found that a variety of markers for cancer risk improved.[35] In a 2001 Finnish study, sixteen participants provided with a raw vegan diet experienced an 18 percent drop in total cholesterol and a 21 percent drop in LDL cholesterol after one month on the test diet.[36] The percentage of calories from fat was not specified in this study; however, the diet was described as a strict, uncooked, vegan diet containing plenty of nuts and seeds. A previous study by the same research group reported fat intakes ranging from 37 to 38 percent of calories using a similar type of diet.[38] An earlier 1995 Finnish study compared the antioxidant status of raw-food vegans consuming 42 percent of calories from fat to omnivores consuming 39 percent of calories from fat.[37] The researchers found that the raw-food vegans had significantly better levels of beta-carotene, vitamin C, and vitamin E, and better overall antioxidant status compared with the omnivores in the study.

Higher-fat diets have been reported to reduce the conversion of essential fatty acid to the more biologically active highly unsaturated fatty acids compared to lower-fat diets,[30] although we don't know if these findings would apply to raw diets containing a better balance of healthful fats.

CONCLUSION: Concentrated fats and oils are among the least nutrient-dense foods in the diet, providing very few nutrients (apart from essential fatty acids and vitamin E) and a lot of calories. These foods may crowd out more healthful foods, making it challenging to meet recommended intakes for many nutrients, especially those that are already marginal in raw vegan diets. For this reason, an upper limit of 7 percent of calories from added fats and oils is suggested, with lower intakes being preferable.

A good dietary goal is to maximize nutrients and other protective dietary constituents in every calorie consumed. This is particularly important in raw diets, as calorie intakes are often relatively low, making it especially challenging to meet nutritional requirements. No more than 7 percent of calories from added fat allows for one tablespoon of fat or oil in a 2,000-calorie diet. (To be precise, 7 percent of 2,000 calories works out to 16 grams of added fat.) For lower-calorie diets, minimize your intake of added oils, and rely on whole foods for most of your fat. If you do use oils, select those that contribute to omega-3 fatty acid intake (see table 7.2 and pages 129–132).

Ensuring Optimal Intakes
of Essential Fatty Acids

Not all fats are villains. In fact, the essential fatty acids (EFAs) and their derivatives, the highly unsaturated fatty acids (HUFAs), are necessary for our survival. They serve as raw materials for building our brain, nervous system, and cell membranes. A lack of these important fatty acids can have devastating consequences for health, increasing the risk of a multitude of diseases and disorders.[39, 40] The essential fatty acids include the parent of the omega-6 fatty acid family, linoleic acid (LA), and the parent of the omega-3 fatty acid family, alpha-linolenic acid (ALA). Our bodies cannot make these fats; we must get them from our food supply.

One of the greatest concerns about essential fatty acid nutrition is that the natural balance of these two essential fatty acids (as found in a whole-food diet) has been greatly altered over the last century. Experts estimate that up until 100–150 years ago, the ratio of omega-6 to omega-3 fatty acids ranged from 1:1 to 2:1 (meaning that there were equal to double the amount of omega-6 fatty acids relative to omega-3 fatty acids).[40, 41] Since that time, vast changes in our food supply have pushed the ratio to 10:1 or higher.[40, 41] In conventional vegan diets, the balance is even more precarious, with reported intake ratios ranging from 10:1 to 20:1.[33] The blame is placed squarely on the food-processing industry and the use of omega-6-rich oils in food preparation. Omega-3-rich oils are largely avoided in food manufacturing due to their poor stability. Simply put, most of us eat too many omega-6 fatty acids and not enough omega-3 fatty acids.

Raw vegan diets have important advantages over conventional vegan diets where essential fatty acid intake and balance is concerned. This is because most raw vegan diets contain plenty of fresh foods, few processed foods, and low to moderate amounts of oil—the dietary constituents that tip the balance in favor of omega-6 fatty acids. Raw-food adherents who do use concentrated oils often select those that are rich in monounsaturated fats (such as olive oil) or omega-3 fatty acids (such as flaxseed or hempseed oil). Raw vegan diets also reduce our exposure to essential fatty acids that have been damaged by food-processing techniques such as high-temperature heating and hydrogenation.[39, 42] While raw vegan diets may offer an advantage in terms of the essential fatty acids they provide, care should be taken to ensure the intake and balance are optimal.

THE IMPORTANCE OF MAINTAINING OPTIMAL
OMEGA-3 TO OMEGA-6 FATTY ACID RATIOS

Omega-6 and omega-3 fatty acids compete for the enzymes that are necessary for the conversion of essential fatty acids to highly unsaturated fatty acids (see figure 7.1, page 124). Three of these highly unsaturated fatty acids are precursors for hormonelike substances called eicosanoids: two omega-6 fatty acids—dihomo-gamma-linolenic acid (DGLA) and arachidonic acid (AA)—and one omega-3 fatty acid, eicosapentaenoic acid (EPA). These eicosanoids help to control many body systems, such as inflammation and immunity, and act as central nervous system messengers. There are four families of eicosanoids: prostaglandins, prostacyclins, thromboxanes, and leucotrienes. For each of these eicosanoid families, a different series of compounds are formed from the highly unsaturated fatty acid precursors. For example, from DGLA, series 1 prostaglandins (PG1) are formed; from AA, series 2 prostaglandins (PG2) are formed; and from EPA, series 3 prostaglandins (PG3) are formed.

Each series of prostaglandins has different effects on the body. Generally speaking, those formed from AA tend to promote inflammation and several other risk factors for heart disease, hypertension, immune-inflammatory disorders, type 2 diabetes, neurological disorders, and possibly certain cancers.[39, 40, 42] While we need some of these eicosanoids for "fight and flight" type responses, when they are overexpressed in the body, they consistently produce negative health consequences. Those formed from EPA tend to have the opposite effect, thereby reducing our risk for disease, as do those from DGLA, although somewhat less strongly. Conversion enzymes usually favor omega-3 fatty acids; however, with high intakes of LA, the scale tips in favor of the omega-6 family. This increases the production of AA in the body, and the inflammatory eicosanoids formed from AA increase as well. For these reasons,

Sources of Essential Fatty Acids and Highly Unsaturated Fatty Acids

The primary sources of the two essential fatty acids, linoleic acid (LA) and alpha-linolenic acid (ALA), are plants, both on land and in the sea. The richest sources are seeds and walnuts. The most common sources of the highly unsaturated fatty acids, which are made from these parent EFAs—arachidonic acid (AA), eicosapentaenoic acid (EPA), and docosahexaenoic acid (DHA)—are animal products (although DHA and EPA are also available from sea plants). Table 7.2, page 130, lists specific amounts of these fatty acids in a variety of foods.

SOURCES OF OMEGA-6 FATTY ACIDS (listed in descending order of omega-6 concentration)

- Linoleic acid (LA): seeds and seed oils (grapeseed, safflower, sunflower, pumpkin, hemp, cottonseed, sesame), nuts and nut oils (walnuts, butternuts, pine nuts), grains and grain oils (corn, wheat germ), and soybeans and soybean oil

- Gamma-linolenic acid (GLA): borage oil, black currant oil, echium oil, primrose oil, spirulina, and hempseed oil (GLA is a precursor of DGLA, as shown in figure 7.1, page 124)

- Arachidonic acid (AA): meat, poultry, dairy products, and eggs

SOURCES OF OMEGA-3 FATTY ACIDS (listed in descending order of omega-3 concentration)

- Alpha-linolenic acid (ALA): seeds (chia, flax, hemp, and canola), nuts (walnuts and butternuts), green leafy vegetables, broccoli, and sea vegetables

- Eicosapentaenoic acid (EPA) and Docosahexaenoic acid (DHA): EPA- and DHA-rich microalgae (not blue-green algae), fish (especially cold-water fish), eggs (especially those from chickens fed fish oil, microalgae, or flaxseed oil), breast milk, and sea vegetables

it is important that the ratio of LA to ALA promotes a favorable balance of eicosanoid production.

There is another highly unsaturated omega-3 fatty acid called DHA that can be negatively affected by a poor ratio of LA to ALA. DHA does not serve as a precursor for eicosanoids; however, it's a critical structural component of cell membranes and is necessary for the proper development and functioning of the brain and central nervous system.

ADEQUATE INTAKES FOR ESSENTIAL FATTY ACIDS

Adequate Intakes (AI) for essential fatty acids are made both as a percentage of total calories and as a specific quantity to be consumed each day. The Institute of Medicine has set AI for LA (an omega-6 EFA) at 12 grams per day for women and 17 grams per day for men. The AI for ALA (an omega-3 EFA) are 1.1 grams per day for women and 1.6 grams per day for men.[1] (There is inadequate information regarding our needs for essential fatty acids to set a Recommended Dietary Allowance [RDA] for healthy individuals. Adequate Intakes are not based on optimal intakes but instead are set based on the median intakes of linoleic acid and alpha-linolenic acid in the United States.) The World Health Organization recommends that 5–8 percent of calories comes from omega-6

FIGURE 7.1 Metabolism of essential fatty acids*

Omega-6 family	Omega-3 family
Linoleic acid (LA) (grapeseed, safflower, sunflower, corn, hempseed, and sesame oils; walnuts; grains)	Alpha-linolenic acid (ALA) (chia seeds, flaxseeds, echium oil, hempseeds, walnuts, greens)
Gamma-linolenic acid (GLA) (borage, black currant, echium, and evening primrose oils; spirulina; hempseeds)	Stearidonic acid (SDA) (echium oil, hempseeds, blue-green algae)
Dihommogamma-linolenic acid (DGLA) Series 1 eicosanoids (PG1)	Eicosapentaenoic acid (EPA) Series 3 eicosanoids (PG3) (microalgae, fish, sea vegetables, breast milk)
Arachidonic acid (AA) Series 2 eicosanoids (PG2) (animal fats)	Docosahexaenoic acid (DHA) (microalgae, fish, eggs, breast milk)

Sources: Data from references 43–45.

*Food sources are listed in descending order of omega-6 and omega-3 concentration.

fatty acids and 1–2 percent of calories comes from omega-3 fatty acids.[24] Both sets of recommendations are meant for the general population and assume that people are getting some direct intake of the highly unsaturated omega-3 fatty acids, EPA and DHA (from fish, eggs, or DHA-rich microalgae).

For vegans who consume little if any direct sources of EPA and DHA, a ratio of omega-6 to omega-3 fatty acids ranging from 2:1 to 4:1 has been suggested as being optimal to ensure maximum conversion of alpha-linolenic acid to EPA and DHA.[46–48] More recent research suggests optimal conversion is achieved with a ratio of 1:1, although this is significantly more difficult to achieve.[49]

While it's not common, it's possible to overconsume omega-3 fatty acids. If a person eats a very low-fat diet, avoiding nuts, seeds, avocados, and concentrated oils (except for very rich sources of omega-3 fatty acids, such as flaxseed oil), the resulting omega-6 to omega-3 ratio could be less than 1:2, potentially leading to an omega-6 fatty acid deficiency.

ESSENTIAL FATTY ACID INTAKE AND THE STATUS OF RAW-FOOD VEGANS

To date, only one study has examined the essential fatty acid status of raw-food vegans. In 1995, a team of researchers from Finland compared fatty acids in the diet, serum (blood), and cell membranes (red blood cells and platelets) of vegans eating a living-food diet with those of nonvegetarians.[38] The ratios of omega-6 to omega-3 fatty acids were similar in both groups (about 5:1 for the raw-food vegans and 4.5:1 for the omnivores) and considerably better than is reported for most nonvegetarians and vegans. However, the living-food group consumed little EPA or DHA (although they would have consumed small amounts of EPA if sea vegetables were included among their choices), while the control group averaged 310 milligrams per day. The blood and tissue levels of EPA and DHA in the living-food group were only 29–36 percent and 49–52 percent, respectively, of those in the nonvegetarian group. It's interesting to note that their levels of AA were similar, indicating no difficulty with the conversion of LA to AA in the raw-food group. (AA comes directly from meat and dairy, so direct intake is very low in vegan diets.) These findings are comparable to those reported for people eating conventional vegan diets.[50–54]

One U.S. study reported on intakes of essential fatty acids in adherents to the Hallelujah Acres diet.[55] Omega-6 fatty acid intakes averaged approximately 10 grams per day, while intakes of omega-3 fatty acids averaged 5 grams per day. This provided a very favorable 2:1 ratio of omega-6 to omega-3 fatty acids. Unfortunately, the fatty acid status (blood and tissue levels) of this population was not assessed, so we do not know whether the improved essential fatty acid intakes resulted in better long-chain omega-3 fatty acid status. The study participants consumed some concentrated oils, including flaxseed oil, and had a low to moderate intake of nuts and seeds. The inclusion of flaxseeds and flaxseed oil increased the omega-3 fatty acid intake in this study group beyond what is generally observed within vegan populations. In addition, only

55 percent of total calories came from raw foods, and grains were the second largest source of calories (after fruits). These intakes differ significantly from those of typical raw-food eaters.

ESSENTIAL FATTY ACID CONVERSION

While highly unsaturated fatty acids (HUFAs), such as arachidonic acid (AA), eicosapentaenoic acid (EPA), and docosahexaenoic acid (DHA), are extremely important to health, they aren't generally considered "essential" because they can be manufactured in your body from essential fatty acids. When you eliminate fish and eggs from your diet, few direct sources of HUFAs remain. Therefore, you must depend on your body's conversion of the essential fatty acids from plants to make highly unsaturated fatty acids.

Unfortunately, the enzymes that create HUFAs are easily disrupted and this conversion is often inefficient, depending on your genetics, age, and overall health. In addition, poorly designed diets can impair the conversion process. High intakes of omega-6 fatty acids can have a profound effect on omega-3 fatty acid conversion, reducing it by as much as 40–50 percent.[56, 57] Too much fat (especially trans-fatty acids), saturated fats, and cholesterol can inhibit conversion. Fasting, which is practiced by some raw-food adherents,[58] and protein deficiency can decrease the activity of conversion enzymes, as can too much sugar or alcohol.[42] Deficiencies of several vitamins and minerals can also inhibit the process.[42, 59, 60] Conversion enzymes may not function as well in people with diabetes, metabolic syndrome, hypertension, or certain metabolic disorders, and in those who inherit a limited ability to produce these enzymes (a possibility in populations where fish has been a major component of the diet for generations).[41, 42]

One study found that diets providing 20 percent of calories from fat were associated with significantly greater conversion of omega-3 fatty acids compared with diets providing 45 percent of calories from fat.[30] (The same number of calories was provided by each diet.) The lower-fat diet improved the fatty acid status in a way that is comparable to eating direct sources of AA, EPA, or DHA, such as DHA-rich microalgae. The authors surmised that the fewer fats that are consumed, the more conversion enzymes would work to convert omega-3s. Although the percentages of various fatty acids were fairly constant in the diets, the absolute amount of saturated fat was slightly more than double in the high-fat diet compared to the low-fat diet. While trans-fatty acid intakes were not listed, several items included in the high-fat diet (such as chips, high-fat muffins, and crackers) could have contained trans-fatty acids. These factors may also have reduced the efficiency of the conversion enzymes. This study doesn't prove that ALA conversion will be lower in whole-food, high-fat, raw vegan diets. However, evidence suggests that high-fat diets reduce conversion, while lower-fat, lower-calorie diets enhance conversion.[42] In the previously mentioned study, the ratios of omega-6 to omega-3 fatty acids were similar, and both were unfavorable (11:1 in the low-fat diet and 12:1 in the high-fat diet). It's possible that as fat intake increases, an even lower ratio is required for optimal conversion.

There is evidence that omega-3 conversion is enhanced when sources of stearidonic acid (SDA) are consumed. SDA is formed in the first step of the conversion of alpha-linolenic acid (ALA) to eicosapentaenoic acid (EPA). It has been shown to produce many of the favorable effects reported for EPA and has also been shown to raise both EPA and DHA concentrations more effectively than ALA.[45] While stearidonic acid is not found commonly in foods, about 2 percent of the oil in hempseed is SDA, as is 12–14 percent of the fat in echium oil.[44, 61] (Echium oil is from a plant called purple viper's bugloss, which is native to parts of Europe but invasive in the United States and Australia.) Small amounts of SDA are also present in blue-green algae.

Direct sources of EPA/DHA are sometimes advised for those with increased needs (for example, pregnant and lactating women) or those who are at greater risk of poor conversion (such as people with diabetes or hypertension, those with neurological disorders, premature infants, and the elderly). While there is considerable speculation regarding the benefits for vegans during pregnancy and lactation, evidence is lacking. On one hand, it would appear that conversion is excellent during these life stages,[62] while on the other hand, EPA and DHA levels in the blood, tissues, and breast milk of vegans have been reported to be only about half that of omnivores.[53] This may be explained, at least in part, by inadequate intakes of omega-3 fatty acids by these vegans and a poor balance of omega-6 to omega-3 fatty acids in their diets. At this time, we don't know if an optimal status could be achieved by correcting intakes and the balance of essential fatty acids without the use of direct sources of DHA.

While the conversion of LA to AA is usually efficient, the conversion of ALA to EPA and DHA tends to be less efficient. It's commonly estimated that 5–10 percent of ALA is converted to EPA, but less than 2–5 percent of it is converted to DHA.[56, 57, 63] There is evidence that the conversion is significantly better in young women than in men.[62, 64] One study found that young women converted 21 percent of ALA to EPA, 9 percent to DHA, and 6 percent to an intermediary highly unsaturated fat called DPA.[62] Accordingly, a remarkable 36 percent of alpha-linolenic acid was converted to highly unsaturated fatty acids. In men, the conversion was 8 percent for EPA, 8 percent for DPA, and zero for DHA, bringing the total conversion to 16 percent.[64] The high conversion rates reported in young women are most likely nature's way of preparing for the increased needs of pregnancy and lactation, as DHA is necessary in the formation and development of the brain, nervous system, and retina of the fetus and newborn.[65, 66]

Women beyond their childbearing years and men convert long-chain omega-3 fatty acids less efficiently than young women. For this reason, some people wonder if these groups would benefit from direct sources of DHA, and possibly EPA. While direct sources may provide benefit for some individuals, it's very likely that conversion is reduced because less is needed. DHA is the most highly unsaturated fat in the diet and also the most unstable (meaning it is easily oxidized by free radicals in the blood). Oxidized fats are bad news; they contribute to all sorts of disease processes, including cardiovascular disease. It's possible that our bodies are smart enough not to bother making DHA when it's not needed. In addition, it's possible that when DHA is in our bloodstream, it's rapidly transported to locations where it's needed and incorporated into tissues, such as the brain and the retina of the eyes.

Although HUFA conversion is slow and incomplete, it appears to be sufficient to meet the needs of most healthy people if ALA intake is sufficient.[49,] [67] The obvious question that arises is whether or not the conversion process provides adequate EPA and DHA for optimal health or just enough to avoid deficiency. We don't know if the health status of vegans would be improved with more direct sources of highly unsaturated fatty acids. However, we do know that reduced omega-3 status can have negative health consequences, so it makes sense to take the necessary steps to optimize conversion.

ACHIEVING OPTIMAL ESSENTIAL FATTY ACID INTAKES IN RAW VEGAN DIETS

In order to ensure a healthful balance of essential fatty acids and their derivatives, we need to adjust our dietary intakes to ensure optimal conversion of alpha-linolenic acid (ALA) to eicosapentaenoic acid (EPA) and docosahexaenoic acid (DHA), and in some cases, we may wish to consider adding a direct source of these two highly unsaturated fatty acids. To achieve the recommended ratio of omega-6 to omega-3 (between 2:1 and 4:1), raw-food vegans are advised to aim for 4–8 percent of calories from omega-6 fatty acids and 1–2 percent from omega-3 fatty acids. Individuals with increased needs or decreased capacity for conversion may need to boost their intake of omega-3 fatty acids to 2.0–2.5 percent of calories. In practical terms, if you consume a 2,000-calorie diet, aim for 9–18 grams of omega-6 fatty acids and 2.2–4.4 grams of omega-3 fatty acids. To achieve a ratio of 1:1, you would need to further reduce omega-6 fatty acids, increase omega-3 fatty acids, or both. Intakes of omega-6 fatty acids would need to drop to 3–4 percent of calories, while intakes of omega-3 fatty acids would rise to 3–4 percent of calories. However, from a practical perspective, this very low omega-6 intake is extremely difficult to achieve and does not appear necessary for healthful conversion rates. (See table 7.2, page 130, for information on the quantities of EFAs in various raw foods.)

Balancing essential fatty acids is not so difficult when you build your diet on whole foods and you know what type of fats predominate in these foods. Among raw plant foods, the primary source of saturated fat is coconut. Avocados, nuts (except for butternuts, pine nuts, and walnuts), and olives are concentrated sources of monounsaturated fat. Seeds are the principle sources of polyunsaturated fats. Grains, fruits, legumes, and vegetables are generally very low in fat, so they make fairly minor contributions. The fat in grains is largely omega-6 fatty acids, while greens provide mostly omega-3 fatty acids. Legumes and fruits contain mainly polyunsaturated fat, with some being higher in omega-6 fats and others in omega-3 fatty acids. Excluding extremes (such as chickpeas, which are mainly omega-6), most legumes average a ratio of omega-6s to omega-3s of about 2:1. The average ratio for fruit rests between 1:1 and 2:1, with apples at about 5:1 and papaya at about 1:5.

Recognizing that you want to consume 5–10 percent of your calories from polyunsaturated fats, and you want a ratio of omega-6s to omega-3s between 2:1 and 4:1, getting the right balance can be relatively simple. If you're eating a very low-fat diet, you need to be sure to include enough seeds to meet your needs for essential fatty acids. If you're eating a diet that includes more liberal amounts of fat, focus on the foods rich in monounsaturated fats (such as avocados and nuts), with the addition of some more concentrated omega-3-rich foods. There is also room for fresh or dried coconut, which is almost exclusively saturated fat with little omega-6 and no omega-3 fatty acids, and a few omega-6-rich seeds, such as pumpkin, sunflower, and sesame seeds.

The following guidelines will help you put together a diet that ensures an excellent intake and balance of essential fatty acids:

1. Make monounsaturates your primary dietary fat. This means avocados, nuts, and olives. If you're consuming less than 15 percent of your calories from fat, this does not apply, as most of your fat should come from polyunsaturated fats. If fat intake is higher, as is the case in most raw diets, monounsaturated fatty acids should predominate. Making monounsaturates the primary fat puts a lid on omega-6 fatty acids. How many avocados and nuts you should be eating depends on how much fat you'd like your diet to provide. If you decide to cap your fat intake at 35 percent of calories, and you eat 2,000 calories per day, you can eat about 78 grams of fat per day. Here is how you can calculate this:

2,000 calories x 35% (.35) = 700 calories from fat

Fat has 9 calories per gram, so 700 ÷ 9 = 78 grams

If you're eating fewer calories or aiming for more or less fat, you can use the same formula—just adjust the numbers. It's important to note that no food contains only monounsaturated fats; all plant foods contain a mixture of saturated, monounsaturated, and polyunsaturated fats. (See table 7.2, page 130, for the fatty acid content of oils and high-fat foods.) Avocados and nuts contain both saturated and polyunsaturated fats, although the polyunsaturated fats are predominately omega-6. If you get all of your fat from whole foods, you could get 78 grams of fat by eating one medium avocado (about 3.5 ounces/100 grams), 2 ounces of nuts, and 1 ounce of seeds, plus the fats from other lower-fat whole foods. If you include concentrated oils in your diet, you could consume one medium avocado (3.5 ounces/100 grams), 1 ounce of nuts, 1 ounce of seeds, and 1 tablespoon of oil. (This could be flaxseed oil, hempseed oil, or olive oil, depending on whether your nut and seed choices provided omega-3 fatty acids.)

2. Include good sources of ALA (omega-3 fatty acids from plants) daily. The richest sources of ALA are seeds (chia seeds, flaxseeds, flaxseed oil, hempseeds, and hempseed oil) and walnuts. Aim for at least 2.2–4.4 grams per day if you're eating a 2,000-calorie diet. (This is 1.1–2.2 grams per 1,000 calories consumed.) While most of the fat in leafy greens is omega-3, the total fat content is very low, so to get 1 gram of ALA from greens, you would need to eat

TABLE 7.2 Fatty acid composition of selected foods

Food	Total fat % of total calories	Saturated fat % of fatty acids	Mono. fat % of fatty acids	Omega-6 % of fatty acids	Omega-3 % of fatty acids	Omega-3 fatty acids		
						ALA mg	EPA mg	DHA mg
OILS (1 Tbsp/15 ml)								
Canola oil	100	7	61	21	11	1.3	0	0
Coconut oil	100	91	7	2	0	0	0	0
Corn oil	100	13	29	58	0	0	0	0
Cottonseed oil	100	26	22	52	0	0	0	0
Flaxseed oil	100	9	18	16	57	8.0	0	0
Grapeseed oil	100	6	17	77	0	0	0	0
Hempseed oil	100	8	11	61	20	2.8	0	0
Olive oil	100	15	75	9	1	0.8	0	0
Palm oil	100	51	39	10	0	0	0	0
Palm kernel oil	100	87	11	2	0	0	0	0
Peanut oil	100	19	48	33	0	0	0	0
Safflower oil	100	6	14	75	0	0	0	0
Safflower oil, high oleic	100	6	75	14	0	0	0	0
Sesame oil	100	14	42	44	0	0	0	0
Soybean oil	100	15	24	54	7	0.9	0	0
Sunflower oil	100	11	20	69	0	0	0	0
Sunflower oil, high oleic	100	10	86	4	0	0	0	0
Walnut oil	100	9	23	53	13	1.7	0	0
NUTS, SEEDS, AND WHEAT GERM (1 oz/30 g, about 3.2 Tbsp/48 ml, unless otherwise specified)								
Almonds	77	8	66	26	0	0	0	0
Butternuts	84	2	19	63	16	2.5	0	0
Cashews	72	21	61	18	0	0	0	0
Chia seeds	72	21	61	18	0	0	0	0
Flaxseeds, whole (2 Tbsp/30 ml/ 20.6 g)	41	9	18	16	57	5.2	0	0
Flaxseeds, ground (2 Tbsp/30 ml/14 g)	41	9	18	16	57	3.8	0	0

Food	Total fat % of total calories	Saturated fat % of fatty acids	Mono. fat % of fatty acids	Omega-6 % of fatty acids	Omega-3 % of fatty acids	Omega-3 fatty acids		
						ALA mg	EPA mg	DHA mg
Hazelnuts	87	7	78	15	0	0	0	0
Hempseeds (2 Tbsp/30 ml)	56	8	11	61	20	1.2	0	0
Macadamia nuts	95	17	81	2	0	0	0	0
Peanuts	76	15	52	33	0	0	0	0
Pecans	94	8	63	28	1	0.3	0	0
Pine nuts	85	9	33	58	0	0.05	0	0
Pistachios	72	12	56	32	0	0	0	0
Pumpkin seeds	76	19	31	45–50	0–5	0–0.7	0	0
Sesame seeds	78	15	39	45	1	0.1	0	0
Sunflower seeds	79	10	40	50	0	0	0	0
Walnuts	90	7	15	63	15	2.6	0	0
Wheat germ (2 Tbsp/30 ml)	24	18	16	58	8	0.1	0	0
SEA VEGETABLES, RAW (3.5 oz/100 g, unless otherwise specified)								
Irish Moss	<1	33	14	7	46	.001	46	0
Kelp	12	58	23	17	2	.004	4	0
Spirulina	13.5	50	12	23	15	0.2	0	0
Wakame	13	32	14	8	46	0.001	186	0
FRUITS AND VEGETABLES								
Avocados (1 medium)	86	17	69	13	1	0.25	0	0
Greens (1 c/250 ml)	12–14	28	5	11	56	0.1	0	0
Olives (10 large)	84	14	77	8	0.1	0.02	0	0
ANIMAL PRODUCTS (for comparison)								
Cod (3 oz/90 g)	7	31	22	1	46	0	54	111
Egg (1 large)	61	37	48	14	0.4	.02	5	51
Salmon, wild Atlantic (3 oz/90 g)	40	18	40	3	39	0.1	517	948

Source: Data from references 68, 69.

about 10 cups. For most omnivores, this would seem an impossible task, but for raw-food eaters, it's entirely doable. Flaxseeds are a rich and economical source of omega-3 fatty acids. However, they're hard little seeds and tend to go through the intestinal tract undigested if they're not ground. The whole seeds do a great job of increasing stool bulk, but they don't provide much in the way of omega-3 if eaten intact, so use ground flaxseeds instead. (See table 7.3, below, for the EFA content of selected plant foods.) If you use concentrated oils for salad dressings, your best choices are those rich in omega-3 fatty acids, such as flaxseed oil and hempseed oil. (See Liquid Gold Dressing, page 276, and Lemon-Tahini Dressing, page 275.)

3. Reduce your intake of omega-6 fatty acids if it is excessive. It is easy to overdo omega-6 fatty acids, especially if you use omega-6-rich oils, such as corn, grapeseed, safflower, sesame, and/or sunflower oil. Of course, if you eat a lot of seeds that are low in omega-3 fatty acids, such as pine nuts (although pine nuts are technically considered tree nuts, they are high in polyunsaturated fatty acids, making them more similar to seeds), pumpkin seeds, sesame seeds, and sunflower seeds, your intake of omega-6 fatty acids could also be quite high, though you will be getting plenty of other nutrients. One ounce of omega-6-rich seeds provides 6–9 grams of omega-6 fatty acids. Recall that we are aiming for 4–8 percent of calories from LA, so in a 2,000-calorie diet, the upper limit for omega-6 fatty acids would be about 18 grams. Of course, if your caloric intake is higher, the upper limit for omega-6 intake would increase proportionally. For example, if you eat 2,800 calories per day, your

TABLE 7.3 The ALA content of selected plant foods

Food	Serving size	ALA % of fatty acids	LA % of fatty acids	Ratio of omega-6 to omega-3	ALA g/serving
Chia seeds	2 Tbsp/30 ml (20 g)	61	20	0.33:1	4.0
Flaxseed oil	1 Tbsp/15 ml (14 g)	57	16	0.28:1	7.8
Flaxseeds, ground	2 Tbsp/30 ml (14 g)	57	16	0.28:1	3.2
Flaxseeds, whole	2 Tbsp/30 ml (20.6 g)	57	16	0.28:1	4.8
Greens (mixed)	1 c/250 ml (50–60 g)	56	11	0.19:1	0.1
Hempseed oil	1 Tbsp/15 ml (14 g)	20	61	3:1	2.8
Hempseeds	2 Tbsp/30 ml (20 g)	20	58	3:1	1.2
Walnuts (English)	1/4 cup/60 ml (28 g)	14	58	4:1	2.6

Source: Data from references 68, 69.

upper limit for omega-6 fatty acids would be 25 grams. While the fats from most avocados and nuts are mainly monounsaturated, those foods contain far more omega-6 than omega-3 fatty acids and contribute to omega-6 intakes. The best way to ensure that omega-6 fatty acids are kept under control is to avoid omega-6-rich oils and keep your intake of omega-6-rich seeds to about an ounce per day.

DIRECT VERSUS INDIRECT SOURCES OF EPA AND DHA

It's difficult to say whether any one individual needs a direct source of the highly unsaturated omega-3s. We do know that low levels of EPA and DHA have been associated with a variety of negative health outcomes. We also know that vegans, including raw-food vegans, appear to have lower EPA and DHA levels than omnivores. However, the health consequences of these differences are uncertain. The most convincing evidence for direct consumption of highly unsaturated omega-3 fatty acids is in the prevention and treatment of coronary artery disease. While it appears that fish consumption protects people who are at high risk of coronary artery disease, it does not appear to reduce the risk in people with health-supporting lifestyles who are at low risk.[70] Studies have not yet compared the health of vegans who take supplemental EPA and DHA to those who don't. However, incorporating direct sources of EPA and DHA may be worth considering, particularly for those who have a reduced conversion ability or increased needs (see page 126).

The most commonly consumed sources of EPA and DHA are fish and seafood. The only plant sources of long-chain omega-3 fatty acids are plants from the sea—microalgae and sea vegetables. Sea vegetables are even lower in fat than most land vegetables, although they do contain small amounts of highly unsaturated omega-3 fatty acids. A 100-gram serving of raw sea vegetables provides, on average, about 100 milligrams of EPA but little DHA. Sea vegetables do not contribute significantly to EPA intakes in the Western world, but they are significant sources in countries where people use large quantities of sea vegetables on a daily basis (such as Japan and other parts of Asia). Some sea vegetables may provide too much iodine if they are consumed in excessive quantities (see table 9.3, page 189, for more information).

Microalgae are the most promising plant sources of ecologically sustainable highly unsaturated omega-3 fatty acids. Unlike fish, cultured microalgae provides an entirely renewable resource, free of environmental contaminants. In the DHA-rich microalgae *Schizochytrium* (a member of the kingdom Chromista and the phylum Heterokonta), 37.4 percent of the fatty acids are DHA and 0.5 percent are EPA. In yellow-green algae (also a member of the kingdom Chromista and the phylum Heterokonta), 27 percent of the fatty acids are EPA and 2.8 percent are DHA.[71] At the present time, DHA-rich microalgae (which may or may not contain appreciable amounts of EPA) are being cultured for commercial use; consequently, vegan supplements generally contain no EPA or very small amounts of EPA. When taking DHA directly, 100–300 milligrams per day is commonly recommended. Some vegan supplements also include small amounts of EPA in combination with DHA. (For sources, do an Internet search for "vegan DHA" or "vegan DHA and EPA.")

Blue-green algae (spirulina and Aphanizomenon flos-aquae) are low in highly unsaturated omega-3 fatty acids. Spirulina is rich in gamma-linolenic acid (GLA), a beneficial omega-6 fatty acid, while 40–50 percent of the fat in Aphanizomenon flos-aquae (AFA) is omega-3 ALA. Although blue-green algae is not a significant source of EPA or DHA, some research indicates that it may promote more efficient omega-3 conversion than what is commonly seen with land plants.[72]

Fats that Provide the Greatest Health Advantages

The dietary fats that are most strongly linked to adverse health consequences are trans-fatty acids from processed foods and saturated fats from animal products. Fats that tend to be neutral or beneficial to health are the monounsaturated fats and polyunsaturated fats, both of which are concentrated in plants.

The highest-quality fat is naturally present in avocados, fresh nuts and seeds, olives, and other lower-fat plant foods. If the oils are extracted from these foods, what is left behind are fiber, minerals, protein, vitamins, unrefined carbohydrates, and a host of protective antioxidants, phytochemicals, and plant sterols. Even unrefined organic vegetable oils pale in comparison to the whole foods from which they were extracted. Of course, there's no contest between the fats found in unrefined organic oils and the chemically altered fats found in margarine, shortening, and other hydrogenated vegetables oils.

Whole foods come packaged by nature to protect them from damaging light, heat, and oxygen, so they're less prone to the ravages of free radicals than concentrated oils. To preserve the quality of fats in foods, it's important to store them appropriately. Nuts and seeds will keep in their shells for up to a year or longer if stored in the refrigerator (between 32 and 45 degrees F/0 and 7.2 degrees C). Most nuts will keep for four to six months in their shells at room temperature, although cooler temperatures will extend the storage time. However, once their shells have been removed, nuts and seeds are best refrigerated or frozen.

If you try to find a single study that suggests that avocados, fresh nuts and seeds, and olives are harmful to health, you'll likely come up empty-handed. Conversely, if you search the scientific literature for evidence of the health benefits associated with their consumption, you'll be completely overwhelmed. There are literally thousands of research studies that attest to the powerful health effects of these foods. The following notes simply scratch the surface.

AVOCADOS

Like other fat-rich plant foods, avocados offer some unexpected surprises. While most people know avocados are rich in protective monounsaturated fats, they are less aware of their high levels of nutrients and phytochemicals. Avocados contain more folate and potassium per ounce than any other fruit (60 percent more than bananas) and are good sources of vitamins C and E. They also contain 76 milligrams of beta-sitosterol per 100 grams of fruit—more than four times that of other commonly eaten fruits and double the amount in other whole foods. Plant sterols, such as beta-sitosterol, can inhibit cholesterol absorption from the intestine, helping to reduce blood cholesterol levels and possibly inhibit tumor growth. Avocados are also among our richest sources of glutathione, a powerful antioxidant. Another little known fact about the avocado is that it's a very high-fiber food, with 13.5 grams of fiber per average fruit (200 grams).[68]

NUTS

Nuts are proof positive that fat can be a good thing. During the past decade, research studies have consistently confirmed the health benefits of these extraordinary foods.[73-74] Regular nut consumption has been associated with an average risk reduction in coronary artery disease of 30–50 percent in several large study groups.[75-82] Numerous clinical studies have observed the beneficial effects of nuts on blood cholesterol levels.[83] Not only do nuts and seeds lower bad LDL cholesterol and raise good HDL cholesterol, but they also appear to normalize the more harmful, small, dense LDL particles, which damage the cells that line the blood vessels. (The larger, fluffy LDL particles are less harmful.)[84] In addition to their impressive cardioprotective benefits, nuts appear to reduce the risk of stroke,[85] type 2 diabetes,[86] dementia,[87] advanced macular degeneration,[88] and gallstones.[89] Calculations suggest that people who eat nuts daily gain an extra five to six years of life free of coronary disease[90] and that regular nut eating increases longevity by about two years.[91] The frequency of nut consumption has been found to be inversely related to all causes of death in several population groups.[92] Maximum benefits appear to occur with intakes of 1–2 ounces (30–60 grams) per day.

Due to the high caloric content of nuts (approximately 800 calories per cup), it is best to eat them in moderation. That said, epidemiological studies suggest an inverse association between the frequency of nut consumption and body fatness.[93] Clinical trials reveal little or no weight change when various types of nuts are included in the diet over a period of one to six months. These rather surprising findings are explained by how easily nuts make us feel full, which appears to compensate for the estimated 65–75 percent of calories from fat they provide. Evidence also suggests that we aren't very efficient at extracting all of the calories nuts provide. To top it off, it seems that nut consumption may favorably affect our metabolic rate.

While nuts are loaded with protective dietary components, the combined effect of these components has not been adequately measured. They include the following:

- Antioxidants, including selenium and vitamin E (possibly reducing LDL oxidation), plant protein, and fiber
- Arginine, an amino acid that preserves the elasticity and flexibility of our blood vessels, helping to improve blood flow
- Copper and magnesium, both shown to protect against heart disease
- Ellagic acid, lignans, phytosterols, and other phytochemicals shown to have anticarcinogenic potential[94, 95]

Nuts are warehouses of healthful fats, mainly monounsaturated fat (except for pine nuts and walnuts, both of which are high in polyunsaturated fats). They are low in saturated fat and free of trans-fatty acids and cholesterol.

Most of the population studies don't distinguish between raw and roasted nuts. Both types of nuts have been shown to afford protection. However, roasted nuts may contain acrylamide (see page 67) and products of oxidation that could reduce their beneficial effects.[96] The formation of acrylamide in almonds begins when the internal temperature of the nuts reaches approximately 266 degrees F (130 degrees C).[97] The temperatures commonly used for roasting nuts commercially are between 285 and 300 degrees F (140 and 150 degrees C).[98] By contrast, soaking (or soaking and sprouting) nuts increases their protective components, such as antioxidants and phytochemicals, and improves nutrient availability.[99, 100]

OLIVES

Olives contain many protective dietary components including phytosterols (plant sterols) and polyphenolic compounds.[101, 102] Oleuropein, the major polyphenol in olives, is a potent free radical scavenger, inhibiting oxidative damage and protecting heart tissue.[103] Both olives and olive oil also contain phytochemicals with known anticancer effects, including lignans, squalene, and terpenoids.[104] The concentration of these protective compounds depends on the processing techniques used.

Raw olives are cured in order to leach out an alkaloid that makes them bitter and unpalatable. Various solutions can be used in this process, including brine, lye, seasoned oil, or water. The olives can also be dry cured by layering them with dry rock salt in barrels, baskets, burlap sacks, or jars. These processes can take from a few days to a few weeks. Canned and jarred olives are often heated to high temperatures and cured in lye, making them unacceptable to raw foodists. It's not easy to know which olives in the bulk bins in supermarkets are truly raw; however, many natural food supermarkets avoid lye-cured and pasteurized olives in their olive bars. Raw olives and sundried olives are available in some natural food markets and online.

SEEDS

Seeds are the life-giving part of a plant, responsible for the survival of their species. Less research has been conducted on seeds than most other plant foods, and their value in human nutrition is sorely underestimated. These concentrated foods are our most plentiful sources of essential fatty acids. Hempseeds, poppy seeds, pumpkin seeds, sesame seeds, and sunflower seeds are all rich in LA (omega-6). Chia seeds, flaxseeds, and hempseeds are all rich in ALA (omega-3). Seeds vary in their protein content from about 12 percent of calories to over 30 percent of calories. This compares to only 4–15 percent of calories from protein in nuts. Seeds are among our richest sources of vitamin E and provide an impressive array of other vitamins, minerals, phytochemicals, and fiber.

The fatty acids in flaxseeds have a remarkable omega-6 to omega-3 ratio of 0.28:1 (approximately 1:4) and average about 57 percent ALA. For these reasons, flaxseeds can go a long way toward helping correct an imbalance of essential fatty acids. Flaxseeds are very high in soluble fiber (the type of fiber that lowers cholesterol) and are one of the richest known sources of boron. Studies show that flaxseeds can help reduce blood cholesterol levels[105] and improve a number of other markers of coronary artery disease.[106–108] Flaxseeds are the richest-known source of lignans, and preliminary evidence suggests they may help to reduce the growth of human cancer cells.[109, 110]

Chia seeds, both whole and sprouted, are rapidly gaining popularity in raw cuisine. Most people associate these seeds with Chia Pets, the clay figurines that are adorned with chia seeds to produce "hair" on the pets. Little did we know that the nutritional value of the "hair" surpassed most, if not all, of the food sitting in our cupboards! Chia seeds are the only food that is higher in omega-3 fatty acids than flaxseeds, with the oil containing about 63 percent omega-3 fatty acids.[111] Packed with antioxidants, a mere 2 tablespoons (30 milliliters) of chia seeds contains 3.3 milligrams of iron and 142 milligrams of calcium. Chia seeds are grown in Australia, Mexico, and several countries of Central and South America.

Hemp could very well be considered the "greenest" crop on the planet. It takes only about a hundred days to grow, can be planted year after year, and requires no pesticides or fertilizers. All parts of the plant can be used to make over 25,000 different products, including biodegradable plastics, cardboard, carpet, cosmetics, diapers, fuel, nets, paper, rope, shoes, textiles, and of course, food. The nutritional value of hempseeds is no less than remarkable. About 20 percent of their calories comes from easily digestible, high-quality protein,[61] and they provide an impressive array of phytochemicals, trace minerals, and vitamins. Hempseed oil provides an excellent balance of omega-6 to omega-3 fatty acids with a ratio of 3:1. It's one of the few foods that provides both stearidonic acid (SDA), an omega-3 fatty acid, and gamma-linolenic acid (GLA), a particularly beneficial omega-6 fatty acid. There is evidence that when stearidonic acid is consumed directly, conversion to EPA is much more efficient than that from ALA.[69]

Coconut Oil: Menace or Miracle?

here are few foods that have been at once maligned and acclaimed as much as coconut oil. Some view it as a notorious health villain because it's the most concentrated source of saturated fat in the diet—even higher than butter or lard. Not surprisingly, it rests at the very top of the list of foods that must be strictly avoided in many heart-healthy diet programs. At the other end of the spectrum are those people who view coconut oil as a fountain of youth and the greatest health discovery in decades. These coconut advocates claim that coconut oil can provide therapeutic benefits for cancer, diabetes, digestive disturbances, heart disease, high blood pressure, HIV, kidney disease, osteoporosis, and overweight. So what is the truth? Is coconut oil a menace or a miracle where health is concerned?

The primary criticism of coconut oil is that over 90 percent of its fat is saturated. Saturated fat is known to increase blood cholesterol levels. When coconut oil is blacklisted, it's almost exclusively because of this extreme saturated-fat content. While many people imagine saturated fat as a single tyrant that clogs arteries, there are actually several different types of saturated fats. These fats contain between 4 and 28 carbons, and depending on the length of their carbon chain, they have very different effects on blood cholesterol levels. The saturated fats that are most plentiful in the diet are lauric acid (12 carbons), myristic acid (14 carbons), palmitic acid (16 carbons), and stearic acid (18 carbons). Their main sources are outlined in the sidebar on page 139.

Saturated fatty acids, with 12–16 carbons, increase blood cholesterol levels, while stearic acid does not. When stearic acid reaches the liver, it's converted to oleic acid (an 18-carbon monounsaturated fat), which may help to explain why it doesn't raise cholesterol. As a result, consumers are often advised not to be concerned about their intake of stearic acid. However, cholesterol is not the only marker for heart disease, and adverse effects of stearic acid have been reported. In one large study, stearic acid increased coronary artery disease risk more than lauric, myristic, or palmitic acid.[90] Apparently, stearic acid may reduce good HDL cholesterol, increase Lp(a), which is another risk factor for heart disease, increase certain blood-clotting factors, and result in lipemia (excess fat in the blood) after eating.[2, 112] In a critical review of dietary fats and coronary artery disease, the authors of the review advised that stearic acid not be distinguished from other saturated fats when providing dietary advice to reduce coronary artery disease.[2]

As it happens, coconut oil is about 50 percent lauric acid, 18 percent myristic acid, and 8 percent palmitic acid. This adds up to 76 percent of the fat in coconut oil being the kind that raises cholesterol. Case closed? Well, not exactly. The predominant fat, lauric acid, does raise total cholesterol, but it appears to raise good HDL cholesterol to an even greater extent than bad LDL cholesterol. The effect on the ratio of total to HDL cholesterol is consistently favorable.[113, 114, 115] Myristic and palmitic acid do not have this effect. Does the 50 percent lauric acid in coconut oil cancel out the 26 percent myristic and palmitic acids?

We don't really know. We do have evidence that fats rich in lauric acid, such as coconut oil, result in more favorable blood cholesterol levels than hydrogenated vegetable oils laden with trans fats.[113] Trans-fatty acids not only raise bad LDL cholesterol, but they also decrease good HDL cholesterol. We also know that coronary artery disease risk is reduced most effectively when trans-fatty acids and saturated fatty acids are replaced with unsaturated fatty acids.[2] The effect of coconut oil, rich in lauric acid, remains somewhat uncertain. However, we cannot ignore the fact that in many parts of the world where coconut and coconut oil are staples in indigenous diets, rates of chronic disease, including coronary artery disease, are low.[116–118] There is one major caveat. The benefits seem to apply only when coconut products are consumed along with a diet that is unprocessed and rich in high-fiber plant foods. When the indigenous diet gives way to a more processed, Western-style diet laden with white flour, sugar, and fatty animal products, disease rates escalate even when coconut continues to be consumed.

> ## Sources of Saturated Fatty Acids with 12 to 18 Carbon Atoms
>
> Lauric acid: coconut, coconut oil, palm kernel oil
>
> Myristic acid: coconut, dairy products, nutmeg oil, palm kernel oil, palm oil
>
> Palmitic acid: animal fats, palm oil
>
> Stearic acid: beef, butter, cocoa butter, lard, mutton

It is worth noting that most of the fatty acids in coconut, particularly lauric acid, are known to have significant antimicrobial properties.[119–122] Virgin coconut oil also contains a variety of protective phytochemicals, including phenolic acids, which are largely eliminated through the refining process.[123, 124]

Another important attribute of coconut fat is its stability. It is so highly saturated that it is not easily oxidized or otherwise damaged.[28] Plant foods that grow close to the equator have a higher quantity of saturated fatty acids in order to protect themselves from the ravages of oxidation that occur in warm temperatures. Foods that grow in cold climates generally contain higher amounts of unsaturated fats, such as omega-3 fatty acids. Once again, this is necessary for the survival of the plant and its seeds; certain fluids in the plant need to remain liquid, even in very cold temperatures. The saturated fat that comes from whole plant foods, such as coconut, may in fact turn out to be of benefit for vegans. Vegan diets sometimes contain excessive amounts of unsaturated fats, which are more prone to oxidation, while the saturated fats in coconut are very stable fats with a low risk of oxidation. While we want to keep our total intake of saturated fat low, we don't want to completely eliminate it (an impossible task on any diet).

It turns out that coconut oil is neither a menace nor a miracle food. Coconut should be treated in much the same way as other high-fat plant foods—enjoyed primarily as a whole food. As such, it is loaded with fiber, vitamin E, and healthful phytochemicals. As a bonus, it has powerful antimicrobial properties. On the other hand, coconut oil should be viewed the same way as other concentrated oils: a food that provides a lot of calories with very few nutrients.

When your diet is high in concentrated fats, it can be difficult to meet your needs for other nutrients. It's okay to use some coconut oil when preparing special-occasion treats, but don't rely on it as part of your daily fare. Base your diet on whole plant foods, and when you do use coconut oil, make sure it is organic and virgin.

CONCLUSION: Moderate amounts of higher-fat whole plant foods make the foods you eat more pleasurable and increase the nutritional quality of your diet. Minimize your use of concentrated oils. If you use oils, stick mainly to those that are rich in omega-3 fatty acids. Concentrated oils contain few nutrients besides fat, so when too many calories in the diet come from oil, the amount of vitamins and minerals you eat may fall below desirable levels.

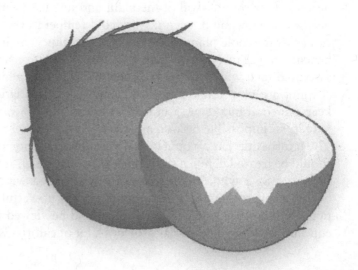

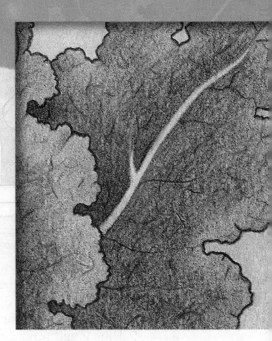

CHAPTER 8

Vitamins: Inviting Vitality

When it comes to vitamin content, a raw or high-raw diet can be a winner over other styles of eating. You can expect health benefits, providing your diet plan includes a variety of foods and reliable sources of vitamins B$_{12}$ and D, plus an adequate fat intake for good absorption of the fat soluble vitamins. In this chapter, we examine the roles of vitamins and explore a wide range of options for meeting your recommended intakes.

Though the total weight of the fourteen essential vitamins is only one-half gram per day, these powerful substances are essential to life. (One-half gram is the weight of one-sixth of a garlic clove or one-eighth of a Brazil nut.) Vitamins are impressive team players in several arenas, including, among others, protection from free radical damage, detoxification, and the production of energy from the carbohydrates, fat, and protein in foods.

Protection by Antioxidants from Free Radical Damage

Moderate quantities of free radicals are formed by the body's normal metabolism, or operating processes. Smoking, consuming foods that are cooked at high temperatures, or drinking alcohol further burden the system. With exposure to environmental pollutants, solvents, or radiation, the quantities of free radicals generated multiply, along with the damage that these rampaging molecules can do to cell membranes, genetic material (DNA), and the essential proteins in cells.

Our rescuers, heroes, and protectors come from three tribes: phytochemicals; certain enzymes that contain the minerals copper, manganese, selenium, and zinc; plus the antioxidant vitamins C and E and the carotenoids that our bodies can convert to vitamin A. The B vitamin riboflavin also has a protective role against free radical damage. If the body becomes depleted of these, the cells are more vulnerable to damage, disease, and aging. As we get older, an antioxidant-rich diet assumes even greater importance. With a well-chosen raw vegan diet, our cells are furnished with a steady supply of the defensive ammunition that can effectively block free radical damage. Raw food, juices, and sprouts provide spectacular amounts of the antioxidant vitamins.[8, 12–19]

Antioxidants are team players. For example, vitamin C promotes the activity of vitamin E, and vitamin E protects beta-carotene from oxidation. A lively field of research concerns the roles of antioxidants in reducing the risk of cancer, cardiovascular disease, cataracts, macular degeneration, diseases of the nervous system (such as Alzheimer's and Parkinson's), and premature aging of the skin due to ultraviolet light. Getting antioxidants from raw plant foods, where a multitude of helpful substances are present, is proving to be far more effective than using supplements. It is well recognized that individual antioxidants in pill form do not provide the same protection from disease as does the diverse and balanced supply of antioxidants that we find in plant foods, which humans have relied on for millennia, before the advent of highly processed foods.[13–16, 20–22]

The Body's Detoxification System

o locate your liver, put your hand over the lowest ribs on your front right side. Just inside those ribs is the busiest hive of activity in your body. One of the liver's functions is to detoxify, or rid the body of poisons and substances that are potentially damaging, such as aflatoxin (a toxic compound found in moldy peanuts and grains), caffeine, dioxin, drugs, exhaust fumes, paint vapors, pesticides, and tobacco smoke. Such activity also occurs in other parts of the body; however, the liver is a primary location. Toxins that are not water-soluble are not readily eliminated through urine or bile. Fortunately, by using some remarkable processes, the body can effectively recognize, transform, and eliminate dangerous molecules, rendering them harmless. Liver detoxification involves two steps: Phase I and Phase II. The enzyme activities of these two phases must be well coordinated, because intermediary compounds that form during Phase I can be even more troublesome than the original toxin. If these intermediary compounds are not quickly processed in Phase II, damage, such as cell injury or the development of cancer, can ensue.

A simplified summary of liver detoxification is shown in figure 8.1, page 143. During Phase I, detoxification enzymes give the toxin an electrical charge, which creates a type of chemical handle that can attach to another molecule during Phase II. In receiving the charge, toxins can change into highly reactive and potentially dangerous molecules. If all is well, as is usually the case, the reactive molecule quickly passes into Phase II, where a large, water-soluble molecule

FIGURE 8.1 Detoxification pathways in the liver and supportive nutrients

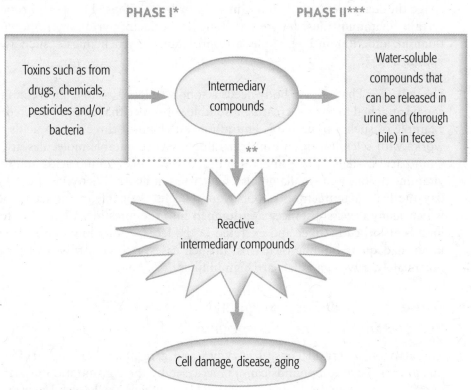

Sources: Data from references 13, 14, 23–25.

*The nutrients needed for Phase I include the B vitamins (folic acid, niacin, pyridoxine, riboflavin, and vitamin B_{12}), iron, specific amino acids, and phytochemicals (flavonoids).

**The nutrients needed to protect against cell damage from reactive intermediary compounds and free radicals include the vitamins A (beta-carotene), C, and E; the minerals copper, manganese, selenium, and zinc; and the phytochemicals found in cruciferous vegetables.

***The nutrients needed for Phase II include choline, riboflavin, selenium, sulfur, and specific amino acids (cysteine and methionine).

is attached, creating a water-soluble complex that the body can quickly and safely dispose of through urine or bile.

DIET AND DETOXIFICATION

Diet and lifestyle choices affect the sequence of flow through Phases I and II in many ways. Knowing the nutrient teamwork that is involved in the body's detoxification process helps us better understand why a varied diet of plant foods goes far beyond supplements in keeping us healthy. Here are some examples.

Phase I. The body's first line of defense is a superfamily of enzymes that the body builds from protein (including the sulfur-containing amino acid cysteine) and iron (called the P450 cytochrome enzyme family). These enzymes carry electrons, or charges, from one spot to another, work in the presence of oxygen, and create a highly reactive form of oxygen that can rearrange the structure of toxic molecules. In order for Phase I to work properly, certain B vitamins must be present (folic acid, niacin, pyridoxine, riboflavin, thiamin, and vitamin B_{12}), along with protective phytochemicals, such as flavonoids.[7, 14, 23]

Phase II. For Phase II, the body needs a supply of large, soluble molecules that can be attached to toxins, creating a soluble substance that can be excreted. An example of such a molecule is glutathione, a chain of three amino acids that works with selenium (found in Brazil nuts). Other suitable molecules are the amino acid cysteine or the mineral sulfur. Several other amino acids and the B vitamins choline and riboflavin also have roles in Phase II detoxification. Each day the liver manufactures about a quart (a liter) of bile, a carrier through which many toxic substances are dumped into the intestine, where this toxic load is absorbed by fiber and excreted in the feces. A diet low in fiber results in an inadequate binding of toxins; in such cases, toxins may be reabsorbed. Fortunately, raw vegan diets are high in fiber.[14, 23, 26–28]

Causes for the Buildup of Highly Reactive Intermediary Compounds

The activity of certain Phase I enzymes and a resultant buildup of dangerous intermediary compounds can be increased by the consumption of alcohol or polycyclic aromatic hydrocarbons (PAHs), which are harmful substances that are created by cigarette smoke or when foods are barbecued (for more information, see chapter 4, page 70). If toxin exposure is very high, overloading enzyme defenders with potentially carcinogenic substances can trigger the initial steps along the path to cancer. Protection can be insufficient when there is a shortage of antioxidants, for example from diets centered on supersized portions of refined, highly processed, and overcooked foods, soda pop, and alcohol instead of fresh fruits and vegetables. Either Phase I or Phase II or both can be inefficient or overloaded with toxins, leading to an imbalance between Phases I and II.[13, 14, 23, 29–31] If the critical nutrients needed for Phase II detoxification or for antioxidant protection are depleted, the buildup of highly toxic activated intermediates can increase the susceptibility to cancer or other diseases.[14, 23–25, 30, 32]

Protection from Highly Reactive Intermediary Compounds

When reactive intermediary compounds and free radicals start to accumulate, the body relies on various substances to block destructive chain reactions: antioxidant vitamins A (beta-carotene), C, and E; enzymes (built from protein plus the minerals copper, manganese, selenium, or zinc); and phytochemicals (such as those from cruciferous vegetables). This remarkable defense system protects DNA, cell membranes, and the proteins in our cells from damage.[13, 14, 23, 24] The supply of protective nutrients and phytochemicals is present in fruits, vegetables, seeds, and nuts.[15, 23, 27, 33–36] Sprouted foods can be a valuable addition. Though there was limited backing from the scientific community decades ago, Ann Wigmore (1909–1994) and other raw-food pioneers recognized the health potential of sprouts, juices, and other raw plant foods.[37] Today, scientists in many parts of the world acknowledge the contribution that such foods can make to our well-being.[28, 33, 38] For example, Isabella Calzuola, an Italian cellular microbiologist who examined the effectiveness of free radical fighters in sprouted wheat, stated that "the cocktail of wheat sprout antioxidant molecules is especially powerful on the scavenging of oxygen superoxide."[39]

VITAMIN A AND CAROTENOIDS

Raw Research

In raw vegan diets, vitamin A comes from beta-carotene and two other carotenoids found in yellow, orange, red, and green vegetables and fruits. The Giessen study of forty-three German adults who had followed a vegan diet that was 98 percent raw for at least two years found that their high-fruit diet provided vitamin A intakes that were about triple the DRIs (see table 8.1, page 146).[4] On average, they consumed 262 grams (about a half pound) of vegetables and 942 grams (about 2 pounds) of fruits daily. Most of these people achieved high plasma levels of beta-carotene, which are associated with a reduced risk of cardiovascular disease.[11, 20, 40] Yet the average beta-carotene levels were not as high as might have been expected. In fact, 15 percent of those studied had low plasma beta-carotene levels, despite eating this quantity of fruits and vegetables. Insights may come from a look at the rest of their diets. The main factor that predicted the participants' plasma carotenoids levels was their fat intake. A lesson from this research is that the body can absorb fat-soluble carotenoids more readily if there is a little fat in the intestine at the same time. All that's needed is a teaspoon (3–5 grams) of fat. Choosing a mono diet, in which just one type of food is eaten at a time, seems to work against carotenoid absorption.[4, 11, 20, 38, 41] You will absorb carotenoids better if you munch on a few seeds or nuts while drinking your juice. Or simply add some avocado or sunflower seeds to soup (such as Garden Blend Soup, page 273), and include a tahini-based dressing (such as Lemon-Tahini Dressing, page 275) or a flaxseed-based dressing (such as Liquid Gold Dressing, page

Antioxidant and Fat-Soluble Vitamins: DRIs and Intakes on Raw Diets

Table 8.1, page 146, summarizes the recommended intakes known as Dietary Reference Intakes (DRIs) for adults for vitamins A, C, E, K, and D (all of these except vitamin C are fat-soluble).[1, 2, 3] These DRIs are guidelines for adults on any diet; no unique guidelines for people on raw diets have been developed. Table 8.1 also shows intakes on raw and mainly raw diets from studies in Germany, the United States, and Finland.

TABLE 8.1 Vitamins A, C, E, K, and D: adult Dietary Reference Intakes and intakes on raw and high-raw diets

	Vitamins				
	A (mcg)*	C (mg)	E (mg)	K (mcg)	D (mcg)†
DRIs for a woman‡	700	75	15	90	5 to 15
DRIs for a man	900	90	15	120	5 to 15
STUDY, COUNTRY, YEAR, PARTICIPANTS, REFERENCES					
Giessen Study, Germany, 2001, 2005, 43 vegans[4, 5]	2,400	424	19	...	3.2
Hallelujah Acres diet, USA, 2001, 87 women[6]	6,740	442	14.9	326	0.3
Hallelujah Acres diet, USA, 2001, 54 men[6]	8,110	481	17	406	0.5
Living-food diet, 1996, Finland, 19 women and 1 man[7]	1,972	183	25	...	0.1
Living-food diet, Finland, 1993, 13 adults (mostly women) with rheumatoid arthritis[8]	1,100	213	21.8	...	...
Living-food diet, Finland, 1992, 9 vegans[9]	...	...	11.1	...	...
Raw vegan diet, USA, 2005, 7 women and 11 men[10]	...	...	...	...	0.4

*Amounts of vitamin A are listed in retinol activity equivalents (RAE), which include vitamin A from carotenoids. Vitamin A intakes from beta-carotene were calculated by dividing by 12.[1, 11]

†The DRI for vitamin D is 5 mcg for adults to age 50, 10 mcg for adults from age 50 to 70 years, and 15 mcg for adults above 70 years of age.[1] Intakes include supplementary vitamin D. Significant increases in recommended intakes for vitamin D are expected.

‡These DRIs apply to women who are not pregnant or lactating.

276) with your salad. As well as being tasty, small amounts of these high-fat foods support good nutrition.

In a U.S.–based study, people on the high-raw Hallelujah Acres diet had intakes of vitamin A that were about nine times the DRIs. Two-thirds of these intakes came from the carotenoids in the nearly 2 cups (460 milliliters) of carrot juice each participant consumed each day.[6] Although high intakes of vitamin A from animal liver or supplements can be toxic, this is not the case with plant foods. If you drink a lot of carrot juice or eat a diet that is particularly high in carotenoid-rich vegetables and fruits, your skin may develop a yellow tinge; however, this temporary condition is harmless.[2, 42]

Another type of raw dietary pattern was studied among Finns, whose living-food diet provided intakes of vitamin A (from carotenoids) that were about 2.5 times the recommended intakes (see table 8.1, page 146). Along with daily carrot juice and wheatgrass juice, this vegan diet contained moderate amounts of seeds and nuts in dressings and nondairy milks, so that the calories from fats averaged 42 percent, similar to that of the control diets. Those on the living-food diet consumed 1.5 times as much vitamin A as nonvegetarian controls who were similar in age, gender, social status, and residence. The high carotenoid intakes on the living-food diet were reflected in serum beta-carotene levels that were triple the levels of the controls.[16] Yet laboratory tests reflecting protection against DNA damage (as an indicator of protection against cancer) showed some benefit from the living-food diet, though not as much as would have been expected.[44] The researchers have offered insights based on the fact that our well-being involves a great many nutrients acting in concert with each other.

CONCLUSION: When people switch to raw diets, they may feel healthier, lighter, less bloated, more rested, and energetic. They may be free of troublesome reactions to gluten, dairy, or other common triggers, if they have food sensitivities. These welcome changes are usually attributed to the elimination of a great many unhealthful or problematic foods. Beyond avoiding harmful foods, it is highly important to focus on getting all of the nutrients we need. Finnish researchers recognized that the tremendous health advantages provided by raw diets—specifically the high intakes (and resultant high blood levels) of the antioxidants beta-carotene and vitamins C and E—can be offset by deficiencies of vitamin B_{12}, the antioxidant selenium, or inappropriate amounts of iodine, for example. Because nutrients work as a team, all team members must be present to do their part![16, 44, 45]

FUNCTIONS OF VITAMIN A AND CAROTENOIDS

Vitamin A is essential for normal vision, growth, reproduction, cell maturation, and immune system protection. Carotenoids act as antioxidants, may protect against several cancers (especially the beta-carotene in raw foods) and macular degeneration, and support communication between cells in the body.[11, 12, 20]

DIETARY SOURCES OF CAROTENOIDS

Carotenoids provide the gorgeous hues seen in apricots, chiles, guava, mangoes, papaya, persimmons, pink grapefruit, pumpkin, squash, sweet peppers, sweet potatoes, tomatoes, and watermelon. They are also in broccoli, collard greens, green beans, kale, and spinach, where their presence deepens the green from chlorophyll. Red sweet peppers have significantly more carotenoids and antioxidant activity than other shades of sweet peppers, and mature leaves of endive and lettuce contain more carotenoids than young, pale leaves on the same head.[20, 46, 47] (For additional sources of vitamin A, see table 8.2, page 154.)

Science shows mixed results when it comes to cooked versus raw sources of carotenoids. Although there can be losses during cooking, the loss is less with steaming. On the other hand, the body seems to absorb some carotenoids more effectively from cooked foods.[20, 47, 49–55]

Shredded raw carrots that were washed with commercial sanitizing solutions to preserve them and prevent discoloration have been shown to lose 50–65 percent of their beta-carotene after being refrigerated for twenty-one days.[56]

Lycopene, the carotenoid that is linked with a reduced risk of prostate cancer, is better absorbed from a cooked food, such as tomato paste or ketchup, rather than from raw tomatoes (which also are sources.)[57] In one study, three-quarters of the German raw-food participants had low plasma levels of lycopene compared with levels of the general population.[11, 132] In addition to raw tomatoes, raw lycopene sources include guava, pink grapefruit, and watermelon.

MAXIMIZING CAROTENOIDS

Certain carotenoids are more readily absorbed from foods that have been juiced, blended, or puréed because the plant matrix is disrupted and cells are broken. These foods and beverages should be consumed soon after their preparation, as antioxidant activity decreases quickly.[17, 20, 38, 41, 54, 58] Also include fat sources, at least in small amounts, when consuming carotenoid-rich foods.

Vitamin C (Ascorbic Acid)

RAW RESEARCH

On raw diets, intakes of vitamin C are two to six times the minimum recommended levels, affording good antioxidant protection (see table 8.1, page 146).[4, 6, 16] Researchers in Finland found that adults on living-food diets had blood concentrations of vitamin C that were about 13 percent higher than those of nonvegetarian controls.[16, 43]

FUNCTIONS OF VITAMIN C

Vitamin C is a highly effective antioxidant; and it may regenerate its team member, vitamin E. Vitamin C is required for the formation of numerous compounds, such as norepinephrine (a neurotransmitter), carnitine (a chaperone to conduct fats to where they are needed), and collagen (a fibrous protein in blood vessel walls, scar tissue, cartilage, tendons, and bone). This vitamin helps the body to resist disease and infection. It also greatly increases the body's absorption of iron when foods rich in iron and vitamin C are consumed at the same time.[42, 59, 60]

DIETARY SOURCES OF VITAMIN C

A few of the excellent sources of vitamin C are broccoli, cantaloupe, citrus fruits, leafy greens, mangoes, papayas, peppers, strawberries, tomatoes, and vegetables in the cabbage family.[2, 61] (Also see table 8.2, page 154.) The vitamin C content of sweet peppers increases as the peppers mature.[62] The process of sprouting starts vitamin C production in seeds and mung beans.[63, 64]

MAXIMIZING VITAMIN C

Choose raw, fresh, organic plant foods that are grown in sunlight. Vegetables show seasonal changes in their vitamin C content; for example, the values for vitamin C in fall crops of broccoli were almost double those from spring crops of the same variety.[65] Organic crops tend to be higher in vitamin C compared to nonorganic.[65] Vitamin C is destroyed when cells are broken and the vitamin is exposed to oxygen, so freshly squeezed orange juice, finely chopped red sweet pepper, or sliced strawberries start to lose this vitamin quickly. Vitamin C is vulnerable to heat and is soluble in cooking water. When broccoli was boiled for five minutes, one-quarter of the vitamin C was lost.[51] Less loss of vitamin C occurs with steaming broccoli than with boiling.[51] Broccoli lost 18 percent of its vitamin C after being refrigerated at 43 degrees F (6 degrees C) for one to two weeks, and lost 38 percent after three weeks. Freezing broccoli led to losses of only 10 percent after two months.[66]

Vitamin E (Alpha-Tocopherol)

RAW RESEARCH

In a study of Finns on a living-food diet of germinated seeds and nuts, sprouts, berries, fruits, and vegetables, vitamin E intakes were triple the DRIs. The participants' blood levels of vitamin E were about 20 percent higher than for nonvegetarians of the same sex, age, and social status.[16, 43] (See table 8.1, page 146.)

Most participants on the Hallelujah Acres diet ate a variety of plant foods, including cooked and sprouted grains, other sprouted foods, nuts, and seeds. A subgroup followed diets that were centered on fruits, vegetables, and carrot juice, with few plant foods that are high in fat or fat-soluble vitamin E. The result was caloric intakes for the subgroup that were between 30 and 60 percent of recommended amounts and shortages of minerals and many vitamins, including vitamin E. A researcher observed, "Attempting to follow the Hallelujah Acres diet but eating very little food (less than 60 percent of the recommended daily intakes) will result in a high risk of compromising one's health." He advised increasing calories and rounding out the diet with nuts, seeds, sprouts, and other plant foods, plus adding supplements for vitamins B_{12} and D.[6, 67]

The Giessen study showed a similar pattern. For the group as a whole, average intakes of many nutrients were adequate. Yet a significant number of people had very low intakes of calories, vitamin E, and many other nutrients.[4]

FUNCTIONS OF VITAMIN E

Vitamin E is a powerful antioxidant that protects vitamin A and polyunsaturated fatty acids from destruction and has roles in the prevention of many diseases. It stabilizes cell membranes and prevents their disintegration.[2, 68] Food sources of vitamin E are preferable to supplements, and high doses of supplemented vitamin E should be avoided.[69] (For more on this, see page 57.)

DIETARY SOURCES OF VITAMIN E

Excellent sources of vitamin E include avocados, nuts, olives, and seeds. If fat is restricted, it becomes difficult to meet recommended intakes of this fat-soluble vitamin. Vitamin E also is present in sweet peppers (especially orange peppers), quinoa, and the wild plant purslane, which was a favorite of the vegetarian philosopher and mathematician Pythagorus.[46, 70, 71] Sprouting wheat greatly increases its content of vitamin E (along with vitamin C and beta-carotene).[19] (For other sources, see table 8.2, page 154.) Vitamin E is lost in cooking, and losses are significantly greater when the cooking is done in metal pots, such as in stainless steel.[72]

Vitamin K

RAW RESEARCH

In the only study reporting on this vitamin, the vitamin K intakes of people on the Hallelujah Acres diet were three to four times the DRIs.[6]

FUNCTIONS OF VITAMIN K

This vitamin helps to build proteins, regulate blood calcium levels, and reduce the risk of bone fracture. Greens are important bone builders in raw diets, in part because of their abundant supply of vitamin K. The designation "K" is derived from the German word *koagulation* and is related to the vitamin's ability to clot blood, an essential defense during times of injury.[3, 73]

DIETARY AND BACTERIAL SOURCES OF VITAMIN K

Excellent sources of vitamin K include asparagus, broccoli, cabbage, kale and other leafy greens, lentils, peas, pumpkin, and the sea vegetable nori.[61] Friendly bacteria in the large intestine manufacture this vitamin, contributing to the body's supply. To support this intestinal production, avoid using oral antibiotics (which can destroy these bacteria) whenever possible, and reduce your sugar consumption, as sugar sustains microorganisms that compete with these friendly bacteria.[3]

Vitamin D (Calciferol)

RAW RESEARCH

People on raw diets have intakes of vitamin D that are far below recommended levels (see table 8.1, page 146). This problem is not isolated to raw-food practitioners, as North American, European, and Australian surveys that included nonvegetarians and vegetarians showed that many adults have intakes of vitamin D that are far below recommended levels, and many have low serum levels of vitamin D. Particularly at risk are those over age fifty, women, people who are inactive or overweight, and people with dark skin.[74–80] The DRIs for vitamin D are currently under review. When they are revised, they are likely to be substantially increased; many experts suggest at least 25 micrograms (1,000 IU) per day for adults.[75, 80–82]

The low intakes listed in table 8.1 (page 146) include supplementary vitamin D taken by a few participants. Some people on the Hallelujah Acres diet took a supplement known as B-Flax-D, which provides vitamins D and B_{12}, selenium, and omega-3 fatty acids.[6, 67]

A small, raw vegan food study based in Missouri found that seven women and eight men, whose average age was fifty-four and who had strictly followed raw vegan diets for 3.6 years, had relatively high concentrations of serum vitamin D compared to a control group of nonvegetarians of similar age and gender. People on the raw diets were slim, with an average BMI of 20 (compared to a BMI of 25 in the control group), and their bone mass was significantly lower than that of the control group. A person's peak bone mass is built up during the first three decades of life, and it declines slowly or quickly thereafter depending on many physical and lifestyle factors. The raw-food adherents made an effort to spend time in the sun on a regular basis. Many lived in the St. Louis area (with a latitude of 38 degrees north). Their low bone mass could have developed before or early after their adoption of the raw diets. Markers of bone turnover indicated that they were not losing bone mass significantly faster than the controls.[10]

FUNCTIONS OF VITAMIN D

Vitamin D helps us to absorb calcium and phosphorus, maintain critical blood levels of calcium, and limit calcium losses through the urine. Low vitamin D intakes and serum vitamin D levels are associated with an increased risk of colon cancer, hypertension, and autoimmune diseases, such as multiple sclerosis.[6, 42, 75, 83, 84]

SOLAR SOURCES OF VITAMIN D

Though vitamin D is classified as a vitamin (meaning that dietary sources or supplements of it are essential), our bodies can make this substance after the skin is exposed to UV rays. The amount of vitamin D produced depends on the following factors:

- The person's geographic location, skin color, and age
- How much skin is exposed
- The time of year
- The time of day
- The cloud cover
- The length of exposure
- Whether sunscreen is used (as it can block vitamin D production if it is thickly applied)

During winter months, latitudes that are farther than 35 degrees from the equator get very little UV light through the earth's atmosphere. For example, from November through February, Boston (with a latitude of 42 degrees north) does not receive enough UV light for adequate vitamin D production. This is a problem for those who live in the latitudes of Canada, northern United States or Europe, or southern Australia, and who receive little or no vitamin D from foods or supplements. The situation is worse for darker-skinned people, who need significantly more UV exposure in order to make vitamin D. Older or obese people, of all skin colors, have less-efficient vitamin D production. Someone who is seldom outdoors or whose skin is covered with clothing or sunscreen will have little vitamin D production. Use of a tanning bed with ultraviolet light can raise vitamin D levels; however, their use can be carcinogenic and is not recommended.[74, 75, 77, 82, 85, 133]

Past guidelines advised that, for adequate vitamin D production, a light-skinned person requires a daily average of ten to fifteen minutes of warm sunlight on the forearms and face, and that as skin tone deepens, two to six times that amount of sun exposure is required, either in terms of length of time or area of skin exposed.[42, 86] Yet even in sunny climates, sunlight's effects can be hard to predict. Recent studies in Hawaii, Arizona, Australia, and other sunny regions have shown inadequate vitamin D production among residents.[74, 77, 78, 80, 87–89] Currently, no reliable prescription exists for a minimum length of sun exposure that would meet the vitamin D requirements. Overexposure to UV light carries the potential risks of premature wrinkling, loss of skin elasticity, sunburn, and skin cancer.[75] Raw foodists often tend to be sun lovers, and for some people, this is a suitable solution.[10] One promising combination is to use a vitamin D supplement or a calcium or multivitamin supplement that includes vitamin D during gray, sunless periods and to spend a moderate amount of time outdoors in the sun, taking care to avoid overexposure.[67, 75, 79, 80]

DIETARY SOURCES OF VITAMIN D

Raw vegan diets do not provide safe food sources of vitamin D. Although certain mushrooms that have been exposed to ultraviolet (UV) light (from the sun or UV lamps) contain small amounts of vitamin D, raw mushrooms contain carcinogens or other types of toxins. (For more on this, see chapter 11, page 231.) Although marinating and dehydrating mushrooms may reduce the toxins, these processes will not eliminate them. The quantity of irradiated mushrooms needed to meet vitamin D requirements is variable and uncertain, and raw mushrooms may remain unsafe even when they have been marinated and dehydrated. When grown on manure, mushrooms can contain other pathogens. Although the toxins in some mushrooms are destroyed by cooking, raw mushrooms are not recommended for our daily dose of vitamin D.[74, 77, 80, 90–97]

Fortified vegan foods vary from one country to another depending on legislation. Examples of foods that are not raw but provide vitamin D include fortified nondairy milks, juices, and breakfast cereals.[61, 77, 80]

VITAMIN D SUPPLEMENTS

Vitamin D is commonly taken in multivitamin-mineral supplements and in supplements that contain vitamin D plus calcium and perhaps magnesium.[80] Recommended intakes of Vitamin D are expressed in micrograms (mcg or µg) of vitamin D_3 and are shown in table 8.1, page 146. One microgram is equivalent to 40 International Units (IU) of vitamin D. Vitamin D_3 (cholecalciferol) comes from animal sources, such as fish, animal hides, or wool. Vitamin D_2 (ergocalciferol) is not of animal origin and is vegan. To locate a source, do an Internet search for "vegan vitamin D." Although research offers a variety of perspectives, the two forms of vitamin D have been shown to be equally effective.[80, 82, 87]

Vitamins in Raw Foods

Table 8.2, pages 154–160, shows the vitamin content of a variety of foods, with typical portions of 1 cup (250 milliliters) of food or one unit (such as one apple). You can find nutrient data at the U.S. Department of Agriculture website.[61]

Note that while tables and databases list an exact number, nature is much more variable. For example, plants that are grown in plenty of sunshine contain much more vitamin C than those grown with less light.[98] There also are differences between organic produce and produce grown with pesticides, though there is still much research to be done in this area.[65, 99–101, 139–142]

TABLE 8.2 Vitamins in raw foods

Food	A, RAE, mcg	C, mg	E, mg	K, mcg	Thiamin, mg	Riboflavin, mg	Niacin, mg	Pyridoxine (B₆), mg*	Folate, mcg	Pantothenic Acid, mg	Biotin, mcg
DRI for a woman	700	75	15	90	1.1	1.1	14	1.3 to 1.5	400	5	30
DRI for a man	900	90	15	120	1.2	1.3	16	1.3 to 1.7	400	5	30
FRUITS											
Apple, chopped (1 c/125 g)	4	6	0.2	2.8	0.02	0.03	0.1	0.05	4	0.1	2
Apple, medium, each	4	6	0.2	3	0.02	0.04	0.1	0.06	4	0.1	2
Apples, dried (1c/86 g)	0	3	0.5	3	0	0.1	0.8	0.11	0	0.2	...
Apricot, medium, each	34	4	0.3	1	0.01	0.01	0.3	0.02	3	0.1	...
Apricots, dried (130 g)	234	1.3	5.6	4	0.02	0.1	3.4	0.2	13	0.7	...
Apricots, sliced (1 c/165 g)	158	16	1.5	5	0.05	0.07	1.4	0.09	15	0.4	...
Banana, dried (1c/100 g)	12	7	0.4	2	0.18	0.24	2.8	0.44	14	0.3	3
Banana, medium, each	4	10	.1	1	0.04	0.09	1	0.43	24	0.4	3
Banana slices (1 c/150 g)	4.5	13	0.2	1	0.05	0.11	1.2	0.55	30	0.5	4
Blackberries (1c/144 g)	16	30	1.7	29	0.03	0.04	0.9	0.04	36	0.4	1
Blueberries (1c/145 g)	4	14	0.8	28	0.05	0.06	0.7	0.08	9	0.2	...
Cantaloupe/Muskmelon, diced (1c/156 g)	264	57	0.1	4	0.06	0.03	1.2	0.11	33	0.2	...
Cherimoya (1c/156 g)	1	18	...	...	0.14	0.19	0.9	0.33	28	0.4	...
Coconut, dried (1c/116 g)	0	2	0.5	0.3	0.07	0.12	2.1	0.35	10	0.9	...
Coconut milk (1c/240 g)	0	7	0.4	0.2	0.06	0	2.8	0.08	38	0.4	...
Crab apple slices (1c/110 g)	2	9	0.6	...	0.03	0.02	0.2	...	...	...	...
Currants, red/white (1c/112 g)	2	46	0.1	12	0.04	0.06	0.1	0.08	9	0.1	5
Currants, European/black (1c/112 g)	13	203	1.1	...	0.06	0.06	0.3	0.07	4	0.4	5
Currants, Zante, dried (1c/144 g)	6	7	0.2	5	0.23	0.20	2.3	0.43	14	0.1	...
Dates, chopped (1c/178 g)	1	1	0.1	5	0.09	0.12	2.6	0.29	34	1	...
Durian, chopped (1c/243 g)	5	48	...	...	0.91	0.49	2.6	0.77	87	0.6	...
Fig, fresh, medium, each	4	1	0.1	2	0.03	0.02	0.2	0.06	3	0.2	...
Figs, dried (1 c/199 g)	1	2	0.7	31	0.17	0.16	1.9	0.21	18	0.9	...
Gooseberries (1 c/150 g)	22	42	0.6	...	0.06	0.04	0.7	0.12	9	0.4	1
Grapefruit, medium, each	143	77	0.3	0	0.11	0.08	0.5	0.13	32	0.6	2
Grapefruit juice, pink (1 c/247 g)	54	94	0.1	...	0.1	0.05	0.5	0.11	25	0.5	2
Grapefruit juice, white (1 c/247 g)	5	94	0.5	0	0.1	0.05	0.5	0.11	25	0.5	2
Grapefruit sections (1 c/230 g)	106	79	0.3	0	0.08	0.05	0.7	0.1	23	0.6	2
Guava (1 c/165 g)	51	303	1.2	4	0.08	0.08	2.2	0.24	23	0.2	...

Food	A, RAE, mcg	C, mg	E, mg	K, mcg	Thiamin, mg	Riboflavin, mg	Niacin, mg	Pyridoxine (B₆), mg*	Folate, mcg	Pantothenic Acid, mg	Biotin, mcg
DRI for a woman	700	75	15	90	1.1	1.1	14	1.3 to 1.5	400	5	30
DRI for a man	900	90	15	120	1.2	1.3	16	1.3 to 1.7	400	5	30
Honeydew melon, diced (1 c/170 g)	5	31	0.0	5	0.06	0.02	0.9	0.15	32	0.3	...
Huckleberries (1 c/145 g)	4	14	0.8	28	0.05	0.06	0.7	0.08	9	0.2	...
Kiwi fruit, diced (1 c/177 g)	7	164	2.6	...	0.05	0.04	1.0	0.11	44	0.3	...
Kiwi fruit, medium, each	3	70	1.1	71	0.02	0.02	0.4	0.05	19	0.3	...
Loganberries (1 c/144 g)	16	30	1.7	29	0.03	0.04	0.9	0.04	36	0.4	1
Mango, medium, each	79	57	2.3	7	0.12	0.12	1.5	0.28	29	0.3	...
Mango, sliced (1 c/165 g)	63	46	1.8	9	0.1	0.09	1.2	0.22	23	0.3	...
Orange, medium, each	14	70	0.3	1	0.11	0.05	0.6	0.08	40	0.3	1
Orange juice (1 c/248 g)	25	124	0.1	0	0.22	0.07	1.1	0.1	74	0.5	1
Orange sections (1 c/180 g)	19	96	0.4	2	0.15	0.07	0.8	0.11	55	0.4	2
Papaya, cubed (1 c/140 g)	77	87	1	4	0.04	0.04	0.7	0.03	53	0.3	...
Papaya, mashed (1 c/230 g)	126	142	1.7	6	0.06	0.07	1.1	0.04	87	0.5	...
Peach, sliced (1 c/170 g)	27	11	1.2	4	0.04	0.05	1.7	0.04	7	0.2	0.3
Peach, medium, each	16	6	0.7	3	0.02	0.03	1	0.02	4	0.1	0.2
Pear, sliced (1 c/165 g)	2	7	0.2	7	0.02	0.04	0.3	0.05	12	0.1	0.3
Pear, medium, each	2	8	0.2	8	0.02	0.04	0.3	0.05	12	0.1	0.3
Pears, dried (1 c/180 g)	0	13	0.1	37	0.01	0.26	2.5	0.13	0	0.3	...
Pineapple, diced (1 c/155 g)	5	56	0	1	0.12	0.05	0.9	0.17	23	0.3	0.5
Plum, each	8	6	0.2	4	0.02	0.02	0.3	0.02	3	0.1	...
Plums, sliced (1 c/165 g)	26	16	1	11	0.07	0.16	0.8	0.13	4	0.3	...
Prunes, dried (1 c/174 g)	68	1	0.8	104	0.09	0.32	3.3	0.36	7	0.7	...
Raisins, seedless, packed (1 c/165 g)	0	4	0.2	6	0.17	0.21	2.6	0.29	8	0.2	3
Raisins, seeded, packed (1 c/165 g)	0	9	1.2	...	0.18	0.30	2.1	0.31	5	0.1	3
Raspberries (1 c/123 g)	2	32	1.1	10	0.04	0.05	0.7	0.07	26	0.4	2
Strawberries, whole (1 c/144 g)	1	85	0.4	3	0.03	0.03	0.7	0.07	35	0.2	2
Watermelon, diced (1 c/152 g)	43	12	0.1	0.2	0.05	0.03	0.4	0.07	5	0.3	2
VEGETABLES											
Asparagus, sliced (1 c/134 g)	51	8	1.5	56	0.19	0.19	1.8	0.12	70	0.4	0.5
Asparagus spear, medium, each	6	1	0.2	7	0.02	0.02	0.2	0.02	8	0.1	...
Avocado, all types, sliced (1 c/146 g)	45	12	2	29	0.16	0.18	3.3	0.41	90	1.4	5
Avocado, all types, puréed (1 c/230 g)	70	18	3.1	46	0.25	0.28	5.2	0.64	142	2.2	8
Avocado, all types, medium, each	61	16	2.7	40	0.22	0.25	4.6	0.56	124	2	7

Food	A, RAE, mcg	C, mg	E, mg	K, mcg	Thiamin, mg	Riboflavin, mg	Niacin, mg	Pyridoxine (B$_6$), mg*	Folate, mcg	Pantothenic Acid, mg	Biotin, mcg
DRI for a woman	700	75	15	90	1.1	1.1	14	1.3 to 1.5	400	5	30
DRI for a man	900	90	15	120	1.2	1.3	16	1.3 to 1.7	400	5	30
Avocado, California, puréed (1 c/230 g)	16	20	4.5	48	0.17	0.33	5.4	0.66	143	3	8
Avocado, California, medium, each	12	15	3.4	36	0.13	0.25	4	0.5	107	2.5	6
Avocado, Florida, puréed (1 c/230 g)	16	40	6.1	...	0.05	0.12	2.6	0.18	80	2	...
Avocado, Florida, medium, each	21	53	8.1	...	0.06	0.16	3.5	0.24	106	2.8	...
Basil, fresh, chopped (1 c/42 g)	56	8	0.1	176	0.01	0.03	0.7	0.05	27	0.1	...
Beans, snap, green (1 c/110 g)	38	18	0.5	...	0.09	0.12	1.2	0.08	41	0.1	1
Beans, snap, yellow (1 c/110 g)	6	18	0.1	16	0.09	0.11	1.2	0.08	41	0.1	1
Beets, sliced (1 c/136 g)	3	7	0.1	0.3	0.04	0.05	0.9	0.09	148	0.2	...
Beet greens (1 c/38 g)	120	11	0.6	152	0.04	0.08	0.4	0.04	6	0.1	...
Bok choy, shredded (1 c/70 g)	156	32	0.1	25	0.03	0.05	0.5	0.14	46	0.1	1
Broccoli (1 c/71 g)	55	66	1.2	146	0.05	0.08	0.8	0.11	50	0.4	0.4
Brussels sprouts (1 c/88 g)	33	75	0.8	156	0.12	0.08	1.2	0.19	54	0.3	...
Cabbage, green, chopped (1 c/89 g)	8	29	0.1	53	0.04	0.03	0.5	0.09	38	0.1	2
Cabbage, pe tsai or napa, chopped (1 c/76 g)	12	21	0.1	33	0.03	0.04	0.3	0.18	60	0.1	2
Cabbage, red, chopped (1 c/89 g)	50	51	0.1	34	0.06	0.06	0.5	0.19	16	0.1	2
Cabbage, red, shredded (1 c/70 g)	39	40	0.1	27	0.05	0.05	0.4	0.15	13	0.1	1
Carrot, chopped (1 c/128 g)	771	8	0.8	17	0.08	0.07	1.5	0.18	24	0.3	6
Carrot, medium, each	433	4	0.5	8	0.05	0.04	0.8	0.1	14	0.2	4
Carrot juice (1 c/236 g)	258	9	2.7	37	0.22	0.13	0.9	...	...	0.2	...
Cauliflower (1 c/100 g)	1	46	0.1	16	0.06	0.06	1	0.22	57	0.7	2
Celery, diced (1 c/120 g)	26	4	0.3	35	0.03	0.07	0.6	0.09	43	0.3	0.1
Celery, rib, large, each	14	2	0.2	19	0.01	0.04	0.3	0.05	23	0.2	0.1
Celery root, diced (1 c/156 g)	0	12	0.6	64	0.08	0.09	1.4	0.26	12	0.5	...
Chiles, hot green (1 c/150 g)	88	364	1	21	0.14	0.14	2.1	0.42	34	0.1	...
Chiles, hot red (1 c/150 g)	72	216	1	21	0.11	0.13	2.5	0.76	34	0.3	...
Cilantro (1 c/46 g)	141	16	0.9	...	0.03	0.08	0.6	0.06	29	0.3	...
Collard greens, chopped (1 c/36 g)	120	13	0.8	184	0.02	0.05	0.5	0.06	60	0.1	...
Corn, white (1 c/154 g)	0	10	0.1	0.5	0.31	0.09	3.2	0.08	71	1.2	...
Corn, yellow (1 c/154 g)	15	10	0.1	0.5	0.31	0.09	3.2	0.08	71	1.2	...
Cucumber, peeled, each	8	6	0.1	14	0.06	0.05	0.1	0.10	28	0.5	...

Food	A, RAE, mcg	C, mg	E, mg	K, mcg	Thiamin, mg	Riboflavin, mg	Niacin, mg	Pyridoxine (B₆), mg*	Folate, mcg	Pantothenic Acid, mg	Biotin, mcg
DRI for a woman	700	75	15	90	1.1	1.1	14	1.3 to 1.5	400	5	30
DRI for a man	900	90	15	120	1.2	1.3	16	1.3 to 1.7	400	5	30
Cucumbers, peeled, sliced (1 c/119 g)	5	4	0	9	0.04	0.03	0	0.06	17	0.3	...
Cucumbers, peeled, chopped (1 c/133 g)	5	4	0	10	0.04	0.03	0	0.07	19	0.3	...
Cucumbers, with peel, sliced (1 c/104 g)	11	6	0.1	...	0.02	0.03	0.3	0.04	14	0.2	0.9
Dandelion greens (1 c/55 g)	136	19	2.6	151	0.10	0.14	0.4	0.14	15	0	0.2
Eggplant, cubed (1 c/82 g)	1	2	0.3	3	0.03	0.03	0.7	0.07	18	0.2	...
Garlic clove (1 c/136 g)	0	42	0	2	0.27	0.15	2.4	1.68	4	0.8	...
Garlic cloves, medium, each	0	1	0	0	0.01	0	0.1	0.04	0	0	...
Jerusalem artichokes, sliced (1 c/150 g)	2	6	0.3	0	0.3	0.09	2	0.12	20	0.6	...
Kale (1 c/67 g)	515	80	0.6	547	0.07	0.09	1.1	0.18	19	0	0.3
Kale, scotch (1 c/67 g)	104	87	0.6	...	0.05	0.04	1.3	0.15	19	0	...
Kelp, Japanese, chopped (1 c/80 g)	5	2	0.7	53	0.04	0.12	1	0	144	0.5	...
Leeks, chopped (1 c/89 g)	74	11	0.8	42	0.05	0.03	0.5	0.2	57	0.1	1
Lettuce, butterhead, chopped (1 c/55 g)	91	2	0.1	56	0.03	0.03	0.3	0.05	40	0.1	1
Lettuce, iceberg, chopped (1 c/55 g)	9	2	0	13	0.02	0.01	0.1	0.03	31	0.1	1
Lettuce, leaf, chopped (1 c/56 g)	207	10	0.2	97	0.04	0.05	0.3	0.05	21	0.1	1
Lettuce, red leaf, chopped (1 c/28 g)	105	1	0	39	0.02	0.02	0.1	0.03	10	0	...
Lettuce, romaine, chopped (1 c/56 g)	162	13	0.1	57	0.04	0.04	0.3	0.04	76	0.1	1
Mushroom, shiitake, dried, each	0	0	0	0	0.01	0.05	0.5	0.04	6	0.8	...
Mushrooms, shiitake, dried (1 c/145 g)	1	4	0.2	1	0.44	1.84	21.2	1.4	236	31.7	...
Mustard greens (1 c/56 g)	294	39	1.1	278	0.04	0.06	0.7	0.1	105	0.1	...
Okra, sliced (1 c/100 g)	19	21	0.4	53	0.2	0.06	1.3	0.21	88	0.2	...
Olives, green (1 c/160 g)	24	0	4.8	...	0	0	0	0.02	1	0	...
Onion, green, each	8	3	0.1	4	0.01	0.01	0.1	0.01	10	0	0.5
Onions, green, chopped (1 c/100 g)	50	19	0.6	28	0.06	0.08	0.9	0.06	64	0	4
Onions, red/yellow/white (1 c/160 g)	0	10	0	1	0.08	0.04	0.6	0.23	30	0.2	6
Parsley (1 c/60 g)	253	80	0.4	984	0.05	0.06	1.2	0.05	91	0.2	...
Parsnips, sliced (1 c/133 g)	0	23	2	30	0.12	0.07	1.2	0.12	89	0.8	0.1
Peas, green, cup (1 c/145 g)	55	58	0.2	36	0.39	0.19	3.9	0.25	94	0.2	0.7

Food	A, RAE, mcg	C, mg	E, mg	K, mcg	Thiamin, mg	Riboflavin, mg	Niacin, mg	Pyridoxine (B₆), mg*	Folate, mcg	Pantothenic Acid, mg	Biotin, mcg
DRI for a woman	700	75	15	90	1.1	1.1	14	1.3 to 1.5	400	5	30
DRI for a man	900	90	15	120	1.2	1.3	16	1.3 to 1.7	400	5	30
Pea pods, snow (1 c/63 g)	34	38	0.2	16	0.09	0.05	0.7	0.1	26	0.5	...
Pepper, bell, green, medium, each	21	96	0.4	9	0.07	0.03	0.8	0.27	13	0.1	...
Peppers, bell, green, chopped (1 c/149 g)	27	120	0.6	11	0.09	0.04	1	0.33	16	0.2	...
Pepper, bell, red, medium, each	187	226	1.9	6	0.06	0.10	1.4	0.35	21	0.4	...
Peppers, bell, red (1 c/149 g)	234	283	2.4	7	0.08	0.13	1.8	0.43	27	0.5	...
Peppers, bell, yellow (1 c/149 g)	15	273	1	...	.04	.04	1.7	0.25	39	0.2	...
Radish, daikon (1 c/88 g)	0	19	0	...	0.02	0.02	0.2	0.04	25	0.1	...
Radish, daikon, medium, each	0	74	0	...	0.07	0.07	0.8	0.16	95	0.5	...
Radishes, daikon, dried (1 c/116 g)	0	0	0	...	0.31	0.79	4.8	0.72	342	2.2	...
Radish, medium, each	0	1	0	0.1	0	0	0	0	1	0	
Radishes, sliced (1 c/116 g)	0	17	0	2	0.01	0.05	0.4	0.08	29	0.2	
Radish sprouts (1 c/38 g)	8	11	...	...	0.04	0.04	1.1	0.11	36	0.3	...
Rutabaga, chopped (1 c/140 g)	0	35	0.4	0.4	0.13	0.06	1.3	0.14	29	0.2	0.1
Spinach, chopped (1 c/30 g)	141	8	0.6	145	0.02	0.06	0.4	0.06	58	0	0
Squash, acorn, cubed (1 c/140 g)	25	15	0.2	...	0.20	0.01	1.2	0.22	24	0.6	
Squash, all varieties winter, cubed (1 c/116 g)	79	14	0.1	1	0.03	0.07	0.9	0.18	28	0.2	...
Squash, butternut, cubed (1 c/240 g)	1,277	50	3.5	3	0.24	0.05	3.4	0.37	65	1	...
Squash, crookneck, cubed (1 c/130 g)	10	11	0.1	...	0.07	0.06	0.8	0.14	30	0.1	...
Squash, hubbard, cubed (1 c/116 g)	79	13	0.1	...	0.08	0.05	1.1	0.18	19	0.5	...
Sweet potato, cubed (1 c/133 g)	967	30	0.3	2	0.10	0.08	1.2	0.28	19	1.1	...
Tomato, cherry, each	7	2	0.1	1	0.01	0	0.1	0.01	3	0	0.7
Tomato, chopped (1 c/180 g)	76	23	1	14	0.07	0.03	1.2	0.14	27	0.2	7
Tomato, green, chopped (1 c/180 g)	58	42	0.7	18	0.11	0.07	1.2	0.15	16	0.9	...
Tomato, medium, each	63	19	0.8	12	0.06	0.03	1.0	0.12	22	0.1	6
Tomato, Roma, each	26	8	0.3	5	0.03	0.01	0.4	0.05	9	0.1	2
Tomato, sun-dried (1 c/54 g)	24	21	0	23	0.28	0.26	5.8	0.18	37	1.1	...
Tomato, yellow, chopped (1 c/139 g)	0	13	...	...	0.06	0.07	1.8	0.08	42	0.2	...
Turnip, cubed (1 c/130 g)	0	27	0	0.1	0.05	0.04	0.7	0.12	20	0.3	0.1
Turnip greens, chopped (1 c/55 g)	0	33	1.6	138	0.04	0.06	0.6	0.14	107	0.2	...
Yam, cubed (1 c/150 g)	10.5	26	0.6	4	0.17	0.05	1.1	0.44	34	0.5	...

Food	A, RAE, mcg	C, mg	E, mg	K, mcg	Thiamin, mg	Riboflavin, mg	Niacin, mg	Pyridoxine (B₆), mg*	Folate, mcg	Pantothenic Acid, mg	Biotin, mcg
DRI for a woman	700	75	15	90	1.1	1.1	14	1.3 to 1.5	400	5	30
DRI for a man	900	90	15	120	1.2	1.3	16	1.3 to 1.7	400	5	30
Zucchini, baby, each	0	4	0	...	0	0	0.1	0.02	2	0	...
Zucchini, cubed (1 c/124 g)	12.4	21	0.1	5	0.06	0.18	0.8	0.27	36	0.2	...
NUTS AND SEEDS											
Almond butter (1 c/256 g)	0	2	52	...	0.34	1.56	17.3	0.19	166	0.7	...
Almonds (1 c/142 g)	1	...	37	...	0.3	1.2	10	0.2	62	0.6	97
Brazil nut, large, each	0	0	0.3	0	0.03	0	0.1	0	1	0	...
Brazil nuts (1 c/140 g)	2	1	8	0	0.86	0.05	3.4	0.14	31	0.3	...
Cashew butter (1 c/256 g)	0	0	4	...	0.80	0.48	14.6	0.65	174	3.1	...
Cashew nuts (1 c/130 g)	0	1	1.2	44	0.55	0.08	7	0.54	32	1.1	...
Chia seeds, dried (1 c/160 g)	...	25	...	...	1.39	0.27	26.3	1.11	182	1.5	...
Flaxseeds, ground (1 c/112 g)	0	1	0.4	5	1.8	0.18	3.4	0.53	97	1.1	...
Hazelnuts, dried (1 c/135 g)	1	9	20.3	19	0.87	0.15	6.6	0.76	153	1.2	103
Pecans (1 c/108 g)	7	2	3.5	...	0.86	0.11	1	0.22	42	1.8	...
Pine nuts, dried (1 c/136 g)	1	1	12.7	73	0.50	0.31	8.2	0.128	91	0.4	...
Pistachio nuts (1 c/128 g)	36	6	2.9	90	1.11	0.20	7.5	2.18	65	0.7	...
Poppy seeds (1 c/141 g)	0	1	2.5	0	1.14	0.23	6	0.6	80	0.5	...
Pumpkin seeds (1 c/138 g)	26	3	0	71	0.29	0.44	11	0.31	80	0.5	...
Sesame butter/tahini (1 c/240 g)	7	0	5.4	...	3.08	1.22	14.2	0.36	235	1.7	...
Sesame seeds, hulled (1 c/150 g)	4	0	0.4	0	1.08	0.13	15.4	0.22	144	1	16
Sesame seeds, with hulls (1 c/144 g)	1	0	0.4	0	1.14	0.36	14.7	1.14	140	0.1	16
Sunflower seed butter (1 c/256 g)	8	7	123	...	0.83	0.73	25.3	2.06	607	18	...
Sunflower seed kernels (1 c/144 g)	4	2	49.7	4	3.30	0.36	14.1	1.11	327	9.7	...
Walnuts, black, chopped (1 c/125 g)	19	4	3.3	...	0.27	0.14	7.2	0.69	82	0.8	24
Walnuts, English, chopped (1 c/120 g)	1	2	0.8	3	0.40	0.18	4.6	0.64	118	0.7	23
Water chestnuts, Chinese, sliced (1 c/124 g)	0	5	1.5	0.4	0.17	0.25	1.2	0.41	20	0.6	...
LEGUMES											
Adzuki beans, dried (1 c/197 g)	4	0	1	...	0.90	0.43	11.5	0.69	1225	2.9	...
Lentils, dried (1 c/192 g)	4	12	0.6	10	0.91	0.47	13.1	1.03	831	3.6	...
Lentil sprouts (1 c/77 g)	2	13	0.1		0.18	0.1	0.9	0.15	77	0.4	...
Mung bean sprouts (1 c/104 g)	1	14	0.1	34	0.09	0.13	1.42	0.09	63	0.4	...

Food	A, RAE, mcg	C, mg	E, mg	K, mcg	Thiamin, mg	Riboflavin, mg	Niacin, mg	Pyridoxine (B₆), mg*	Folate, mcg	Pantothenic Acid, mg	Biotin, mcg
DRI for a woman	700	75	15	90	1.1	1.1	14	1.3 to 1.5	400	5	30
DRI for a man	900	90	15	120	1.2	1.3	16	1.3 to 1.7	400	5	30
Mung beans, dried (1 c/207 g)	12	10	1.1	19	1.3	0.48	4.7	0.79	1294	4.0	...
Pea sprouts (1 c/120 g)	10	12	0	...	0.27	0.19	3.7	0.32	173	1.2	...
GRAINS											
Amaranth, dry (1 c/195 g)	0	9	2	...	0.16	0.41	8.4	0.43	96	2	...
Barley, dry (1 c/184 g)	2	0	1	4	1.19	0.52	14.9	0.58	35	0.5	...
Buckwheat, dry (1 c/170 g)	0	0	1.8	...	0.17	0.72	17.4	0.36	51	2.0	...
Buckwheat sprouts (1 c/33 g)	0	1	0	...	0.07	0.05	1	0.09	13	...	...
Kamut, dry (1 c/186 g)	0	0	1.1	3	1.00	0.33	11.8	0.47	...	1.7	...
Millet, dry (1 c/200 g)	0	0	0.1	2	0.84	0.58	13.4	0.77	170	1.7	...
Oat groats, dry (1 c/156 g)	0	0	...	...	1.19	0.22	1.5	0.19	87	2.1	...
Quinoa, dry (1 c/170 g)	0	0	8.3	...	0.34	0.67	9.1	0.38	83	1.8	...
Rye, berries, dry (1 c/169 g)	2	0	2.2	10	0.53	0.42	11.6	0.5	101	2.5	...
Sprouted wheat bread, slice	0	0	0.1	...	0.11	0.07	1.1	0.03	11	0	1
Wheat berries, hard, red, dry (1 c/192 g)	1	0	1.9	4	0.97	0.21	17.2	0.65	83	1.8	...
Wheat berries, hard, white, dry (1 c/192 g)	1	0	1.9	4	0.74	0.21	13	0.71	73	1.8	...
Wheat sprouts (1 c/108 g)	0	3	0.1	...	0.24	0.17	5.4	0.29	41	1	...
Wild rice, dry (1 c/160 g)	2	0	1.3	3	0.18	0.42	15.5	0.63	152	2	...
OTHERS (NOT NECESSARILY RAW)											
BarleyMax† (1 tsp/2 g)	26	4	0	95	0.01	0.04	0.2	0.04	22	0.1	2
Maple syrup (1 c/322 g)	0	0	0	0	0.01	0.03	0.1	0.01	0	0.1	...
Oil, flaxseed (1 c/218 g)	0	0	38	0	0	0	0	0	0	...	...
Oil, olive (1 c/216 g)	0	0	31	130	0	0	0	0	0	0	...
Red Star Vegetarian Support Formula nutritional yeast (1 c/100 g)	0	0	...	...	63	63	367	60	1,500	6	130
Red Star Vegetarian Support Formula nutritional yeast (1 Tbsp/6 g)	0	0	...	...	4	4	23	4	94	0.4	8
Spirulina sea vegetable, dried (1 c/119 g)	35	12	6	30	2.83	4.37	33.5	0.43	112	4.1	...

Source: Data from references 1–3, 6, 61, 67, 102–104.

Note: Cells with no values indicate that data for those nutrient are not available.

*The DRI for pyridoxine (B₆) is 1.3 for adults to age 50; above the age of 50 it increases to 1.5 for women and 1.7 for men.

†BarleyMax is available from www.hacres.com/products.

Production of Energy from Foods: The B Vitamins

The body uses carbohydrates, fat, and protein as fuel in the production of energy. The tiny workers that make this happen are vitamins and enzymes. In complex sequences that resemble a busy factory's production lines, each of the nine B vitamins assists specific enzymes. Each of these enzymes cannot function without its vitamin assistant, or coenzyme. For energy production, the body requires dietary sources of thiamin, riboflavin, niacin, pantothenic acid, pyridoxine, and biotin. Folate and vitamin B_{12} are required to form new cells that deliver oxygen and nutrients so that the energy production line can run; choline helps this duo. Certain vitamins help regenerate others. The B vitamins also are builders of fats that are needed in cell membranes, of genetic material, of substances that transmit nerve impulses, and of certain hormones. (For more details about vitamin function, see http://lpi.oregonstate.edu/infocenter/vitamins.html, *Becoming Vegan* by Brenda Davis and Vesanto Melina, or *Vitamins and Minerals Demystified* by Steve Blake.) If one vitamin (such as vitamin B_{12}) is lacking, the complex chain of events can come to a halt, with dire health consequences.

Consider Benjamin Franklin's take on a fourteenth-century proverb (he became vegetarian at sixteen years of age):

A little neglect may breed mischief . . .

for want of a nail, the shoe was lost;

for want of a shoe the horse was lost;

and for want of a horse the rider was lost.

When raw diets include enough calories from an assortment of seeds, nuts, vegetables, and fruits, with or without sprouted grains and legumes, they can meet the DRIs for the B vitamins, apart from vitamin B_{12}. (See table 8.3, page 162.) When calories are restricted, for example during a period of weight loss, vitamin intakes can drop below the DRIs, and this can affect energy levels and well-being. Though not a raw food, nutritional yeast is an excellent source of B vitamins that is acceptable to many raw-food enthusiasts; Red Star Vegetarian Support Formula includes vitamin B_{12} and can be a way to boost dietary intake. Because B vitamins are water-soluble, they can be lost in soaking water that is discarded. Dietary sources for each B vitamin are shown in table 8.2, page 154.

THIAMIN (VITAMIN B_1)

Raw Research and Functions

Studies show that reasonable intakes of thiamin are achieved on raw diets (see table 8.3, page 162). Thiamin is sometimes known as "the carbohydrate burner."

TABLE 8.3 B vitamins: adult Dietary Reference Intakes and intakes on raw and high-raw diets

Food	Thiamin mg	Riboflavin mg	Niacin mg	Pyridoxine (B₆), mg†	Folate mcg	Pantothenic acid mg	Biotin mcg	Vitamin B₁₂ mcg*
DRI for a woman	1.1	1.1	14	1.3 to 1.5	400	5	30	2.4
DRI for a man	1.2	1.3	16	1.3 to 1.7	400	5	30	2.4
STUDY, COUNTRY, YEAR(S), PARTICIPANTS, REFERENCES								
Giessen study, Germany, 2001, 2005, 43 vegans[4,5]	...	1.4	...	3.3	518	...	...	0.2
Hallelujah Acres diet, USA, 2001, 54 men (34 vegans)[6]	2.4 (2.2)	2.0*	18.0	4.0	594 (703)	6.4 (6.7)	37.0 (40.6)	0.6 (0.1)
Hallelujah Acres diet, USA, 2001, 87 women (47 vegans)[6]	2.0 (2.2)	1.7	14.8	3.2 (3.6)	487 (523)	5.2 (5.8)	29 (31.4)	0.5 (0.5)
Hallelujah Acres diet, USA, 2001, 20 fibromyalgia patients[106]	2.1	1.7	16.0	3.6	550	...	...	0.6
Living-food diet, Finland, 1995, 1996, 19 women and 1 man [7, 107, 109, 110]	1.9	1.2	13	...	...	...	...	0.1‡
Living-food diet, Finland, 1993, 13 adults (mostly women) with rheumatoid arthritis[8]	2.7	1.8	19.2	...	...	...	...	...
Living-food diet, Finland, 1992, 9 adults[9, 111]	1.7	...	...	2.6	...	...	...	...

*Vitamin B₁₂ intakes include supplements.

†The DRI for pyridoxine for adults up to age 50 is 1.3 mg; for adults over the age of 50 it increases to 1.5 mg for women and 1.7 mg for men.

‡A study of this group showed intakes that included inactive vitamin B₁₂ analogs and did not sustain vitamin B₁₂ over time.[107–110]

Dietary Sources of Thiamin

The top sources of thiamin in raw diets include seeds (such as sesame and sunflower), nuts (such as Brazil and pine nuts), and sprouted grains and legumes. This vitamin is also available in avocados, carrot juice, cherimoyas, corn, dried fruits, durians, peas, and squash. It is found in most raw foods and is easily destroyed by cooking.

RIBOFLAVIN (VITAMIN B₂)

Raw Research and Functions

As with thiamin, intakes on raw diets are reasonable (see table 8.3, page 162). Riboflavin is a team member in energy production and detoxification. If you have taken a vitamin supplement and have an excess of this water-soluble vitamin to excrete, you may notice its fluorescent yellow color in your urine.

Dietary Sources of Riboflavin

Good sources of riboflavin include the following:

almonds	broccoli	green beans	quinoa
asparagus	buckwheat	leafy greens	sea vegetables
avocados	cashews	nutritional yeast	seeds
bananas	durians	peas	sweet potatoes

Sprouting has been shown to increase the riboflavin content of alfalfa seeds and mung beans.[63, 105] The ultraviolet rays of the sun and fluorescent light can destroy riboflavin. For this reason, items such as nutritional yeast, an excellent source of riboflavin (see table 8.2, page 154), should be stored in an opaque container or dark cupboard.

NIACIN (VITAMIN B₃)

Raw Research and Functions

Average niacin intakes were low among Finns on a somewhat low-calorie living-food diet and low among those people on the Hallelujah Acres diet whose caloric intakes were less than 60 percent of recommended levels.[6, 8] Niacin is part of a coenzyme that assists hundreds of enzymes that are active in the production of energy and that support the health of our skin, nervous system, and digestive system.

Dietary Sources of Niacin

Sources of niacin include foods that are also good protein providers, such as the following:

avocados	legumes	quinoa
buckwheat	(including peanuts)	rye
cherimoyas	nutritional yeast	seeds
dried fruits	nuts	wild rice
durians	peas	

The niacin in corn is poorly absorbed unless the corn is soaked in lime, as is the Mexican tradition for making tortillas.[41] When diets provide extra protein, some niacin can be derived from the amino acid tryptophan. If a diet is low in protein, as is typical for some low-calorie raw diets, this can be reflected in low niacin intakes due to limited intakes of the vitamin and of tryptophan. Furthermore, when intakes of riboflavin, vitamin B_6, or iron are low, the conversion of tryptophan to niacin can be impaired because these nutrients are involved in the conversion.

Amounts of niacin shown in nutritional tables typically are expressed in milligrams (mg) of "Niacin Equivalents" and take into account both the vitamin and the conversion from tryptophan (see table 8.2, page 154).[102]

PANTOTHENIC ACID (VITAMIN B₅)

Raw Research and Functions

On low-calorie raw diets, intakes of this vitamin have been shown to fall far below DRIs.[6] As a coenzyme that is found in all living cells, this vitamin plays a central role in helping the body to release energy from carbohydrates, fat, and protein.

Dietary Sources of Pantothenic Acid

The name "pantothenic acid" derived from the Greek word *pantothen*, meaning "from every side." In fact, this vitamin is present "from all sides," at least in small amounts, in whole foods. Avocados and sunflower seeds are particularly high in pantothenic acid; grains, legumes, nuts, and other seeds also are good sources.

PYRIDOXINE (VITAMIN B₆)

Raw Research and Functions

Studies show that pyridoxine intakes tend to be good on raw diets (see table 8.3, page 162). This vitamin is needed for the conversion of amino acids to energy and for building amino acids, fatty acids, and neurotransmitters (substances that transmit nerve impulses). As one of its many functions, pyridoxine helps remove homocysteine, a troublesome compound that is created during certain metabolic processes. Pyridoxine, folate, and vitamin B_{12} convert homocysteine into two amino acids that the body can use in building protein. With shortages of these three B vitamins, homocysteine levels rise, arterial walls can be damaged, and blood clots form, increasing the risk of heart disease. For people over the age of fifty, the DRI for vitamin B_6 increases by about 15 percent.[42, 102]

Dietary Sources of Pyridoxine

Vitamin B_6 is well distributed among plant foods, especially fruits. For example, you can get a day's supply from three bananas. Raw vegan diets provide plenty of sources, such as avocados, legumes, nuts, and seeds. Nutritional yeast also is a good source. This vitamin is easily destroyed by cooking and is lost in soaking water.

FOLATE (FOLIC ACID)

Raw Research and Functions

Folate intakes on raw diets are at reasonable levels (see table 8.3, page 162).[44] The coenzyme form of folate transfers small segments of molecules to sites where they are needed to build the genetic material DNA and amino acids. Folate protects DNA from changes that may lead to cancer and works with vitamins B_{12} and B_6. Requirements are increased during pregnancy, when a great deal of cell division occurs.[112]

Dietary Sources of Folate

The name for this vitamin has the same root as the word "foliage." Given this hint, you may guess that important contributors to raw diets are the leafy greens. (In 1945, folate was first isolated from spinach.) Other sources are:

almonds	berries	legume sprouts	pineapple
apricots	carrots	mango	quinoa
Asian pears	cashews	nectarines	plums
avocados	green peppers	oranges	raisins
bananas	kelp	papaya	seeds
beets	kiwifruit	peaches	squash

Sprouting has been shown to more than double the folate content of seeds, such as rye berries.[112] In order to absorb folate, the body requires adequate intakes of vitamin C and iron. Folate is easily destroyed by boiling, whereas steaming has been shown to cause little or no loss of folate from broccoli or spinach.[113]

BIOTIN

Raw Research and Functions

People on plant-based diets seem to fare well when it comes to this vitamin. Intakes of biotin by raw foodists are likely to be sufficient unless calorie intakes are particularly low.[6, 42] Along with other B vitamins, biotin is involved in the metabolism of amino acids, fats, and carbohydrates.

Dietary Sources of Biotin

Avocados, cauliflower, and raspberries are among the many sources of biotin. This vitamin doesn't hit the headlines because deficiencies are rare. Biotin also can be manufactured by bacteria in the large intestine and absorbed by the body from there, adding to the supply provided from our diets.

CHOLINE

Raw Research and Functions

Choline helps to build cell membranes and transport fats and nutrients into and out of cells.

Dietary Sources of Choline

Because it is a part of all cells, choline is widely distributed in plant foods, though data showing exact amounts is limited. From 3 ounces (100 grams) of each of the following foods, you can expect to get the amounts of choline listed:

> fruits: 5–10 milligrams choline
>
> legumes, cooked: 60–90 milligrams choline
>
> mung bean sprouts: 15 milligrams choline
>
> nuts and seeds: 25–60 milligrams choline
>
> vegetables: 5–20 milligrams choline[114]

Compare these amounts to DRIs of 425 milligrams for women and 550 milligrams for men. Your body can make choline to add to your dietary supply as long as it has sufficient folate, vitamin B_{12}, and the amino acid methionine.

Vitamin B_{12} (Cobalamin, Cyanocobalamin)

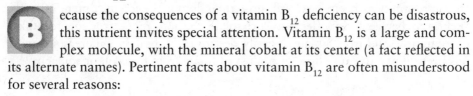

Because the consequences of a vitamin B_{12} deficiency can be disastrous, this nutrient invites special attention. Vitamin B_{12} is a large and complex molecule, with the mineral cobalt at its center (a fact reflected in its alternate names). Pertinent facts about vitamin B_{12} are often misunderstood for several reasons:

- Some deficiency symptoms can be masked for a time by the effects of another vitamin (folate) that is abundant in raw vegan diets.

- Inactive analogs, which are structurally similar vitamin B_{12} "impersonators," are present in certain foods. These inactive analogs show up in certain laboratory analyses as vitamin B_{12}, yet these substances cannot perform the necessary functions of true B_{12}.

- Vitamin B_{12} is produced by bacteria that are present at a few locations along the gastrointestinal tract, but this production cannot be relied on to prevent deficiency.

- Vitamin B_{12} is transported and absorbed by some rather complex mechanisms.[102, 115]

Because of its peculiarities, it's not surprising that there is confusion about safe ways to get this essential nutrient.

Vitamin B_{12} helps to build DNA and is crucial for cells that reproduce rapidly, such as the red blood cells that are produced in bone marrow. Another significant role of this vitamin is the maintenance of protective sheaths that surround nerve fibers. Vitamin B_{12} is part of the team that converts carbohydrates, fat, and protein to useable energy. As one aspect of its work with amino acids, vitamin B_{12} helps to rid the body of homocysteine, a potentially damaging breakdown product of the amino acid methionine that can injure the delicate inner lining of artery walls and be a trigger for heart disease. In cases of vitamin B_{12} deficiency, either from insufficient intake or from inadequate absorption of this vitamin, some combination of the following symptoms can appear.[102, 115] These symptoms are easily avoided by ensuring that you have a reliable source of this essential nutrient.[102, 116, 117]

VITAMIN B_{12} DEFICIENCY SYMPTOMS

Megaloblastic Anemia

Megaloblastic anemia is a condition in which cells fail to divide properly because of improper synthesis of DNA, resulting in the appearance of abnormally shaped, large red cells in the blood. The abnormal red blood cells have a decreased ability to carry oxygen, leading to fatigue, weakness, decreased stamina, shortness of breath, palpitations, and skin pallor.

Nerve Damage

The effects of vitamin B_{12} deficiency on nerve cells, the spinal cord, and the brain can cause mental changes, such as confusion, depression, irritability, mood fluctuations, insomnia, and inability to concentrate, plus physical symptoms, such as tingling and numbness in fingers, arms, and legs, difficulty with balance, lack of sensation, and eventual paralysis.

Deficiencies early in pregnancy have been linked to neural-tube defects in the baby. Breast-fed infants whose mothers have insufficient dietary B_{12}, and other infants whose diets are low in B_{12}, can develop serious and permanent damage to the nervous system. According to James Mills, a senior investigator with the U.S. National Institute of Child Health and Human Development, "Nobody should get pregnant with low vitamin B_{12} levels."

Gastrointestinal Disturbances

Symptoms of a vitamin B_{12} deficiency involving the gastrointestinal tract include a sore tongue, reduced appetite, indigestion, and diarrhea.

Elevated Homocysteine in the Blood

With vitamin B_{12} deficiency, homocysteine increases, atherosclerotic plaque accumulates, and arteries begin to clog, resulting in heart disease and strokes.

LABORATORY TESTING FOR VITAMIN B$_{12}$ STATUS

Several lab tests are used to detect vitamin B$_{12}$ deficiency. (Lab tests are discussed in detail in the the Institute of Medicine's online document.[102])

- **Homocysteine.** High homocysteine levels in the blood can indicate vitamin B$_{12}$ deficiency. This test is more commonly used as an indicator of an increased risk of heart disease, but it is also a possible measure of inadequate B$_{12}$.[42, 102, 118]

- **MCV.** A test that can indicate vitamin B$_{12}$ deficiency is mean corpuscular volume (MCV), an indicator of macrocytic anemia (a condition that occurs when red blood cells are larger than normal). This test doesn't work for people with high intakes of greens, oranges, and other excellent sources of folate, because folate can help prevent macrocytic anemia, even when someone is deficient in vitamin B$_{12}$. Consequently, raw foodists with high intakes of greens, oranges, and other folate sources can have a B$_{12}$ deficiency that remains undetected by an MCV test while the underlying damage to nerves proceeds and homocysteine levels rise.[42]

- **MMA.** A reliable and sensitive test for confirming the adequacy of B$_{12}$ status is a measure of a compound in blood or urine called methylmalonic acid (MMA), which is related to homocysteine. (Physicians and lab technicians may be unfamiliar with this test.) Normal MMA levels should be less than 370 nanomoles per liter (nmol/L) in blood or less than 4 micrograms per milligram (mcg/mg) of creatinine in urine, but with a B$_{12}$ deficiency, MMA accumulates.[42, 102, 118, 119]

- **Serum or plasma vitamin B$_{12}$.** Your blood serum should contain more than 300 picomoles of vitamin B$_{12}$ per liter (pmol/l), or 400 picograms per milliliter (pg/ml). Neither this test nor the test for plasma B$_{12}$ is always a reliable indicator of your vitamin B$_{12}$ status because these tests also detect inactive B$_{12}$ analogs, which cannot perform essential metabolic functions, along with the true vitamin B$_{12}$. Such analogs are similar to true B$_{12}$, but they cannot perform essential metabolic functions. If people consume spirulina or sea vegetables that are high in inactive vitamin B$_{12}$ analogs, the analogs that are present "fool" the blood test, showing lab results within the normal range while levels of the actual vitamin are far lower.[110] Another lab test to consider measures holotranscobalamin.[120–122]

- **Holotranscobalamin.** Another lab test to consider measures holotranscobalamin.[120-122]

MYTHS AND FACTS ABOUT VITAMIN B$_{12}$

The following are a number of common beliefs about vitamin B$_{12}$ that do not stand up to scientific scrutiny. Each is followed by accurate information.

The Naturalist Argument

Myth: Nature provides every nutrient we need. Consuming supplements or fortified foods of any kind is unnecessary if your diet is truly optimal. The supplement-free, natural diets of primates provide solid proof that a natural, plant-based diet is adequate.

Truth: Great apes and other primates consume insects, termites, soil, and even bits of fecal material along with their unwashed fruits, shoots, leaves, and nuts. This contamination contains a host of microbes, some harmful bacteria, and some beneficial vitamin B_{12}-producing bacteria. For a raw diet that is free of pathogenic bacteria, other sources of vitamin B_{12} must be found.[118, 123]

Plant-Food Sources of Vitamin B_{12}

Myth: Fermented foods, sprouts, mushrooms, dulse and other sea vegetables, spirulina, algae, sprouts, and raw plant foods (with or without bits of dirt on them) provide plenty of vitamin B_{12} for people.[108, 110, 119, 123, 124]

Truth: None of the following can be relied on as sources of vitamin B_{12}: fermented foods, mushrooms, sea vegetables, spirulina, sprouts, or raw plant foods, such as fruits, nuts, seeds, or vegetables, dirty or clean. If true B_{12} is present, amounts are too variable to be reliable. You obtain little or no true vitamin B_{12} from these, and you may obtain inactive analog forms that are worse than useless. In fact, MMA levels in people eating large quantities of algae, such as dulse or nori, increased even further, and MCV and deficiency symptoms worsened for people using nori and spirulina. These analog molecules fail to meet human requirements, and they can interfere with the action of true B_{12}. Despite reports from individuals saying that they have relied on one or another of these as their vitamin B_{12} source without ill effect, there are no well-documented scientific studies showing that any of these items have proved to be reliable sources of true B_{12} or that any of them can relieve vitamin B_{12} deficiencies. Instead, studies show that numerous people trying these alternatives have fared less well and eventually developed deficiencies.[42, 102, 107–110, 118, 119, 123, 125, 126, 144] (For information on vitamin B_{12} and *Chlorella* and Klamath brand blue-green algae, see page 172.)

Internal Production of Vitamin B_{12}

Myth: You make plenty of vitamin B_{12} in your mouth and small intestine to supply your daily needs.

Truth: Bacteria in saliva and plaque can produce vitamin B_{12}, especially if you have poor oral hygiene and your teeth are ridden with plaque. However, the quantity produced above the small intestine is variable and typically insufficient. There are far more reliable ways to get this essential nutrient.

Production of Vitamin B$_{12}$ in the Large Intestine

Myth: Some vitamin B$_{12}$ originating from bacteria in the large intestine goes against the current and travels upstream to the absorption site for vitamin B$_{12}$ in the small intestine. Furthermore, if you just work hard enough at healing your intestine, vitamin B$_{12}$ will be produced and utilized.[119]

Truth: Bacteria do indeed make vitamin B$_{12}$ in the large intestine; however, we do not absorb it there. The vitamin goes with the flow, meaning that B$_{12}$ manufactured in the large intestine ends up in the toilet.[102, 119]

Recycling Vitamin B$_{12}$ in the Body

Myth: Some people manage with no reliable dietary or supplementary source of vitamin B$_{12}$.

Truth: The body is adept at recovering and reusing vitamin B$_{12}$, and some people are better recyclers than others. Between 1 and 10 micrograms a day of vitamin B$_{12}$ can be excreted in the bile and then effectively reabsorbed at the specific absorption site for this vitamin in the small intestine. A few people seem to be particularly adept at recycling vitamin B$_{12}$ and manage to avoid deficiency with no obvious dietary source of it for as long as twenty years. An individual who is an efficient recycler might get trace amounts from B$_{12}$-producing bacteria-laden water, food, or dental plaque. A lab test for MMA or homocysteine can provide inside information about vitamin B$_{12}$ status. Most people do not recycle the vitamin this efficiently. Adult supplies typically last for a year or two, although some become deficient in a matter of months. Without a reliable source, vitamin B$_{12}$ stores diminish, blood cells become abnormal and start to malfunction, and the sheaths around nerve cells fail to be maintained. Deficiency symptoms include fatigue, paleness, anorexia, mental confusion, delusions, paranoia, numbness and tingling in fingers and toes, walking difficulties, weight loss, and respiratory problems. The damage can be dramatic and, in a few unfortunate cases, irreversible.

RAW RESEARCH: VITAMIN B$_{12}$ INTAKES AND STATUS OF PEOPLE ON RAW VEGAN DIETS

In the Giessen study that included thirty-nine people who had been on a raw vegan diet for at least two years, every participant who did not take a vitamin B$_{12}$ supplement was deficient in vitamin B$_{12}$ as defined by low plasma B$_{12}$ (their average was 126 pgmol/L) and high homocysteine levels (18.5 µmol/L). Twelve percent also had developed an increased MCV, indicating macrocytic anemia (see page 168). The four people who used some vitamin B$_{12}$ supplements had higher plasma B$_{12}$ levels and less of the potentially damaging homocysteine than did the thirty-nine who took no supplements.[5] The raw diets had many health-supportive features, yet their long-term health was at risk due to potentially damaging homocysteine levels.

A study of forty-nine American adults who had followed the Hallelujah Acres diet for two to four years without vitamin B_{12} supplementation showed that three-quarters of the participants had serum B_{12} or MMA levels indicating a vitamin B_{12} deficiency. The deficiencies were in the early stages, and participants were unaware of any deficiency symptoms. Some participants believed they were receiving adequate intakes of vitamin B_{12} from raw fruits and vegetables, probiotics, fermented foods, dried greens, dulse, nori, blue-green algae, and/or spirulina, or from intestinal production; however, this proved not to be the case.[6, 67, 119] Though some participants believed chlorinated water might be a factor affecting B_{12} status, exposure to chlorinated water did not have any effect on whether people were deficient in vitamin B_{12}. In a follow-up study, twenty-five of those with vitamin B_{12} deficiency continued the Hallelujah Acres diet but with an important adjustment. The participants were divided into three groups: one group added sublingual supplements of vitamin B_{12}, one group consumed Red Star brand Vegetarian Support Formula nutritional yeast on a regular basis, and the third group took probiotics. The vitamin B_{12} supplements proved to be powerfully beneficial in quickly reversing deficiency. Nutritional yeast had a strong effect, but it was found to be less reliable than supplements (which contain specified quantities), as one person's deficiency was not completely remedied within the three-week time period. The probiotics were ineffective at reversing vitamin B_{12} deficiency.[6, 67, 119]

Twenty Finns who had been on a living-food diet for an average of five years assumed that the substantial amounts of fermented foods they ate would provide plenty of vitamin B_{12}, that the diet would modify their intestinal bacteria to provide more vitamin B_{12}, and that nori and *Chlorella* algae also would provide vitamin B_{12}. Their average vitamin B_{12} intakes are shown in table 8.3, page 162. These individuals were deficient in vitamin B_{12}, with serum B_{12} levels averaging 193 picograms/milliliter (with a range of 35–408 picograms/milliliter), 62 percent of the levels of nonvegetarians who were matched for age, gender, social status, and residence.[107] As it turned out, the fermented foods did not help with vitamin B_{12} status. Questions remained about the value of sea vegetables, and researchers checked the vitamin B_{12} status of nine of these people two years later.[107] Eight consumed nori, with or without other sea vegetables. Lab tests showed a slow and consistent decrease in their average vitamin B_{12} status, indicating that these sea vegetables could not supply enough B_{12} to maintain human health over the long term. One woman relied on quantities of *Chlorella*; she had vitamin B_{12} levels that were within the normal range, though the test used was serum B_{12} rather than the more reliable MMA or homocysteine. Researchers noted that high intakes of sea vegetables are accompanied by excessive iodine intakes, which could be harmful (see page 189), though opinions vary on this and other relevant points.[107, 109, 110, 127]

A 1982 study in the United States reported that serum levels of B_{12} were assessed for vegans who attended a natural hygiene conference. These people ate raw fruits, vegetables, nuts, seeds, and minimal amounts of grains and legumes. They took no supplements and believed that their intestinal bacteria would supply the necessary B_{12}. They were found to be deficient in vitamin B_{12}. Whereas 400 picograms per milliliter is a minimum for good health, 93 percent had serum B_{12} levels of less than 200 picograms per milliliter and 53 percent were severely deficient, with serum B_{12} levels that were lower than 100 picograms per millileter.[123, 128]

VITAMIN B_{12} AT DIFFERENT STAGES OF LIFE

Taking a reliable or supplementary source of vitamin B_{12} is especially important during pregnancy and lactation, as well as during infancy and early childhood, when young ones have not yet built up their reserves of this nutrient.

Some people on raw diets include raw animal products in an effort to get vitamin B_{12}. With age, the body's ability to absorb the form of vitamin B_{12} that is present in animal products diminishes. In animal products, vitamin B_{12} is attached to a protein, and as people get older, production of the stomach acid that can split this complex of vitamin B_{12} and protein diminishes. The recommendations for vitamin B_{12} take into account that up to one in three of all individuals age fifty and older have low stomach-acid secretion. The form of vitamin B_{12} that is present in fortified foods and supplements is not attached to protein; therefore, its absorption is not affected by a change in acid production. It is recommended that people over the age of fifty, regardless of their diet choice, rely either on foods fortified with vitamin B_{12} or supplements to meet their recommended intakes. In addition to changes in gastric acidity, approximately 2 percent of older adults (regardless of diet) do not produce enough of a carrier (intrinsic factor) that is part of the complex process of vitamin B_{12} absorption. To detect such a problem, people should have their vitamin B_{12} status tested every five years starting after age fifty. For individuals in whom absorption is impaired by lack of the intrinsic factor, monthly injections of vitamin B_{12} can be an effective solution.[42, 102, 129, 130]

CHLORELLA

It is possible that *Chlorella* (a cobalt-containing green algae) may be considered a source of vitamin B_{12}. Though a 1968 U.S. study failed to detect vitamin B_{12} in *Chlorella*, Finnish research raised the possibility that *Chlorella* might be a source of vitamin B_{12}, and several recent studies have detected true vitamin B_{12} in *Chlorella*. Until *Chlorella* is tested on a significant number of humans to determine whether it can lower MMA levels and reverse deficiency, and its availability to the body is confirmed, it should not be considered a reliable source of vitamin B_{12}.[108–110, 123, 127, 131, 134–136] Human trials have not been conducted with the related algae *Pleurochrysis carterae*.

APHANIZOMENON FLOS-AQUAE (AFA)

A small Italian study involving fifteen vegan participants found that Klamath brand blue-green algae (Aphanizomenon flos-aquae, or AFA), a particular type of blue-green algae, improved the vitamin B_{12} status of some but not all of the group. Participants took six capsules of AFA per day. Improved vitamin B_{12} status was measured by a significant reduction of blood homocysteine levels in some participants.[125]

FORTIFIED FOODS

Although fortified foods, such as nondairy beverages or breakfast cereals, are not raw, some people following a mostly raw diet choose to get their vitamin B_{12} from them. Research has shown that 17 percent of the vitamin B_{12} is lost from a fortified breakfast cereal after the cereal has been stored for a year.[138]

Scientifically Proven Approaches for Getting Vitamin B_{12}

Regardless of whether your diet is raw, vegan, vegetarian, or nonvegetarian, or whether you choose fortified foods or a supplement, the most dependable source of vitamin B_{12} is typically bacteria. To be safe, use a trusted source of vitamin B_{12} before deficiency symptoms appear. Here are several ways to obtain a reliable supply of this essential nutrient, either daily or once a week.

EVERY DAY

Take a supplement daily. Choose a vitamin or multivitamin mineral supplement that includes at least 10 micrograms (mcg) of vitamin B_{12} (cobalamin or cyanocobalamin). Most provide at least this amount. When you take your day's supply all at once, you absorb a little less. That is why the recommendation is 10 micrograms rather than 2.4 micrograms.

Alternatively, instead of a supplement, you can take Red Star Vegetarian Support Formula nutritional yeast. This yeast is grown on a vitamin B_{12}-enriched medium. Several reports show the yeast to be less reliable than a supplement because the amount of vitamin B_{12} in the yeast can vary from one batch to another and can be affected by storage factors, such as exposure to heat and light.[42, 102, 123, 126, 137, 138]

To meet the adult recommended intake of 2.4 micrograms vitamin B_{12} with Red Star Vegetarian Support Formula nutritional yeast, take 5 grams of this yeast. This is about 1 tablespoon (15 milliliters) of mini flakes or 1½ tablespoon (22 milliliters) of large flakes. Either choice will supply about 2.4 micrograms of vitamin B_{12}. For tasty ways to incorporate this nutritional yeast into your diet, see the recipes on pages 268, 269, 272, 275, 276, 279, 281, and 285.

ONCE A WEEK

Take 2,000 micrograms (mcg) of vitamin B_{12} sublingually (under the tongue) or in supplement form. This amount is much larger than the recommended daily intake (multiplied by seven) because most of a large dose is excreted. (Still, this "large" dose is only 0.002 grams!)

CHAPTER 9

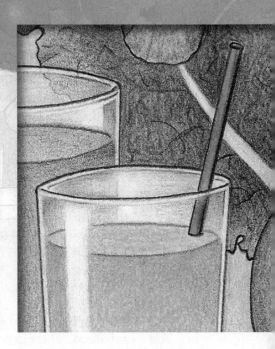

Acid-Base Balance, Bones, and Minerals

Minerals are elements that come from the earth or the sea. They enter the body through plant foods (even the minerals in animal products can be traced back to plant sources or drinking water), and once inside, they stay until they are excreted (for example, in urine, feces, or perspiration). A mineral can perform one role in the body and then another, yet it remains the same mineral. Iron is iron, though it becomes part of various compounds, like a magician wearing a series of cloaks or assuming different characters. Minerals are part of dynamic systems in our bones, fluids, and nerves. While reading this and later when you sleep, you are remodeling bones and creating new red blood cells. For these purposes, you need a steady supply of building materials.

Though they also can settle out in hard little crystals, minerals are water-soluble and some (calcium, magnesium, and sodium) are found in drinking water, depending on the geographic locale. Filtration systems remove minerals, along with unwanted chemicals. Due to the solubility of minerals, when foods are boiled, these elements are leached into the cooking water, which is generally disposed of. Steaming leads to fewer losses; of course, retention is greatest in foods that remain raw. When nuts, seeds, and other raw foods are soaked and the soaking water is discarded, a small proportion of minerals is lost, though big gains are made in terms of how well the body can absorb the minerals that remain. The availability of minerals is increased immensely by preparation practices that have been recognized for decades in raw-food communities. At long last, the wisdom behind soaking, sprouting, blending, and juicing is being recognized and given credit by scientific research.

In this chapter, you will learn how to create a mineral-rich diet (including tips about mineral absorption), discover how diet can help to maintain the precise pH balance between acid and base in body fluids that is necessary to sustain life, and see how this balance affects bone health. For the essential minerals, you will find the functions of each and a wide range of delicious raw foods that can be your sources.

Acid-Base Balance and Bones

ACID-BASE BALANCE

One task of our hard-working kidneys, in partnership with our lungs, is to maintain the acidity, or pH, of our body fluids within a very narrow range (7.35 to 7.45). A pH between 0 and 7 is acidic (with the lowest numbers being more acidic); values above 7 indicate pH levels that are increasingly alkaline. Diet has a powerful influence on this system. Meat and other flesh foods, milk and dairy products, and grains are acid-forming, meaning that they influence body fluids and the urine to be acidic after these foods are consumed, digested, and metabolized. This effect is related to the amounts of phosphorus, sulfur, and protein in these foods. In contrast, vegetables and fruits tend to be alkali-forming, or base-forming, counterbalancing the effects of animal products and grains. Though many sour tasting fruits such as citrus fruits are acidic, this acidity is quickly disposed of during digestion. The end result on the body of the breakdown of both fruits and vegetables is linked to the presence of calcium, magnesium, and potassium, and the alkaline effect of these minerals. When we look at family meals, restaurant menus, and shopping-cart contents, it is easy to see why the standard Western diet tips the scales in an acid-forming direction.[1-4]

Though Paleolithic diets included wild game, it is estimated that two-thirds or more of the calories in these diets came from leafy greens, fruits, nuts, seeds, and other parts of uncultivated plants. (Naturally, diets varied greatly from one region to another.) The wild fruits eaten by early humans (and by primates) were higher in minerals and protein and were lower in sugars than the cultivated fruits we find in supermarkets today.[5, 6] In a few situations, as with the the !Kung tribe of the African Kalahari Desert and the Hazda of Australian Tanzania, as much as 95 percent of their calories came from plant parts that they gathered. Grains and dairy products were not part of the diet. The traditional Hopi diet was centered on plant foods, such as purslane and other wild greens, corn, a mineral-rich plant-ash preparation, beans, and dried melon and peaches.[7] Along with greens, gourds, and other plant foods, nuts and seeds were an important part of the earliest crops in eastern North America.[8] Humans evolved on a diet that was much more alkali-forming than the diets eaten today. When humans switched from hunter-gatherer diets to diets containing grains plus large quantities of animal products, they greatly increased the amount of acid-forming foods that must be processed by the kidneys and other organs of the body.[5, 6, 9-14]

Table 9.1, page 177, shows an approximate prediction of the effect of various food groups on the acidity of the urine, called the potential renal acid load

TABLE 9.1 Estimated potential renal acid load (PRAL) of food groups

Food group (per 100 g)	PRAL
Meat	9.5
Eggs	8.2
Fish	7.9
Milk and dairy products	1.0 to 23.6*
Grains and grain products	3.5 to 7.0
Nuts and seeds	5.0 to 20.0
Legumes	2.6
Oil (olive, sunflower)	0
Vegetables	-2.8
Coconut	-2.9
Fruits and fruit juices	-3.1

Source: Data from references 3, 4, 13, 19, 20.

*The PRAL is particularly high for processed and low-fat cheeses.

(PRAL). These values are based on quantities of protein, potassium, magnesium, and phosphorus in 100 grams of food. The positive numbers above zero indicate foods that acidify our bodies and place a greater load on our kidneys. The negative numbers make our system more alkaline and decrease the amount of acid that our kidneys need to excrete. As you can see, a diet providing plenty of vegetables and fruits is highly important in maintaining the slightly alkaline pH that is essential to life and health.[3, 4, 13, 15]

A few fruits—cranberries, plums, prunes, rhubarb, and sour cherries— are acid-forming because they contain organic acids (oxalic or benzoic acid), which are not completely broken down to bicarbonate in the body. Though the body's required pH range of 7.35 to 7.45 is just slightly more alkaline than the neutral point of 7, this does not mean that acidic foods must be entirely avoided. The general idea is to get an assortment of foods, ending up with an overall mix that is just slightly alkaline. The body manages best when it has plenty of vegetables and fruits with a negative PRAL to offset the acid-forming foods with a positive PRAL that are used in smaller amounts, such as nuts and seeds and perhaps some legumes and grains. Buckwheat and quinoa, which are pseudo cereal grains, are less acid-forming than true grains.[3, 16]

Contemporary Western diets are off balance in that they contain an excess of acid-forming foods (over alkali-forming foods). The consequences of this excess acid load on the kidneys, and of keeping our cells in an environment that is a little too acidic, include the wasting of muscles, the formation of kidney stones, kidney damage, and the dissolution of bone. As we age, such diets lead to a mild but slowly increasing metabolic acidosis.[9, 13, 14, 16, 17]

ACID-BASE BALANCE, MUSCLE WASTING, AND AGE

Glutamine is an amino acid that is present in significant amounts in our muscle protein and that has the ability to neutralize a mildly acidic environment. The body may counteract acidosis by breaking down muscle and, in the process, liberating glutamine plus other amino acids that can be converted to glutamine. Amino acids from this muscle breakdown are then excreted, causing an overall loss of muscle protein. A shift in diet toward fruits and veggies may minimize or slow these losses by neutralizing the acid environment.[21, 22] For some people, mild acidosis, possibly due to a decline in kidney function or to dietary changes, seems to worsen with age, and this may explain some of the muscle loss (and bone loss) that can occur.[23]

AN ACIDIC ENVIRONMENT, BONES, AND KIDNEYS

In order to neutralize a mildly acidic environment, the body also draws on calcium that is stored in bone, because calcium is a strong alkali. As a result, bone mineral content decreases, bones are weakened, and more calcium may be lost from the body than is consumed. The urine contains high levels of calcium, and there is a tendency for calcium salts to settle out in the form of kidney stones.[9,18, 21, 24-27]

FACTORS THAT INFLUENCE BONE LOSS

Metabolic Acidosis

High intakes of dietary protein, especially from meat, cheese, other animal proteins, and grains, can lead to calcium losses, because the kidneys rid themselves of excess sulfur from the breakdown of these proteins and calcium is excreted in the process. Women whose overall diets had the greatest PRAL scores were shown to have more indicators of bone loss. (Processed and low-fat cheeses have PRAL scores as high as 29! In cheese production, the more alkali-forming whey is discarded, leaving cheese that is highly acid-forming.) When we simply take calcium supplements in an attempt to slow bone loss, it's like turning on the faucet in a bathtub but failing to put in the plug. In this case, the "plug" that could decrease urinary calcium loss is creating a less acidic body environment.[3, 4, 18, 19, 25, 28, 29, 88]

Sedentary Lifestyles

When our bones are not subjected to the impact of weight-bearing exercise, they start to shrivel up and we lose bone mass. This has been observed in immobilized hospital patients, in astronauts, and in couch potatoes. According to Eckhardt Schönau of the University of Cologne, "A short-term 'peak' [bone mass] in youth is easily cancelled out by a lifetime of sloth." [30]

High Salt Intakes

When the diet is high in salty foods and ingredients (whether the sodium chloride is in the form of table salt or comes from tamari or Nama Shoyu), excess sodium chloride passes out through the urine, and along with it goes calcium. This happens because sodium increases our volume of urine, taking calcium with it; at the same time, sodium decreases our kidneys' ability to reabsorb calcium as it flows out.[9, 15, 31, 32]

Insufficient Protein

While our bones can lose calcium if our dietary protein is excessively high, low protein intakes also are linked with bone loss because protein is an essential part of bone structure.[29] For people with low protein intakes (as is the case in many raw diets), an increase in dietary protein can result in increased bone density.[19]

FACTORS THAT INFLUENCE BONE-LOSS PREVENTION

Potassium-Rich Foods

The alkaline effect from a potassium-rich diet centered on vegetables and fruits tends to protect against hip fractures. Countries with the greatest ratio of plants to animal products in the diet have the lowest incidence of hip fractures. Of course, numerous other bone-building nutrients in fruits and vegetables help too.[9, 28]

Weight-Bearing Exercise

When muscle pulls on bone, the result is denser, stronger bone. Exercise helps to build bone before age twenty-five or thirty and also helps to maintain bone density later in life. The best activities for these purposes are weight-bearing exercises: weight lifting, jogging, hiking, stair climbing, step aerobics, dancing, racquet sports, and power walking (in a manner that involves an impact). A good goal is an hour each day, at least six days a week.

ADEQUATE PROTEIN INTAKE

For several decades, scientists have been perplexed by the effects that extremely low- or high-protein intakes can have on bone health. Whereas low-protein diets fail to provide the protein building blocks that are fundamental to our bone structure, studies show that very high-protein diets increase our acid load, and this mildly acidic environment leads to bone loss. Consequently, very high-protein diets are also detrimental. Research guides us to the middle path, revealing that protein intakes that meet or somewhat exceed Recommended Dietary Allowances are beneficial in building and maintaining strong bones.

Bone Nutrition

For lifelong bone health, the World Health Organization advises us to do the following:

- Consume a calcium intake close to the DRI (see table 9.2, page 185).
- Optimize vitamin D status through adequate exposure to summer sunshine and, when needed, take supplementary vitamin D.
- Be physically active.
- Avoid smoking.
- Limit alcohol intake.
- Restrict salt intake.
- Consume plenty of fruits and vegetables.[29]

Advertising has misled many people to believe that their intake of dairy products is the single most important predictor of bone health, and that without dairy foods it is almost impossible to meet calcium requirements. Also, the dairy industry's marketing campaigns often depict calcium as the sole superstar in the osteoporosis equation. Not so!

Bone formation and maintenance require every member of the bone team. We need boron, calcium, copper, magnesium, manganese, phosphorus, potassium, and zinc. Minerals are embedded in a protein matrix, so protein is a fundamental requirement. In supporting roles are the B vitamins and vitamins C, D, and K. Bone building requires the full nutritional team, not just one or two players.[29, 35] In order to provide the nutrients required for good bone health, a raw diet needs to be nutrient dense, with few added oils, sweeteners, and similar foods that have little nutritional value beyond calories.

Although the research may seem contradictory, the truth is that we require the recommended protein intakes (see chapter 5), which supply our vast array of protein needs, including the amino acids for building bone matrix. Simultaneously, we need a diet rich in vegetables and fruit that reduces the burden on the kidneys. A well-planned raw vegan diet can fit the bill with enough protein, but not too much.[23, 24, 32–34, 89] (See the menus in chapter 12.)

Mineral Absorption

INORGANIC AND ORGANIC FORMS OF MINERALS

In nutritional science, the word "organic" refers to compounds that are derived from plants or animals and therefore contain carbon. (In farming practices, the word "organic" relates to the use of fertilizers that are derived from plants or animals, rather than chemical fertilizers.) In plants and in the body, both inorganic and organic forms of minerals have specific functions and are necessary for life. Minerals occur as inorganic free ions (such as sodium in the fluids between cells); as a compound with other minerals (such as the calcium phosphate in bones); and as part of larger, carbon-containing (organic) molecules. Examples of the latter are cobalt as a part of vitamin B_{12}, iodine as a part of thyroid hormones, iron as a part of hemoglobin, sulfur as a part of the amino acids cysteine and methionine, and, in plants, magnesium as a part of chlorophyll.[36]

Whether the body more readily absorbs minerals in their organic or inorganic form varies from one mineral to another and is dependent on a variety of complex factors. Some minerals are absorbed primarily in their organic state. Others must be released from their organic carrier molecule so that the smaller, inorganic mineral can pass through the intestinal wall and into the bloodstream; in this instance, absorption depends on how easily this release occurs.

Consider the absorption of calcium from several foods and supplements where the mineral can be bound in a number of different organic or inorganic forms. Calcium must be released from these complexes if it is to be absorbed. Where calcium is bound to oxalate, preparation techniques have little effect on absorption. Where calcium is bound to phytate, the complex is more easily broken and some types of food preparation enable this release.

The exact absorption figures vary depending on the amount of calcium in the portion, meal, or supplement; other compounds that are present; a person's state of deficiency (the greater the deficiency, the more will be absorbed); and other factors. Vitamin D is required for calcium absorption.[36, 37]

This brief glimpse illustrates a few factors that can affect mineral absorption and demonstrates some of the complexity of the process. In plant-based diets, the presence of fiber, phytate, and oxalate can hinder mineral absorption. Some of these disadvantages can be counterbalanced by practices that greatly increase mineral availability, such as soaking, sprouting, and fermenting foods.[38, 39] The fat present in foods such as avocados, nuts, olives, salad dressings, and seeds may help us to absorb minerals, such as calcium, iron, manganese, and zinc. In contrast, the very low fat content of some raw diets may hinder the absorption of minerals.[40, 41]

Calcium Absorption from Different Sources

- Although spinach contains plenty of calcium (in the form of organic calcium oxalate), only about 5 percent of the calcium is absorbed, despite various food preparation practices. (For the purpose of comparison, we absorb 30–32 percent of the calcium from tofu and from cow's milk.[42–45])

- From almonds, which contain calcium phytate and oxalate, we absorb between 14 and 21 percent of the calcium. After almonds are soaked for 8–12 hours, much of the calcium is released from the phytate and we can expect better absorption.[46–48]

- From the forms in various supplements—calcium carbonate, calcium citrate, calcium lactate, or calcium phosphate—we generally find absorption to be in the range of 30 to 40 percent, with calcium citrate malate (found in supplements and fortified juices) leading the pack.[36, 37]

- From low-oxalate greens, such as bok choy, broccoli, dandelion greens, kale, mustard greens, napa cabbage, turnip greens, and watercress, we can absorb 40 percent or more of the calcium present. (These figures are based on cooked greens. Unfortunately, data on raw greens is not available.)[42, 45]

MINERALS, HEAT, AND REFINING

Cooking does not destroy minerals. In fact minerals survive very high temperatures and form the ash that remains from a fire. The Hopi Indians traditionally used ash from burnt corn cobs, bean vines, juniper bushes, and other plants in their food preparation. This ash became an important dietary ingredient and a source of calcium, copper, iron, phosphorus, and zinc in their mainly plant-based diets.[7]

Even with less-extreme cooking temperatures, minerals can become more available for absorption. Various methods of cooking beans have been shown to break down some of the phytate (see page 183), releasing minerals for absorption.[47] Yet with boiling, 30–40 percent of the minerals are lost into the cooking liquid, which is then discarded.[49] Food processing also can result in significant loss of minerals. When whole grains are milled to make white flour, the germ and bran are removed, leaving a refined flour that lacks most of its original minerals.[47]

MINERALS IN RAW FOODS

There are a number of reasons why the mineral content in raw foods can vary widely. Due to differences in soil content, kale grown in one location can have several times the calcium of kale from another field. The number listed in a table is an average, but not necessarily what you'd get from analyzing the kale from your supermarket or garden. As it matures, a red sweet pepper gains minerals. The mineral content of organic produce can be higher than that of produce grown with pesticides, though this is not always the case.[50–57]

OXALATES (OXALIC ACID)

The presence of oxalates greatly decreases our absorption of calcium, iron, and magnesium from some otherwise rich food sources of these minerals. Oxalates occur naturally in plants (especially leaves), where oxalic acid is tightly bound together with one of these minerals, forming an oxalate salt that resists being broken down during food preparation and digestion. Beet greens, chives, lamb's quarters, parsley, purslane, quinoa, sorrel, spinach, star fruit (carambola), Swiss chard, whole sesame seeds, and yams are among the most oxalate-dense plant foods. (For specific amounts in several foods, see the U.S. Department of Agriculture's list "Oxalic Acid Content of Selected Vegetables" online.[58] Much smaller amounts of oxalates are present in almonds, berries and several other fruits, black tea, cashews, chocolate, and green beans. Although oxalates will lower calcium absorption from certain calcium-rich greens, these greens still contribute calcium to the diet; for example, about 5 percent of the calcium present may be absorbed from a bowl of spinach. In addition, you will get plenty of beta-carotene, folate, vitamin K, and numerous other nutrients and protective phytochemicals that are not affected by oxalate, and generally there is no need to avoid nutritious foods that contain oxalates in a diet that is varied.

Some oxalates can be lost when foods are soaked and the soaking water is discarded, though calcium and other minerals that are bound to the oxalates are lost at the same time. Research has shown that boiling reduces the total oxalate content in spinach by 60 percent and in lentils by 16 percent. Total calcium absorption is low from both raw and boiled spinach compared to kale or other very low-oxalate foods.[43, 47, 59-63]

Oxalates are found in body fluids; however, when they become too concentrated, for example in the kidneys, the result can be the most common type of kidney stone. People with certain types of kidney or gallbladder problems or rheumatoid arthritis may be advised to limit their intakes of high-oxalate foods. An important aspect of kidney stone prevention is to avoid dehydration; drink plenty of water to maintain dilute urine (so crystals do not settle out).

PHYTATES (PHYTIC ACID)

In plant foods, most of the phosphorus is packaged in compounds known as phytates, which have some similarities to oxalates. They bind minerals, such as calcium, iron, magnesium, and zinc, and the phytate-mineral complex is not broken down during digestion. Yet a significant difference exists because common practices that are used to prepare raw foods—soaking, sprouting, fermenting, juicing, or blending—can break down the phytate-mineral complex. Then, when the food reaches the intestine, the minerals are easily extracted and absorbed.

For example, when raw seeds, nuts, mung beans, or lentils are soaked or sprouted, the phytases (phytate-splitting enzymes) that are naturally present in the dry food become active; also, some phytases are formed. Mung beans that were soaked for twelve hours and then sprouted for forty-eight hours lost 37 percent or more of their phytates. Swedish scientists discovered that soaking or sprouting lentils at 115 F (45 C) for ten hours led to a significant reduction in phytate. (Raw lentils are already low in phytate, having only about 25 percent as much phytate as soybeans or kidney beans.) Phytate breakdown also occurs during the fermentation of plant foods through the added action of phytases in bacteria or yeasts. When plant foods are juiced or blended, cells are broken, releasing phytase. All of these processes allow the release of bound calcium, iron, magnesium, and zinc from these phytate-mineral complexes so that our bodies can absorb the minerals. Don't get the impression that phytates are all bad; research shows that these phosphorus-rich compounds can help to lower cholesterol and may provide us with some protection from cancer.[38, 39, 47, 61, 63, 64, 66, 67] According to Gloria Urbano of the University of Granada, the reputation of phytate "has had a roller-coaster ride since its discovery; it has undergone alternate eminence and infamy."[67]

Mineral Intakes on Raw Diets, Their Functions, and Food Sources

 able 9.2, page 185, shows the adult Dietary Reference Intakes (DRIs) for minerals established by the Food and Nutrition Board, Institute of Medicine.[68-70] These are based on a wide range of indi-

viduals consuming a variety of diets. No alternative guidelines for optimal intakes on raw diets have been developed. This table also indicates intakes by people on raw and mainly raw diets from studies in Germany, the United States, and Finland.

CALCIUM

Raw Research

Adult DRIs for calcium are shown in table 9.2, page 185, along with intakes from raw-food studies. The DRI increases from 1,000 to 1,200 milligrams of calcium for people age fifty and older. Among participants on the high-raw Hallelujah Acres Diet, the average calcium intakes were only about two-thirds of the recommended levels. Those with the lowest caloric intakes were particularly low in many bone-building nutrients.[72]

> If people eat a very small amount of food, causing them to be very lean and underweight, they are likely to have trouble with their bones. This is true of people following any diet.
>
> **MICHAEL DONALDSON**, director of research for the Hallelujah Acres diet study

A typical advantage of raw diets is that sodium intakes tend to be low and potassium intakes high, and these factors give some protection against drains on calcium reserves. The plant-derived calcium intake of our big-boned Paleolithic ancestors has been estimated at about 1,500 milligrams of calcium per day in a 3,000-calorie diet. (They were more active, consumed more food than modern humans, and ate wild greens and other calcium-rich plant foods that are not found in supermarkets.[81])

Findings from a small study in St. Louis, Missouri, give a mixed message.[79] The bad news is that bone mass, measured at critical areas in eighteen people who had followed a raw vegan diet for an average of 3.6 years, proved to be significantly lower than that of a control group of people following standard Western diets. Calcium intakes on the raw diets were 50–60 percent of the DRIs. The good news from lab tests is that these raw foodists were not losing bone mass faster than the control group, they did not have indicators of osteoporosis, and they were getting adequate vitamin D though sun exposure to aid in calcium absorption.

Functions of Calcium

Calcium is best known for its structural role in making bones and teeth hard (see Bone Nutrition, page 180). About 1 percent of the calcium in the body has important nonstructural functions: blood clotting (preventing blood loss after an injury), muscle relaxation (without calcium, muscles remain tight after contracting), nerve cell message transmission, and the regulation of cell metabolism (such as the storage of energy as glycogen). Intakes at recommended levels also may help to prevent hypertension.[68, 82]

TABLE 9.2 DRIs for minerals and mineral intakes on raw and mainly raw diets

	Calcium mg	Copper mcg	Iodine mcg	Iron* mg	Magnesium mg	Manganese mg	Phosphorus mg	Potassium mg	Selenium mcg	Sodium mg	Zinc mg
DRIs for a woman	1,000 to 1,200	900	150	8 or 18	310 to 320	1.8	700	4,700	55	1,200 to 1,500	8
DRIs for a man	1,000 to 1,200	900	150	8	400 to 420	2.3	700	4,700	55	1,200 to 1,500	11

PARTICIPANT DESCRIPTIONS AND COUNTRY

	Calcium mg	Copper mcg	Iodine mcg	Iron* mg	Magnesium mg	Manganese mg	Phosphorus mg	Potassium mg	Selenium mcg	Sodium mg	Zinc mg
Giessen study, Germany, 2001, 43 adults [71]	714	...	...	18	618	...	...	...	...	...	8.1
Hallelujah Acres diet, USA, 2001, 87 women [72]	577	1,970	...	14	392	4.95	857	5,420	67	1,220	6.7
Hallelujah Acres diet, USA, 2001, 54 men [72]	687	2,380	...	17	483	6.3	1,100	6,400	54.3	1,510	8.3
Living-food diet, Finland, 1994, 1995, 1996, 19–20 women and 1 man (or subgroup)[73–75]	562	1,800	27 to >900 mcg	18	618	...	...	...	27	...	11
Living-food diet, Finland, 13 adults (mostly women) with rheumatoid arthritis [76]	796	...	...	25.5	...	...	...	5,100	...	1,200	17.9
Living-food diet, Finland, 1992, 7 women and 2 men[77, 78]	520	...	...	23.5	760	...	...	5,040	...	1,220	16.2
Raw vegan diet, USA, 2005, 2007, 7 women and 11 men [79, 80]	579	...	...	...	...	...	...	5,500	...	1,400	...

Source: Data on DRIs from references 68–70

*For postmenopausal women, the DRI for iron is 8 mg; for premenopausal women, the DRI for iron is 18 mg due to menstrual losses. Although the iron DRI for vegetarians was set at 1.8 times the DRI for nonvegetarians (listed above), the higher value is based on research that may be inappropriate for raw vegan diets because the experimental diet that was the basis for this recommendation was centered on very different foods and was far lower in fresh fruits, vegetables, and vitamin C than raw diets.

Dietary Sources of Calcium and Supplements

Calcium is abundant in plant foods, such as almonds, fresh and dried fruits, seeds, and a wide assortment of vegetables, particularly low-oxalate greens (bok choy, broccoli, dandelion greens, kale, mustard greens, napa cabbage, turnip greens, and watercress). A lesson can be learned from big-boned animals, such as cows and elephants, who graze on greens in a leisurely manner every day, consuming large amounts. The low-oxalate greens bok choy, broccoli, and kale contain calcium that is extremely well absorbed by our bodies in the range of 40–61 percent (compared to absorption rates of 30–32 percent from cow's milk and tofu). From high-oxalate greens (such as beet greens, spinach, and Swiss chard) and rhubarb, we absorb only 5–8 percent of the calcium present.[45]

> One farmer says to me, "You cannot live on vegetable food solely, for it furnishes nothing to make bones with," and so he religiously devotes a part of his day to supplying his system with the raw material of bones; walking all the while he talks behind his oxen, which, with vegetable-made bones, jerk him and his lumbering plough along in spite of every obstacle.
>
> **HENRY DAVID THOREAU,**
> Walden, 1852

While we can get 1,000 milligrams of calcium from eleven cups of kale (and absorb it even better than calcium from cow's milk), that is a lot of kale to consume! Another way we might choose to get our day's supply of calcium is from three oranges, a very large salad (three cups each of kale, napa cabbage, and romaine lettuce), three tablespoons of sesame tahini (in salad dressing), one-half cup of almonds, plus five figs. Typically, a wide assortment of raw plant foods contributes to our overall mineral intake, and we can meet our needs in a vast number of tasty ways. (See the menus in chapter 12, pages 244–249.) For calcium sources in raw diets, see table 9.4, page 198.

Calcium supplements can be a wise choice to top up your intake, if you have difficulty consuming enough calcium from foods. No multivitamin-mineral tablet contains 100 percent of the DRI (or DV, for daily value) for calcium; the resulting pill would be too large to swallow. Calcium preparations used as supplements include calcium carbonate, calcium citrate, calcium citrate malate, calcium gluconate, and calcium lactate. To maximize absorption, use a supplement that includes vitamin D. Most calcium supplements should be taken with meals, although calcium citrate and calcium citrate malate can be taken anytime.[37, 83]

CHROMIUM

Raw Research and Functions

Chromium supports the action of the hormone insulin. Without sufficient chromium, syndrome X (also known as metabolic syndrome) can develop, a condition that combines symptoms of insulin resistance, obesity, high blood pressure, high LDL ("bad" cholesterol), high triglycerides, and low HDL ("good" cholesterol). When carbohydrates are refined in the production of white flour and sugar, one of the minerals that is lost is chromium; consequently, it is reasonable to place at least part of the blame for syndrome X on diets that are high in refined carbohydrates. High intakes of glucose and fructose (found in agave syrup and honey) as well as sucrose can deplete chromium.[69, 84] The DRI for chromium for men is 35 micrograms to age 50 years, and 30 micrograms after that; for women it is 25 micrograms to age 50 years, and 20 micrograms after that. Requirements of athletes may be slightly higher than those of nonathletes.[69]

Dietary Sources of Chromium

Chromium is present in nuts, seeds, fruits, vegetables, and sea vegetables. Data showing specific quantities of chromium in foods is very limited and unreliable, and amounts reported for particular foods can vary widely. One reason for the lack of accurate data is that chromium contamination can occur when samples are tested. Also, the amounts in soil vary greatly from one geographical region to another. Nonetheless, a raw diet that meets caloric requirements and is centered on whole plant foods can be expected to provide reasonable amounts of chromium.[69]

COPPER

Raw Research and Functions

Copper intakes of raw foodists, vegans, and other vegetarians tend to meet the DRIs shown in table 9.2, page 185, and are usually higher than those of non-vegetarians. Copper is an integral part of the enzymes that are involved in the utilization of iron, in protecting us from free radicals, and in protein metabolism. It is also used for building connective tissue, bones, and hormones.

Dietary Sources of Copper

We need not worry about copper, as we can meet the DRIs with a daily handful of nuts and seeds. Copper is abundant in Brazil nuts, pecans, other nuts, seeds, sweet potatoes, and fruits, such as bananas, raisins, and prunes (see table 9.4, page 198). High intakes of zinc (for example, when someone consumes zinc as a single mineral supplement in excess of the DRI) can prevent the absorption of copper, resulting in copper deficiency. This problem does not occur with use of a multivitamin-mineral supplement.[36, 69, 85]

IODINE

Raw Research

Iodine is of particular interest to those on raw diets. The recommended intake for adults is 150 micrograms (mcg) of iodine per day, a miniscule amount. However, raw and vegan diets can miss the mark and hit two extremes, with some falling short and others with iodine intakes that are excessive. Finns who had followed living-food diets for three to ten and a half years had iodine intakes (shown in table 9.2) that clustered in two groups: one group had low average intakes of 29 micrograms per day, and the other group, whose sea vegetable intake was high, consumed 900 micrograms per day (which is below the acceptable upper limit, or UL, of 1,100 micrograms). One person also used iodized salt. Diets included moderate amounts of the substances from the cabbage family that can interfere with thyroid function (see page 190); about 1/4 cup (30 grams) per day of sauerkraut was consumed. For Finns at both levels of iodine intake, their laboratory tests showed normal thyroid function.[73–75, 86] Americans on the Hallelujah Acres diet included small amounts of kelp as an iodine source.[72]

Functions of Iodine

Iodine is a part of the thyroid hormones, and most of the organ systems in the body are under the influence of these hormones. Iodine is essential for energy metabolism, and deficiency can result in either depressed or accelerated metabolic function (also known as hypo- or hyperthyroidism, respectively). Insufficient iodine has been linked with fibrocystic breast disease. Iodine exerts its effect through the thyroid gland, which is located in the lower part of the throat. Hypothyroidism can result in a growth called a goiter, in which the thyroid gland becomes greatly enlarged in its efforts to trap iodine; other symptoms are skin problems, weight gain, and increased cholesterol levels, all of which can be reversed in adults with sufficient iodine in the diet.[86, 87]

Iodine intakes of some people on raw diets may be insufficient unless they use either iodized salt, supplements, or sea vegetables. Iodine deficiency is particularly risky during pregnancy, during which the DRI is increased to 220 micrograms.

Iodine deficiency during pregnancy is a different story, as this mineral is essential for normal brain development of the fetus. Its lack causes the most important and most easily preventable cause of mental retardation in children around the world—an irreversible and tragic condition known as cretinism. Thyroid hormones are crucial during pregnancy, while an infant's brain is developing. Adults can survive severe iodine deficiency, but they cannot thrive or reproduce.[85, 90–92]

Iodine in Salt

Prior to the iodization of salt in 1924, goiter and cretinism appeared in many North American regions, such as the Great Lakes area and the Northwest. These conditions still occur in parts of Africa, Asia, Europe, and Latin America, where iodized salt is not used and where people eat locally grown foods with low iodine levels. In order to prevent goiter and cretinism, table salt has been fortified in many countries, so that about 3/8 to 1/2 teaspoon (2 milliliters) of iodized table salt or iodized sea salt delivers the adult DRI of 150 micrograms (see table 9.3, page 189). This action has proved to be powerfully effective. Suppliers of popular noniodized salts advertise the presence of minerals in their products in general terms, yet the amounts of iodine in micrograms are not disclosed or fall far short of DRIs due to losses during the drying process.[86, 93]

TABLE 9.3 Iodine in salt and dried sea vegetables

Iodine source	Amount supplying DRI (150 mcg)	Avoid frequent use of this amount supplying UL (1,100 mcg)
Iodized sea salt or table salt	³/₈ to ½ tsp/2 ml	4 tsp/20 ml
Noniodized sea salt or table salt	Not a reliable source of iodine	...
Commercial preparation of sea salt with sea vegetables	⅛ tsp/0.5 ml	¾ tsp/4 ml
Arame	½ tsp/2 ml	1.2 Tbsp/18 ml
Dulse granules	½ tsp/2 ml	3⅓ tsp/16 ml
Hijiki	¾ tsp/4 ml	1.8 Tbsp/27 ml
Kelp	less than ¹/₁₆ tsp/0.3 ml	0.4 tsp/2 ml
Kombu	one ¹/₁₆-inch-long (1.6-mm-long) piece	one ⅓-inch-long (1-cm-long) piece
Nori	1½ sheets/4g	10½ sheets/26 g
Wakame	1⅛ tsp/6 ml	2¾ Tbsp/41 ml

Source: Data from references 93, 100, 101.

Note: Amounts can vary greatly depending upon where the sea vegetables were gathered and how they were dried and stored. To confirm amounts in salts and sea vegetables, check labels and contact manufacturers.

Dietary Source of Iodine

Nutrient tables lack data on the iodine content of various foods due to the immense variability among crops (or vegetables) from different regions. Amounts in soil vary from one location to another depending on the extent to which flooding, glaciation, or rainfall has leached iodine from the soil, eventually depositing this mineral into the oceans. Some plant foods from the ocean are excellent sources of iodine and other nutrients; in fact, in Japan, where National Seaweed Day (February 6) is celebrated, recommendations for public health advise an increased consumption of sea vegetables.[94] The challenge lies in knowing how much iodine you are getting. Raw and dried sea vegetables (including powders and kelp tablets) are generally high in iodine, though amounts of digestible iodine vary as much as eightfold from one batch to another. Much of this mineral is lost to the air during the drying process. Iodine in dried kelp can vary between 0.1 percent and 0.8 percent of the dry weight. Quantities are higher in sea vegetables that grow near coral reefs. It can be difficult to find a supplier with accurate information about iodine content. Kelp tablets may deliver the stated amounts of iodine, though amounts may be underestimated. Some people use a guideline of ¹/₄ teaspoon (1 milliliter) of kelp every four days to meet their iodine DRI. (See table 9.3, page 189.) It is preferable to consume one's recommended intake of iodine in small but frequent amounts daily or once or twice a week than to consume a large dose less frequently.[85, 86, 90–92, 94, 95] Commercially available hijiki seaweed has been found to contain significant amounts of the toxic and carcinogenic element arsenic, and consumers have been advised to avoid it.[96] (Also see page 233 in chapter 11.)

Substances that Can Interfere with Thyroid Function

Certain very nutritious foods from the cabbage family contain substances known as thiocyanates that interfere with thyroid metabolism *if* iodine is in short supply in your diet. Thiocyanates are naturally present in broccoli, brussels sprouts, cabbages, cauliflower, collard greens, kale, kohlrabi, and flaxseeds; these nutritious foods normally cause no problems if adequate iodine is available from other sources. Fermentation, a food-preservation technique used, for example, in making sauerkraut, eliminates thiocyanates. The water pollutants perchlorate (a by-product of solid fuels) and nitrogen (from fertilizers) also can amplify thyroid problems in people who are iodine deficient or whose intakes are low. For these reasons, you are well advised to get iodine in recommended amounts.[75, 86]

Thyroid and Iodine Tests

Lab tests that assess thyroid status and function typically have "T" in their name, such as "T4" and "TSH." Do-it-yourself skins tests using iodine solutions have not proved to be a valid way to assess iodine deficiency; the rate at which the iodine stain fades from your skin is related to other factors, such as atmospheric pressure and temperature.

Excess Iodine

For iodine, as for many nutrients, an upper level (UL) of intake that is "likely to pose no risk of adverse effects" has been set. For adults this is 1,100 micrograms of iodine. High intakes of sea vegetables or other iodine sources can damage the thyroid gland and cause hyper- or hypothyroidism or thyroid cancer. In the north islands of Japan, where people consume a great deal of sea vegetables, excess iodine intake has resulted in a type of goiter. Scientists estimate that regular and high intakes of kelp—*Laminaria* species, which is adept at picking up iodine and heavy metals from the area where it grows—could cause thyroid problems. Furthermore, a kelp intake of 41 milligrams per day from herbal supplements has been known to deliver toxic levels of arsenic, despite a supplement label stating that it contributes to "vital living and well-being."[69, 85, 86, 93–95, 97–99, 115]

The right dose differentiates a poison and a remedy.

PARACELSUS, the father of toxicology (1493–1541)

IRON

Raw Research

In the Giessen study, iron intakes met the DRIs on average (see table 9.2, page 185), although many individual diets were short of iron. Lab tests showed that the participants' serum iron and ferritin levels were low, and for those who had been on raw diets the longest, 43 percent of the men and 15 percent of the women were anemic. Among all women of childbearing age, 70 percent had menstrual irregularities and 23 percent had stopped menstruating.[40, 71, 102] On the high-raw Hallelujah Acres diet, women over fifty and men of all ages typically met the DRI for iron, while women of childbearing age, whose DRI is usually higher due to menstrual losses of iron, fell short.[72, 103] Finns on a living-food diet had significantly higher intakes of iron (18–25 milligrams). They maintained their hemoglobin levels on diets that included nuts and seeds; sprouted buckwheat, lentils, mung beans, rye, and wheat; fermented cucumber, oats, and red cabbage; fresh and dried fruit; plenty of vegetables; and small amounts of sea vegetables.[74, 76, 78] The various diets previously mentioned provided two to six times the DRIs for vitamin C. This feature, along with many food preparation practices that reduced phytate, gave excellent support for iron absorption when a reasonable amount of iron was present in the foods.

Although the iron DRI for vegetarians has been set at 1.8 times the DRI for nonvegetarians, this is based on research that may be inappropriate for raw diets because the experimental diet that was the basis for this recommendation contains many foods not used in raw diets and was far lower in fresh fruits, vegetables, and vitamin C.[69, 104]

Functions of Iron

Iron, the mineral at the heart of the hemoglobin molecule in blood, plays a central role in transporting oxygen throughout the body, releasing this life-giving substance where it is needed, and carrying away the metabolic waste product carbon dioxide. As part of many enzyme systems, iron also plays key roles in the production of cellular energy, in immune system functioning, and in certain mental processes. Our body does its best to recycle this precious mineral; our intake must replenish losses through perspiration, urine, and cells that are sloughed off from skin and from the intestinal lining. Women of childbearing age lose iron during menstruation, increasing their requirements over those of men. Iron deficiency is the most common nutritional deficiency in North America, occurring most commonly in women and children.[69, 85]

Vegetarians are not more likely than nonvegetarians to have iron-deficiency anemia. Vegetarians often have relatively low amounts of stored iron (as shown by low serum ferritin levels in lab tests), yet this is not accompanied by fatigue or other symptoms. In fact, this could even be an advantage, linked to improved insulin resistance and decreased risk of heart disease, since there is less free iron to act as a pro-oxidant. If one's iron supply is replenished by good dietary choices, low iron stores do not seem to be a problem. To some extent, the body can adjust its absorption efficiency, depending on our need for iron.[85, 105, 106]

When an actual iron deficiency exists, lab tests will show decreases in serum iron and the degree that transferrin (the iron-transport protein) is saturated with iron. Symptoms commonly include fatigue and increased sensitivity to cold. With further depletion, iron-deficiency anemia develops, a condition in which blood hemoglobin falls below the normal range. Since the body's oxygen-delivery system is diminished, people with this condition are likely to feel exhausted, irritable, and lethargic, and may also experience headaches. Due to the dilution of the red hemoglobin molecule in the tiny blood vessels just below the surface of the skin, the skin may appear pale.

Dietary Sources of Iron

To boost iron intakes, raw foodists have access to a wealth of food sources (see table 9.4, page 198). Furthermore, by consuming items that provide at least 25 milligrams of vitamin C (see table 8.2, page 154) at the same meal or snack that we have our iron sources, we can double the amount of iron we absorb. With 50 milligrams or more of vitamin C, we can increase iron absorption by a factor of three to six. The practices of soaking, sprouting, and fermenting foods increase the ease with which the body absorbs the iron present by breaking down phytate. Sprouting generates the production of vitamin C, further increasing iron absorption. Note that when seeds and nuts are soaked, some minerals are leached into the soaking water and then discarded.[38, 85, 95, 105]

MAGNESIUM

Raw Research

Magnesium is at the center of the chlorophyll molecule, so it is not surprising that average intakes on German, American, and Finnish raw diets have been well above the DRIs. In contrast, average dietary intakes of North American women on nonvegetarian diets fall below the DRIs. The DRI for magnesium increases from 400 to 420 milligrams for men age thirty-one and older and from 310 to 320 milligrams for women age thirty-one and older.[68]

Functions of Magnesium

The functions of this mineral are more diverse than those of any other. Magnesium is a structural component for strong teeth and bones. It helps convert the calories from food into useable energy. It is necessary for the transmission of nerve impulses, and it helps to maintain the rhythm of the heart. A magnesium-rich diet (which is typically a diet that is rich in vegetables and fruits) is associated with lower blood pressure and reduced risk of type 2 diabetes, heart disease, and stroke.[46, 107]

Dietary Sources of Magnesium

Greens, colored by chlorophyll, are good sources of magnesium (see table 9.4, page 198). So are other vegetables, nuts, seeds, fruits, legumes, and cacao (and chocolate). Wheatgrass juice, being rich in chlorophyll, is very high in magnesium. Intakes on raw diets tend to be good unless caloric intakes are restricted.[72, 85]

MANGANESE

Raw Research

Intakes of manganese by Americans on the Hallelujah Acres diet were found to be about triple the DRI.[72]

Functions of Manganese

Manganese is required for proper bone formation and wound healing and is part of an important antioxidant in cells. It activates enzymes that produce energy from protein, fat, and carbohydrate.

Dietary Sources of Manganese

Manganese is present in a wide variety of raw foods and deficiency is unlikely.[85]

PHOSPHORUS

Raw Research

Average intakes on the high-raw Hallelujah Acres diet exceeded the DRI by about about 57 percent for men and about 22 percent for women.[72]

Functions of Phosphorus

Phosphorus is the second most abundant mineral in the body after calcium. In its inorganic form, 85 percent of the body's phosphorus, along with calcium, gives strength and rigidity to bones and teeth, whereas protein gives bone some flexibility. Phosphorus is present in blood and in the fluid between cells, where it helps to maintain the body's pH. Our ability to store and release energy requires phosphorus in the compound adenosine triphosphate (ATP). Phosphorus is a component of the genetic material in every cell of humans, animals, and plants. In soft tissues, it is combined with fat in organic complexes called phospholipids.[68, 107]

Dietary Sources of Phosphorus

Phosphorus is widely distributed among plant foods, as shown in table 9.4, page 198. Most of the phosphorus in plant foods is stored in compounds called phytates, where phosphorus-containing phytic acid is bound together with calcium, magnesium, iron, and zinc. Phytates are not easily broken down in the human digestive tract. However, the practices of soaking and fermenting nuts, seeds, legumes, and grains change phytates so that the phosphorus (as inorganic phosphate) and other minerals become more available for absorption. Although phytic acid (or phytate) used to be blacklisted as an antinutrient that blocks mineral absorption, it is now also receiving favorable press as an antioxidant that can help protect us against cancer.[67, 72, 85]

POTASSIUM

Raw Research

When it comes to potassium intakes, raw diets excel, whereas the standard Western diet fails. Potassium intakes on the Hallelujah Acres diet and Finnish living-food diet exceeded the DRIs (see table 9.2, page 185).[72, 76, 77]

Functions of Potassium

Potassium has a role in attracting and holding water inside cells that parallels the role of sodium outside cells. It acts with sodium to create an electrochemical charge across cell membranes that supports the transmission of nerve impulses and the contraction of muscles, including the heart. Potassium acts to blunt a rise in blood pressure when we consume too much sodium. It tips our acid-base balance in an alkaline direction and decreases the recurrence of kidney stones. People whose diets are high in potassium, and who take their habit of eating plenty of fruits and veggies into old age, reduce their risk of bone fractures.[17, 85]

Dietary Sources of Potassium

Potassium is abundant in a wide assortment of fruits and vegetables, so getting enough of this mineral on a raw diet is easily accomplished. Though bananas have somehow become famous as a potassium-rich food, cantaloupes, brussels sprouts, grapefruits, green beans, strawberries, and tomatoes have more potassium per calorie than bananas.

SELENIUM

Raw Research

In the Hallelujah Acres study, diets of 42 percent of the participants met the selenium DRI, while 58 percent of the participants' intakes were below the DRIs.[72] Selenium intakes of the Finns were lower still (see table 9.2, page 185). However, lab tests showed the Finns to have higher levels of antioxidant enzymes that depend on selenium, which the scientists took as an indicator of good absorption of this mineral from the sprouted and fermented foods in the living-food diet.[74]

Functions of Selenium and Absorption

In the body, selenium becomes a part of various enzymes that protect us from "oxidative stress." As part of the antioxidant team (with vitamins C and E), selenium prevents oxidative damage to heart cells, red blood cells, and other cells by transforming free radicals into harmless molecules. Selenium-containing enzymes convert a thyroid hormone to its active form, and thyroid problems can be linked to low selenium intakes. Selenium is best absorbed and utilized in the organic form that is present in foods and where it is linked with the amino acid methionine.[108-110]

Dietary Sources of Selenium

As with iodine, soil levels of selenium vary greatly from one part of the world to another. Soil levels of selenium in Europe and central Asia are low, whereas soil levels and dietary intakes in North America tend to be higher. Some favorite raw-food sources of this mineral are asparagus, cherimoya, most seeds, and the selenium superstar, the Brazil nut (which is botanically a seed, not a nut, and generally comes from Bolivia, not Brazil). Half of a large Brazil nut provides a day's selenium supply! Nutritional yeast and shiitake mushrooms also provide selenium. Cooking does not change selenium from its organic to its inorganic form.[108-110]

SODIUM

Raw Research

Humans evolved on diets that were much lower in sodium than they are today.[9, 111] Over history, salt was not always easy to come by and was highly valued, hence the biblical saying "the salt of the earth." Roman soldiers received salt as part of their pay, and the word "salary" originated from this practice. Now, 10 percent of the sodium consumed by North Americans is from what occurs naturally in foods, 75 percent comes from processed foods, and 15 percent is from salt sprinkled on foods at the table. Average sodium intakes from natural and processed foods exceed the recommended upper limit (UL) and are in the range of 2,320–4,720 milligrams per day—and that's without any added table salt.

Most young adults should keep their daily sodium intake between 1,500 and 2,300 milligrams; however, people over the age of forty, those with hypertension, and all African Americans should limit their sodium intake to 1,500 milligrams. For those age fifty to seventy, the lower limit of the range is 1,300 milligrams per day, and for seventy years of age and older, it is 1,200 milligrams per day. In the raw diets of the people studied, many of whom were over fifty years of age, average intakes of sodium cluster around the lower end of the recommended ranges (see table 9.2, page 185) due to an avoidance of processed foods. The favorable balance between relatively low sodium intakes and high potassium intakes is a positive feature of raw diets.[70, 85]

Functions of Sodium

Due to its ability to attract water, sodium plays an important role in maintaining the proper amount of fluid between the cells of our body. It's a central part of our body's internal communication system, because sodium is essential for the electrical current that allows the transmission of nerve impulses. This mineral is also a part of the digestive secretions from the pancreas.

A sodium deficiency can occur when considerable salt is lost through perspiration over the course of many hours of physical labor or during endurance athletic events, particularly in hot environments. Excess sodium intakes (above 2,400–3,000 milligrams per day) are problematic for older people with established hypertension and for salt-sensitive individuals.

Dietary Sources of Sodium

Sun-dried tomatoes and sea vegetables tend to be rich sources of sodium in raw diets. The raw condiment Nama Shoyu provides 240–282 milligrams of sodium per teaspoon (5 milliliters). Condiments that are not raw but are used in similar ways include tamari (with 233–320 milligrams of sodium per teaspoon) and Bragg Liquid Aminos (with 217 milligrams of sodium per teaspoon). Check the product labels for exact amounts in various brands.

Many people on raw diets find unrefined, unheated sea salts to be preferable to regular table salt that has been refined, heated, and then enriched with iodine. Unrefined salts contain trace minerals in amounts that are miniscule compared with the DRIs, plus they deliver miniscule amounts of heavy metals, such as lead. Unfortunately, unrefined salt lacks iodine, as this is lost in the drying process. Some unrefined salts are mixed with kelp, making them a source of iodine.

ZINC

Raw Research

Studies have shown that adults on raw vegan diets consume less than the recommended amounts of zinc, especially when their calorie intakes are low. In the Giessen study in Germany, average intakes met the DRI for women but not the higher DRI for men (see table 9.2, page 185).[40, 71] In the Hallelujah Acres diet, average zinc intakes fell below the DRIs for 62 percent of the group. In the subgroup, whose low caloric intakes were 60 percent or less of recommended levels, almost no one met the goal for zinc intake.[72, 103] A Finnish study showed average zinc intakes of those on living-food diets to be 92 percent of the DRIs. Lab tests showed the Finns to have higher levels of antioxidant enzymes that depend on zinc, which the scientists took as an indicator of good zinc absorption from the sprouted and fermented foods in the diet.[74]

Functions of Zinc

Zinc takes part in numerous highly important reactions throughout the body. It is essential to cell division and the generation of new cells. Zinc is necessary for the elimination of carbon dioxide, other aspects of respiration, maintaining the acid-base balance in the body, wound healing, immune system functions, and our ability to taste. It helps build protein, blood, and DNA and is crucial at times of growth and reproduction. Symptoms of zinc deficiency include poor appetite, a reduced ability to taste, and a weakened immune system. Certain tissues and fluids in the body contain relatively high concentrations of zinc; these include the iris and retina of the eye, and also the prostate, sperm, and seminal fluid.[69] In fact, men lose about 0.6 milligrams of zinc with each seminal emission—about 5 percent of the recommended intake for the day.[112] (This can be replenished with a handful of almonds, cashews, pine nuts, pistachios, pumpkin seeds, or sunflower seeds.)

Dietary Sources of Zinc

Zinc is concentrated in plant parts that are closely involved with the generation of new plant life—legumes, nuts, seeds, and whole grains. It also is present in berries that have seeds in them, durians, and nutritional yeast. Because nuts and seeds are good sources of zinc, keep a bowl of them handy to snack on, or carry a supply of trail mix. Sprouting lentils and mung beans and soaking nuts, seeds, and whole grains greatly increases our ability to absorb zinc from these foods. These processes break down phytate, allowing our bodies access to the zinc we need for abundant good health.[65, 85, 95, 113]

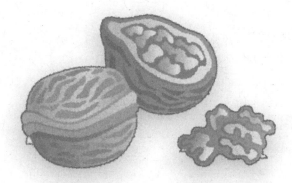

TABLE 9.4 Minerals in raw foods

Food	Calcium mg	Copper mcg	Iron mg	Magnesium mg	Manganese mg	Phosphorus mg	Potassium mg	Selenium mcg	Sodium mg	Zinc mg
DRIs for a woman	1,000	900	8 or 18*	320	1.8	700	4,700	55	1,200 to 1,500	8
DRIs for a man	1,000	900	8	400	2.3	700	4,700	55	1,200 to 1,500	11
FRUITS										
Apple, chopped (1 c/125 g)	8	34	0.2	6	0	14	134	0	1	0
Apple, medium, each	8	37	0.2	7	0	15	148	0	1	0
Apricots, sliced (1 c/165 g)	21	129	0.6	16	0.1	38	427	0	2	0
Apricot, medium, each	5	27	0.1	4	0	8	91	0	0	0
Apricots, dried (1 c/160 g)	79	...	6.2	...	...	...	2,080	...	5	...
Banana, sliced (1 c/150 g)	8	117	0.4	40	0.4	33	537	2	2	0
Banana, medium, each	6	90	0.3	32	0.3	26	422	1	1	0.2
Banana, dried (1 c/100 g)	22	391	1.2	108	0.6	74	1,491	4	0	0.6
Blackberries (1 c/144 g)	42	238	0.9	29	0.9	32	233	1	3	0.8
Blueberries (1 c/145 g)	9	83	0.4	9	0.5	17	112	0	1	0.2
Cantaloupe, diced (1 c/156 g)	14	64	0.3	19	0	23	417	1	25	0.3
Cherimoya, diced (1 c/225 g)	52	...	1.1	...	...	90	...	...	7	...
Coconut, dried (1 c/116 g)	30	924	3.8	104	3.2	239	630	21	43	2.3
Coconut milk (1 c/240 g)	38	638	3.9	89	2.2	240	631	15	36	1.6
Crab apple, sliced (1 c/110 g)	20	74	0.4	8	0.1	16	213	...	1	...
Currants, red/white (1 c/112 g)	37	120	1.1	15	0.2	49	308	1	1	0.3
Currants, black (1 c/112 g)	62	96	1.7	27	0.3	66	361	0	2	0.3
Currants, Zante, dried (1 c/144 g)	124	674	4.7	59	0.7	180	1,284	1	12	1
Dates, chopped (1 c/178 g)	69	367	1.8	77	0.5	110	1,168	5	4	0.5
Durian, chopped (1 c/243 g)	15	503	1.0	73	0.8	95	1,059	...	5	0.7
Fig, medium, fresh, each	18	35	0.2	8	0	7	116	0	0.5	0.1
Figs, dried (1c/199 g)	322	571	4.0	135	1	133	1,353	1	20	1.1
Gooseberries (1 c/150 g)	38	105	0.5	15	0.2	40	297	1	2	0.2
Grapefruit sections (1 c/230 g)	28	108	0.2	18	0	18	320	3	0	0.2
Grapefruit, pink, medium, each	54	79	0.2	22	0	44	332	0	0	0.2

Food	Calcium mg	Copper mcg	Iron mg	Magnesium mg	Manganese mg	Phosphorus mg	Potassium mg	Selenium mcg	Sodium mg	Zinc mg
DRIs for a woman	1,000	900	8 or 18*	320	1.8	700	4,700	55	1,200 to 1,500	8
DRIs for a man	1,000	900	8	400	2.3	700	4,700	55	1,200 to 1,500	11
Grapefruit juice (1 c/247 g)	22	80	0.5	30	0	37	400	0	2	0.1
Grapes (1 c/160 g)	16	0	.6	11	0.1	32	306	0	3	0.1
Guava, diced (1 c/165 g)	33	170	0.5	16	0.2	41	469	1	5	0.4
Honeydew melon, diced (1 c/170 g)	10	41	0.3	17	0	19	388	1	31	0.2
Huckleberries (1 c/145 g)	8.7	82	0.4	9	0.5	17	112	0	1	0.2
Kiwi fruit, diced (1 c/177 g)	60	230	0.5	31	0.2	60	552	0	7	0.2
Kiwi fruit, medium, each	26	99	0.2	13	0	26	237	0	2	0.1
Loganberries (1 c/144 g)	42	238	0.9	29	0.9	32	233	1	1	0.8
Mango, sliced (1 c/165 g)	17	181	0.2	15	0	18	257	1	3	0.1
Mango, medium, each	21	228	0.3	19	0	23	323	1	4	0.1
Mango, dried (1 c/121 g)	242	...	1.1	...	...	...	30	...	61	...
Orange sections (1 c/180 g)	72	81	0.2	18	0	25	326	1	0	0.1
Orange, medium, each	52	59	0.1	13	0	18	237	1	0	0.1
Orange juice (1 c/248 g)	27	109	0.5	28	0	42	496	0	2	0.1
Papaya, cubed (1 c/140 g)	34	22	0.1	14	0	7	360	1	4	0.1
Papaya, mashed (1 c/230 g)	55	37	0.2	23	0	12	591	1	7	0.2
Peach, sliced (1 c/170 g)	10	116	0.4	15	0.1	34	323	0	0	0.3
Peach, medium, each	6	67	0.2	9	0.1	20	186	0	0	0.2
Peach, dried, each	0	...	0.4	...	...	...	123	...	0	...
Pear, sliced (1 c/165 g)	15	135	0.3	12	0.1	18	196	0	2	0.2
Pear, medium, each	20	...	0	...	...		210	...	0	...
Pear, Bartlett, medium, each	15	136	0.3	12	0.1	18	198	0	2	0.2
Pear halves, dried (1 c/180 g)	61	668	3.8	59	0.6	106	959	0	11	0.7
Pineapple, diced (1 c/155 g)	20	153	0.4	19	1.8	12	178	0	2	0.2
Plum, sliced (1 c/165 g)	6.6	71	0.2	12	0.1	16	289	1	0	0.2
Plum, medium, each	0	...	0	...	...	...	110	...	0	...
Prunes, dried (1 c/170 g)	73	478	1.6	70	0.5	117	1,244	1	3	0.7
Raisins, seedless, packed (1 c/165 g)	82	525	3.1	53	0.5	167	1,234	1	18	0.4

Food	Calcium mg	Copper mcg	Iron mg	Magnesium mg	Manganese mg	Phosphorus mg	Potassium mg	Selenium mcg	Sodium mg	Zinc mg
DRIs for a woman	1,000	900	8 or 18*	320	1.8	700	4,700	55	1,200 to 1,500	8
DRIs for a man	1,000	900	8	400	2.3	700	4,700	55	1,200 to 1,500	11
Raisins, seeded, packed (1 c/165 g)	46	498	4.3	50	0.4	124	1,361	1	46	0.2
Raspberries (1 c/123 g)	31	111	0.9	27	0.8	36	186	0	1	0.5
Strawberries, dried (1 c/80 g)	40	...	0.7	...	...	...	...	...	0	...
Strawberries, halved (1 c/152 g)	24	73	0.6	20	0.6	37	233	1	2	0.2
Strawberries, whole (1 c/144 g)	23	69	0.6	19	0.5	35	220	0	1	0.2
Watermelon, diced (1 c/152 g)	11	064	0.4	15	0.1	17	170	1	2	0.2
Watermelon, diced (1 c/152 g)	11	064	0.4	15	0.1	17	170	1	2	0.2
VEGETABLES										
Arugula, chopped (1 c/20 g)	32	0	0.3	9	0.1	10	73	0	5	0.1
Asparagus, sliced (1 c/134 g)	32	253	2.9	19	0.2	70	271	39	3	0.7
Asparagus spear, medium, each	4	...	0.1	...	...	...	46	...	0	...
Avocado, all types, each (1 c/201 g)	22	527	2.0	78	0.5	82	1,204	1	20	0.8
Avocado, all types, puréed (1 c/230 g)	25	603	2.3	90	0.5	94	1,378	1	23	1
Avocado, all types, sliced (1 c/146 g)	16	383	1.5	57	0.3	60	875	1	15	0.6
Avocado, California, medium, each	22	294	1.1	50	0.3	93	877	1	14	1.2
Avocado, California, puréed (1 c/230 g)	30	391	1.4	67	0.3	124	1,166	1	18	1.6
Avocado, Florida, medium, each	30	945	0.5	73	0.3	122	1,067	0	6	1.2
Avocado, Florida, puréed (1 c/230 g)	23	715	0.4	55	0.2	92	807	0	5	0.9
Basil, fresh, chopped (1 c/42 g)	65	122	1.3	34	0.6	30	196	0	2	0.4
Beans, snap green/yellow (1 c/110 g)	41	76	1.1	28	0.2	42	230	1	7	0.2
Beets, sliced (1 c/136 g)	22	102	1.1	31	0.4	54	442	1	106	0.5
Beetroot juice (1 c/236 g)	...	...	...	...	...	68	571	...	472	...
Beet greens, chopped (1 c/38 g)	44	73	1	27	0.1	16	290	0	86	0.1
Bok choy, shredded (1 c/70 g)	74	15	0.6	13	0.1	26	176	0	46	0.1
Broccoli, chopped (1 c/71 g)	34	32	0.6	18	0.2	47	231	2	19	0.3
Brussels sprouts (1 c/88 g)	37	62	1.2	20	0.3	61	342	1	22	0.4
Cabbage, green, chopped (1 c/89 g)	42	20	0.5	13	0.1	20	219	1	16	0.2

Food	Calcium mg	Copper mcg	Iron mg	Magnesium mg	Manganese mg	Phosphorus mg	Potassium mg	Selenium mcg	Sodium mg	Zinc mg
DRIs for a woman	1,000	900	8 or 18*	320	1.8	700	4,700	55	1,200 to 1,500	8
DRIs for a man	1,000	900	8	400	2.3	700	4,700	55	1,200 to 1,500	11
Cabbage, napa (1 c/85 g)	60	...	0	...	...	...	...	...	10	...
Cabbage, pe-tsai, chopped (1 c/76 g)	59	27	0.2	10	0.1	22	181	0	7	0.2
Cabbage, red, chopped (1 c/89 g)	40	15	0.7	14	0.2	27	217	0	24	0.2
Cabbage, red, shredded (1 c/70 g)	32	12	0.6	11	0.2	21	170	0	19	0.2
Carrot, chopped (1 c/128 g)	42	58	0.4	15	0.2	45	410	0	88	0.3
Carrot, medium, each	24	32	0.2	9	0.1	25	230	0	50	0.2
Carrot juice (1 c/236 g)	64	...	...	...	...	73	517	...	123	...
Cauliflower, chopped (1 c/100 g)	22	42	0.4	15	0.1	44	303	1	30	0.3
Celery, diced (1 c/120 g)	48	42	0.2	13	0.1	29	312	0	96	0.2
Celery, rib, medium, each	26	22	0.1	7	0.1	15	166	0	64	0.1
Celery root, chopped (1 c/156 g)	67	109	1.1	31	0.3	179	468	1	156	0.5
Chiles, hot, green, chopped (1 c/150 g)	27	261	1.8	38	0.4	69	510	1	10	0.4
Chiles, hot, red, chopped (1 c/150 g)	21	194	1.5	34	0.3	64	483	1	14	0.4
Cilantro (1 c/46 g)	31	103	0.8	12	0.2	25	235	0	25	0
Collard greens, chopped (1 c/36 g)	52	14	0.1	3	0.1	4	61	0	7	0
Corn, yellow/white (1 c/154 g)	3	83	0.8	57	0.2	137	416	1	23	0.7
Cucumber, with peel, sliced (1 c/104 g)	15	34	0.3	11	0.1	21	150	0	2	0.2
Cucumber, peeled, sliced (1 c/119 g)	17	84	0.3	14	0.1	25	162	0	2	0.2
Dandelion greens, chopped (1 c/55 g)	103	94	1.7	20	0.2	36	218	0	42	0.2
Eggplant, cubed (1 c/82 g)	7	67	0.2	11	0.2	20	189	0	2	0.1
Endive, chopped (1 c/50 g)	26	0	0.4	8	0.2	14	157	0	11	0.4
Garlic cloves (1 c/136 g)	246	407	2.3	34	2.3	208	545	19	23	1.6
Garlic clove, medium, each	5	9	0.1	0.8	0	5	12	0	1	0
Horseradish, grated (1 c/240 g)	252	336	3.4	79	1.1	157	1,330	0	22	3.4
Jerusalem artichoke, sliced (1 c/150 g)	21	210	5	25	0.1	117	644	1	6	0.2
Kale, chopped (1 c/67 g)	90	194	1.1	23	0.5	38	299	1	29	0.3
Kale, Scotch, chopped (1 c/67 g)	137	163	2	59	0.4	42	302	1	47	0.2

Food	Calcium mg	Copper mcg	Iron mg	Magnesium mg	Manganese mg	Phosphorus mg	Potassium mg	Selenium mcg	Sodium mg	Zinc mg
DRIs for a woman	1,000	900	8 or 18*	320	1.8	700	4,700	55	1,200 to 1,500	8
DRIs for a man	1,000	900	8	400	2.3	700	4,700	55	1,200 to 1,500	11
Kelp, Japanese, chopped (1 c/80 g)	134	104	2.3	97	0.2	34	71	1	186	1
Leeks, chopped (1 c/89 g)	53	107	1.9	25	0.4	31	160	1	18	0.1
Lettuce, butterhead, chopped (1 c/55 g)	19	9	0.7	7	0.1	18	131	0	3	0.1
Lettuce, iceberg, chopped (1 c/55 g)	11	14	0.2	4	0.1	12	84	0	5	0.1
Lettuce, leaf, chopped (1 c/56 g)	20	16	0.5	7	0	16	109	0	16	0.1
Lettuce, red leaf, chopped (1 c/28 g)	9	8	0.3	3	0.1	8	52	0	7	0.1
Lettuce, romaine, chopped (1 c/56 g)	18	27	0.5	8	0.1	17	138	0	4	0.1
Mushrooms, shiitake, dried (1 c/145 g)	16	7,490	2.5	191	1.7	426	2,224	197	19	11
Mushroom, shiitake, medium, dried, each	0.4	194	0.1	5	0	11	57	5	0	0.3
Mustard greens, chopped (1 c/56 g)	58	82	0.8	18	0.3	24	198	1	14	0.1
Okra, sliced (1 c/100 g)	81	94	0.8	57	1	63	303	1	8	0.6
Olives, green (1 c/160 g)	98	545	2.6	35	...	27	88	2	3,840	0.1
Onions, green, chopped (1 c/100 g)	72	83	1.5	20	0.2	37	276	1	16	0.4
Onion, green, medium, each	11	12	0.2	3	0	6	41	0	2	0.1
Onions, red/yellow/white, chopped (1 c/160 g)	35	61	0.3	16	0.2	43	230	1	5	0.3
Parsley, chopped (1 c/60 g)	83	89	3.7	30	0.1	35	332	0	34	0.6
Parsnips, sliced (1 c/133 g)	48	160	0.8	39	0.7	94	499	2	13	0.8
Peas (1 c/145 g)	36	255	2.1	48	0.6	157	354	3	7	1.8
Pea pods, snow (1 c/63 g)	27	50	1.3	15	0.2	33	126	0	3	0.1
Pepper, bell, green, medium, each	12	79	0.4	12	0.1	24	208	0	4	0.2
Pepper, bell, red, medium, each	8	20	0.5	14	0.1	31	251	0	2	0.3
Peppers, bell, green, chopped (1 c/149 g)	15	98	0.5	15	0.2	30	261	0	4	0.2
Peppers, bell, red, chopped (1 c/149 g)	10	25	0.6	18	0.2	39	314	0	3	0.4
Peppers, bell, yellow, chopped (1 c/149 g)	16	160	0.7	18	0.2	36	316	0	3	0.2
Radish, daikon, sliced (1 c/88 g)	24	101	0.4	14	0.0	20	200	1	...	0.1

Food	Calcium mg	Copper mcg	Iron mg	Magnesium mg	Manganese mg	Phosphorus mg	Potassium mg	Selenium mcg	Sodium mg	Zinc mg
DRIs for a woman	1,000	900	8 or 18*	320	1.8	700	4,700	55	1,200 to 1,500	8
DRIs for a man	1,000	900	8	400	2.3	700	4,700	55	1,200 to 1,500	11
Radish, medium, each	1	2	0	0	0	1	10	0	2	0
Radish, daikon, medium, each	91	389	1.4	54	0.1	78	767	2	71	1
Radishes, daikon, dried (1 c/116 g)	730	1,892	7.8	197	0.6	237	4,053	1	322	2.5
Radishes, sliced (1 c/116 g)	29	58	0.4	12	0.1	23	270	1	45	0
Radish sprouts (1 c/38 g)	19	46	0.3	17	0.1	43	33	0	2	0
Rutabaga, chopped (1 c/140 g)	66	56	0.7	32	0.2	81	472	1	28	0.5
Spinach, chopped (1 c/30 g)	30	39	0.8	24	0.3	15	167	0	24	0.2
Squash, acorn, cubed (1 c/140 g)	46	91	1	45	0.2	50	486	1	4	0.2
Squash, butternut, cubed (1 c/240 g)	115	173	1.7	82	0.5	79	845	1	10	0.4
Squash, crookneck, cubed (1 c/130 g)	27	133	0.6	27	0.2	42	276	0	3	0.4
Squash, hubbard, cubed (1 c/116 g)	16	74	0.5	22	0.2	24	371	1	8	0.2
Squash, winter, all types, cubed (1 c/116 g)	32	82	0.7	16	0.2	27	406	0	5	0.2
Sweet potato, cubed (1 c/133 g)	40	201	0.8	33	0.3	63	448	1	17	0.4
Tomato, cherry, each	2	10	0	2	0.0	4	40	0	1	0
Tomato, chopped (1 c/180 g)	18	106	0.5	20	0.2	43	427	0	9	0.3
Tomato, green, chopped (1 c/180 g)	23	162	1	18	0.2	50	367	1	23	0
Tomato, medium, each	15	88	0.4	16	0.2	36	353	0	7	0.3
Tomato, Roma, medium, each	6	37	0.2	7	0.1	15	147	0	3	0
Tomato, sun-dried (1 c/54 g)	59	768	4.9	105	1	192	1,851	3	1,131	1.1
Tomato, yellow, chopped (1 c/139 g)	15	140	0.7	17	0.2	50	359	1	32	0
Turnip, cubed (1 c/130 g)	39	110	0.4	14	0.2	35	248	1	87	0.4
Turnip greens, chopped (1 c/55 g)	104	192	0.6	17	0.3	23	163	1	22	0.1
Watercress, chopped (1 c/34 g)	41	0	0.1	7	0.1	20	112	0	14	0
Yam, cubed (1 c/150 g)	26	267	0.8	32	0.6	82	1,224	1	14	0.4
Zucchini, baby, each	2	11	0.1	4	0	10	51	0	0	0.1
Zucchini, cubed (1 c/124 g)	19	63	0.4	21	0.2	47	325	0	12	0.4

Food	Calcium mg	Copper mcg	Iron mg	Magnesium mg	Manganese mg	Phosphorus mg	Potassium mg	Selenium mcg	Sodium mg	Zinc mg
DRIs for a woman	1,000	900	8 or 18*	320	1.8	700	4,700	55	1,200 to 1,500	8
DRIs for a man	1,000	900	8	400	2.3	700	4,700	55	1,200 to 1,500	11
NUTS AND SEEDS										
Almonds (1 c/142 g)	352	1,576	6.1	390	3.6	673	1,034	11	1	4.7
Almond butter (1 c/256 g)	691	2,304	9.5	776	6.0	1,339	1,940	12	28	7.8
Brazil nut, large, each	8	82	0.1	18	0.1	34	31	91	0	0.2
Brazil nuts (1 c/140 g)	224	2,440	6.1	526	1.7	1,015	923	2,684	7	5.7
Cashew butter (1 c/256 g)	110	5,606	12.9	660	2.1	1,170	1,398	29	38	13.2
Cashew nuts (1 c/130 g)	48	2,854	8.7	380	2.2	771	858	26	16	7.5
Chia seeds, dried (1 c/160 g)	1,010	301	16	123	3.5	1,517	256	...	30	5.6
Flaxseeds, ground (1 c/128 g)	320	896	12.8	448	9	832	960	...	59	2.6
Flaxseeds, whole (1 c/176 g)	440	1,232	17.6	616	12.3	1,144	1,320	...	81	3.5
Hazelnuts (1 c/135 g)	154	2,329	6.3	220	8.3	392	918	3	0	3.3
Pecans (1 c/108 g)	...	1,296	2.2	138	...	314	423	13	1	6
Pine nuts (1 c/136 g)	22	1,801	7.5	341	12	782	812	1	3	8.8
Pistachio nuts (1 c/128 g)	137	1,664	5.3	155	1.5	627	1,312	9	1	2.8
Poppy seeds (1 c/134 g)	1,946	2,195	12.6	445	9.2	1,141	941	2	28	13.7
Psyllium seeds, ground (1 c/156 g)	521	...	31.2	80	2.5	98	1,265	2,184	25	3.3
Pumpkin seeds (1 c/138 g)	59	1,914	20.7	738	4.2	1,620	1,114	8	84	10.3
Sesame seeds, hulled (1 c/150 g)	197	2,190	11.7	520	2.1	1,164	610	3	60	15.4
Sesame seeds, unhulled (1 c/144 g)	1,404	5,878	21	505	3.5	906	674	8	16	11.2
Sesame tahini (1 c/240 g)	338	3,864	10.6	228	...	1,896	1,102	4	84	11.1
Sunflower seed butter (1 c/256 g)	312	4,685	12.2	945	5.4	1884	184	200	8	13.5
Sunflower seeds, hulled (1 c/144 g)	167	2,523	9.7	510	2.9	1,015	992	86	4	7.3
Walnuts, black, chopped (1 c/125 g)	72	1,275	3.8	252	5.3	580	655	21	1	4.3
Walnuts, English, chopped (1 c/120 g)	118	1903	3.5	190	4.1	415	529	6	2	3.7
Water chestnuts, Chinese, sliced (1 c/124 g)	14	404	0.1	27	0.4	78	724	1	...	0.6
LEGUMES										
Adzuki beans, dried (1 c/197 g)	130	2,155	9.8	250	3.4	751	2,470	6	10	9.9
Lentil sprouts (1 c/77 g)	19	271	2.5	28	0.4	133	248	0	8	1.2

Food	Calcium mg	Copper mcg	Iron mg	Magnesium mg	Manganese mg	Phosphorus mg	Potassium mg	Selenium mcg	Sodium mg	Zinc mg
DRIs for a woman	1,000	900	8 or 18*	320	1.8	700	4,700	55	1,200 to 1,500	8
DRIs for a man	1,000	900	8	400	2.3	700	4,700	55	1,200 to 1,500	11
Lentils, dried (1 c/192 g)	98	1,636	17.3	205	2.7	872	1,738	16	19	6.9
Mung bean sprouts (1 c/104 g)	14	171	0.9	21	0.2	56	155	1	6	0.4
Mung beans, dried (1 c/188 g)	240	1,770	14.4	355	1.95	690	1,920	15	0	5.0
Pea sprouts (1 c/120 g)	43	326	2.7	67	0.5	198	457	1	24	1.3
GRAINS										
Amaranth, dry (1 c/195 g)	298	1,515	14.8	519	4.4	887	714	...	41	6.2
Barley, hulled, dry (1 c/184 g)	61	916	6.6	245	3.6	486	832	69	22	5.1
Buckwheat, dry (1 c/170 g)	31	1,870	3.8	393	2.2	590	782	14	2	4.1
Buckwheat sprouts (1 c/33 g)	9	86	0.7	27	...	66	56	...	5	0.5
Kamut berries, dry (1 c/188 g)	28	...	5.7	...	...	...	697	...	58	...
Millet, dry (1 c/200 g)	16	1,500	6.0	228	3.3	570	390	5	58	3.4
Oat groats, dry (1 c/164 g)	110	...	6.4	116	...	572	505	...	43	...
Quinoa, dry (1 c/170 g)	102	1,394	15.7	357	3.8	697	1,258		36	5.6
Rye berries, dry (1 c/169 g)	56	760	4.5	204	4.5	632	446	60	10	6.3
Sprouted wheat bread, slice	27	55	0.9	12	0.3	39	52	...	138	0.3
Wheat berries, hard, red (1 c/192 g)	48	787	6.9	238	7.8	637	653	136	4	5.3
Wheat berries, hard, white (1 c/192 g)	61	697	8.8	179	7.3	682	829	152	4	6.4
Wheat sprouts (1 c/108 g)	30	282	2.3	89	2	216	183	46	17	1.8
Wild rice, dry (1 c/160 g)	34	838	3.1	283	2.1	693	683	4	11	9.6
OTHER										
BarleyMax supplement (1 tsp/2 g)†	19.6	23	0.6	11	0.1	10	84	...	8	0.1
Oil, olive (1 c/216 g)	2	0	1.4	0	0	0	2	0	6	0
Spirulina, dried (1 c/119 g)	143	7,259	33.9	232	2.3	140	1,622	9	1,247	2.4
Spirulina, dried (1 c/119 g)	143	7,259	33.9	232	2.3	140	1,622	9	1,247	2.4

Source: Data from references 101, 114.

Note: Foods are fresh unless otherwise indicated. The "vegetables" category includes sea vegetables as well as fruits such as tomatoes that are commonly used as vegetables. Data for nuts and seeds are before soaking. Mineral levels are particularly high in dried foods, such as fruit and shiitake mushrooms, because the minerals become more concentrated when the moisture is removed.

*The DRI for iron is 18 mg per day for women 19 to 50 years of age and 8 mg per day for women 51 years of age or older.

†BarleyMax is available from www.hacres.com/products.

CHAPTER 10

The Great Enzyme Controversy

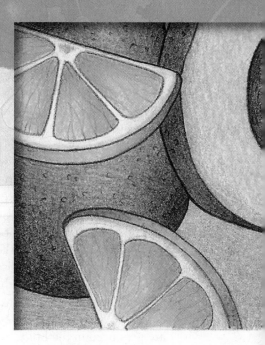

In the raw-food community, food enzymes are commonly considered the single most important dietary component for longevity, disease prevention, and overall well-being. Certainly, vitamins and minerals are recognized for their contributions, but enzymes are viewed as the missing link to health. In the mainstream medical world, food enzymes don't even rate a paragraph in a textbook; they are considered rather irrelevant to human health. When it comes to the enzymes in food, the two schools of thought couldn't be further apart. In this chapter, we'll investigate the roots of the food-enzyme theory (also known as the food-enzyme concept) and scrutinize the scientific literature to try and make sense of this discrepancy.

Understanding Enzymes and Their Functions

Enzymes are biological catalysts—substances that speed up all chemical reactions in living cells. It is said that we can live about three weeks without food and three days without water, but we would likely survive only about three minutes without enzymes! There are thousands of different kinds of enzymes in every single cell, each one being responsible for a specific chemical reaction. Enzymes are almost always proteins made of tens, hundreds, or thousands of amino acids. Like all proteins, enzymes have a limited life span and are constantly replenished by the body. Each enzyme has a unique shape, including a special location, or active site, where reactions occur. A molecule called a substrate attaches itself to the active site like a key fits into a lock. A chemical reaction quickly takes place, and the enzyme releases the product it just created.

The enzyme is unaffected by the reaction, and once the product is released, the enzyme is ready for another substrate and another reaction.

Some molecules can slow down or accelerate the activity of enzymes. Molecules that decrease enzyme activity are called enzyme inhibitors, while molecules that increase enzyme activity are called enzyme activators. Enzymes are designed for very specific internal environments, so if the pH or temperature isn't just right, they won't be able to do their job. Many enzymes also require the presence of a nonprotein cofactor, such as a metal ion like zinc or copper or a vitamin such as thiamin (B_1), riboflavin (B_2), or niacin (B_3), for their activity.

Enzymes are often named after the substrate they react with, but an "ase" is added to the first part of the substrate name. For example, lipase is named after lipids, amylase after the starch amylose, and protease after protein. Some of the enzymes that were discovered before this naming system came into effect have an "in" at the end of their names (for example, chymotrypsin, pepsin, and trypsin). Three types of enzymes are of interest in human health: metabolic, digestive, and food enzymes. The first two (metabolic and digestive enzymes) are produced in the body, and the third (food enzymes) is produced in plants.

METABOLIC ENZYMES

Metabolic enzymes are highly specialized structures trained to run and maintain the body. Every organ, every tissue, and every cell requires metabolic enzymes to initiate and direct the chemical reactions necessary for respiration, regeneration, energy production, and every other biochemical activity that takes place within the body.

DIGESTIVE ENZYMES

Digestive enzymes break down food, enabling nutrients to be absorbed into the bloodstream. There are three main categories of digestive enzymes: amylases, lipases, and proteases. Amylases help to break down starches and are secreted mainly in the mouth and the small intestine. Lipases, which break down fats, are secreted in the mouth (lingual lipase), the stomach (gastric lipase), and the small intestine (pancreatic lipase). Proteases break down proteins. They are secreted in the stomach (pepsin is the only enzyme designed to withstand the acid pH of the stomach) and the small intestine. Within each category are several distinct enzymes with specific jobs. Some are like axes that chop very large molecules into smaller pieces; others are like pruners that reduce the fragments further. Some are like fine shears that snip small molecules into their component parts so they can be absorbed into the bloodstream.

FOOD ENZYMES

Food enzymes are naturally present in all raw plant foods. Enzymes in plants catalyze all the reactions necessary to the life of the plant. They help to harvest energy from the sun, break down the storage forms of energy in seeds to support the growth of a new plant, turn inactive phytochemicals into active metabolites, and enable fruits to ripen. Plant foods are most concentrated in the enzymes that the plant needs to break down the carbohydrates, protein, and fat that were stored for energy. For example, bananas have a lot of amylase because they are mainly carbohydrate, avocados are high in lipase because of their rich fat content, and legumes contain many proteases because they are high in protein. Foods that are especially noted for their high enzyme content are sprouts of all kinds, unripe papayas, and unripe pineapples.

A BRIEF HISTORY OF FOOD ENZYMES IN HUMAN HEALTH

Several early health pioneers understood that there was something in raw plant foods that was lost with cooking. For many centuries, these losses were not ascribed to enzymes, as enzymes had not yet been discovered. Pythagoras, the eminent Greek philosopher and mathematician, was among the first to advocate a vegetarian regimen rich in uncooked foods, which was the daily fare for all pupils in his school of higher learning. Many centuries later, Maximilian Oskar Bircher Benner (1867–1936), a Swiss physician and inventor of the soaked breakfast cereal known as muesli, founded the Bircher-Benner Clinic in Switzerland to heal people of dreaded diseases. His primary therapy was raw vegetable food, which he considered to be the purest and most powerful diet that existed.

In 1897, Eduard Buchner (1860–1917) discovered enzymes when he realized that sugar could be fermented without living yeast cells. He called the enzyme that resulted in the fermentation of sucrose "zymase." Artturi Ilmari Virtanen (1895–1973), a Finnish chemistry Nobel Prize recipient, demonstrated that the enzymes in raw foods are released in the mouth when vegetables are chewed. This did not occur with cooked vegetables. These early enzyme discoveries led some of the health pioneers to the conclusion that what was lost in cooking was enzymes. Of course, it was not until the first half of the twentieth century (between 1912 and 1948) that vitamins were discovered, and not until the 1980s that we began to identify phytochemicals in plants that provide protection to people.

Max Gerson (1881–1959), a German physician who immigrated to the United States in 1936, promoted an enzyme-rich, largely raw vegan diet to reverse cancer and other chronic diseases. Anne Wigmore (1909–1994), co-founder of the Hippocrates Health Institute, promoted a living-food diet with a focus on raw fruits, vegetables, juices, and nuts; sprouted seeds, grains, and legumes; and chlorophyll-rich green juices. Herbert Shelton (1895–1985), a naturopathic physician and champion of the natural hygiene movement, believed that the body's digestive enzymes had limitations and people should be conscious of how all food choices affect the enzymes in our bodies.

While these pioneers helped to shape the beliefs and practices of raw-food advocates, the most celebrated authority on the food-enzyme theory was an

American physician by the name of Edward Howell (1898–1988). The vast majority of raw-food literature concerning food enzymes can be traced back to the theories of Howell, who is widely recognized as the "father of food enzymes." Howell wrote two books, *Enzyme Nutrition* and *Food Enzymes for Health and Longevity*. The later book was actually written in 1939 and published in 1946 under the title *The Status of Food Enzymes in Digestion and Metabolism*.

The Food-Enzyme Theory: Fact and Fiction

 owell's food-enzyme theory contends that food enzymes must be consumed by people for optimal health. The five key points, in theory, are:

1. Food enzymes possess a "vital life force."
2. People have a finite ability to produce enzymes over their lifetimes.
3. Insufficient digestive enzymes lead to poor health, chronic disease, and premature death.
4. Cooking destroys enzymes in food.
5. Food enzymes are important for human digestion.

Over the years, raw-food proponents have gathered evidence to further support these assertions. A rather surprising source commonly cited in raw-food circles is a series of studies on cats by American researcher Francis Pottenger (1901–1967). Pottenger compared varying intakes of raw and cooked animal products in over nine hundred cats. His findings showed tremendous health advantages for cats eating raw animal products compared to those consuming cooked diets. A second fascinating source from the 1930s is the work of Paul Kouchakoff, who proposed that cooked foods cause digestive leukocytosis (a rise in white blood cell count), while raw foods do not.

The most recent academic proponents of food enzymes in human digestion are a team of academics lead by Lawrence J. Prochaska and Walter V. Piekutowski at Wright State University in Dayton, Ohio. Prochaska and Piekutowski released a medical hypothesis in 1994 regarding the synergistic effects of food enzymes and digestive enzymes and, along with two colleagues, released a second medical hypothesis in 2000. In addition to the theories of Prochaska and Piekutowski, scientific research conducted by contemporary enzyme researchers, such as Stephen Rothman, professor emeritus, University of California, San Francisco, and Michael Gardner, retired emeritus professor from the University of Bradford, UK, are often cited as providing proof of the food-enzyme theory.

In the minds of the vast majority of physicians, dietitians, physiologists, and nutrition researchers, food enzymes are of little or no consequence to human health. However, there is a strong belief within the raw-food community, and among a handful of academics, that food enzymes are critical to health and longevity. The material that follows is our concerted effort to make sense of the discrepancy. We will begin by examining each of the five key points that form the basis of the food-enzyme theory and the science that currently exists on either side of the controversy.

THEORY #1: FOOD ENZYMES POSSESS A "VITAL LIFE FORCE."

Howell's food-enzyme theory rests on the premise that enzymes consist of protein carriers charged with a "vital life force" that give off a kind of radiation when they work. He compared enzymes to a battery that consists of metallic plates charged with electrical energy. While science regards enzymes as merely catalysts made of protein, Howell was convinced that they are much more than that. Because of this vital life force, an energy that cannot be created by man, Howell believed that enzymes could be produced only within living organisms.

SCIENTIFIC FINDINGS

Before we can fairly address this theory, it is important to recognize the limitations of science. Science refers to the organized body of knowledge concerning our physical world, both animate and inanimate. If a theory or hypothesis cannot be proved scientifically (that is, it cannot be demonstrated to be false), this does not mean that it is not true, merely that it is not science based. Many cultures embrace the concept of a vital energy that exists in all living things. Good examples are *chi* in the Asian tradition (which also extends to nonliving things, such as spaces) and *prana* in the yogic tradition. Many spiritual beliefs also fall into this category. The claim for a vital force in enzymes cannot be proved false; for this reason, it is not within the realm of science. However, there are certain aspects of the vital life-force theory as it applies to enzymes that are tangible and can be tested. One example is the belief that enzymes can be produced only in a living organism. In fact, several teams of researchers have succeeded in producing synthetic enzymes. One recent example is the development by researchers at the California Institute of Technology (Caltech) of a new group of fifteen highly stable fungal enzymes that efficiently break down cellulose into sugars.[1] Another research team at the University of Washington in Seattle recently designed an enzyme to cleave a bond in a molecule not found in nature.[2]

The term "vital life force" dates back to the seventeenth century. At that time it was universally believed that living organisms contained a mysterious vital life force that was necessary for the formation of organic matter. While scientists could not prove that a vital life force does not exist, they could investigate the claim that a vital life force was necessary to produce organic matter. For decades, the vital-life-force theory stood strong, as scientists were unsuccessful in their attempts at producing organic matter from inorganic matter. However, in 1814, the vital-life-force theory received a serious blow when

Swedish chemist Jöns Jacob Berzelius proved that the basic laws of chemical change applied to organic and inorganic substances equally. Furthermore, in 1828, German chemistry professor Friedrich Wöhler succeeded at producing urea (an organic compound) using two inorganic salts—potassium cyanate and ammonium chloride. This discovery was followed by the formation of numerous organic compounds from inorganic starting materials. By 1850, scientists believed the vital-life-force theory to be essentially dead.[3] Of course, these findings do not really prove that a "vital life force" is nonexistent, but rather that certain measurable aspects of this claim, as they relate to the production of organic matter, are unfounded.

THEORY #2: PEOPLE HAVE A FINITE ABILITY TO PRODUCE ENZYMES OVER THEIR LIFETIMES.

Howell believed that people are born with a finite lifetime "enzyme potential" for manufacturing digestive enzymes. He used the analogy of a bank account we receive at birth that must last us a lifetime. We cannot make any deposits, only withdrawals. Eating raw food helps to conserve our body's enzymes, while cooking food destroys plant enzymes. Howell believed that a diet rich in cooked food would strain our enzyme account, because our body would need to produce more digestive enzymes, thereby using up our precious enzyme potential. This, he asserted, also robs our capacity to manufacture the metabolic enzymes necessary for reactions throughout the body.

SCIENTIFIC FINDINGS

Scientific evidence is lacking to support the theory that humans and other animals have a finite lifetime enzyme potential or that eating cooked food drains our enzyme reserves. According to proponents of the food-enzyme theory, the most compelling evidence in support of this concept comes from a U.S. team of researchers lead by Stephen Rothman. Rothman and his colleagues demonstrated that the body conserves enzymes through a process called enteropancreatic circulation.[4-6] Their original work was published in the mid '70s, with more recent findings published in 2002. In their 2002 report "Conservation of Digestive Enzymes," Rothman and his team explain that the conventional belief that a new complement of digestive enzymes is provided for each meal is incorrect. The traditional thinking has been that because 95–99 percent of all digestive-enzyme activity disappears by the time the half-digested food, or chyme, reaches the large intestine, the enzymes must have been degraded. These researchers provide strong evidence that digestive enzymes are reabsorbed into the bloodstream, returned to the pancreas, and reused, rather than being broken down into amino acids. The authors conclude, "Mechanisms that avoid the need to manufacture an entirely new batch of digestive enzymes for each meal, such as is the case with bile salts, would seem to provide an important advantage for an organism, particularly when food is scarce, as it often is in nature."

The proponents of the finite lifetime enzyme potential hold Rothman's work up as scientific proof that enzymes are being carefully safeguarded by the body because of a limited lifetime supply. While this may seem to be a reasonable conclusion, it is possible that this work demonstrates only that the body is efficient in its enzyme production. We asked Stephen Rothman whether his research supports the finite enzyme theory. The following is his response:

> As we age, most of our functions are diminished, and though I am not aware of a study in humans that shows a decrease in digestive-enzyme secretion with age, it would not be surprising. However, a decrease in the rate of secretion over time and some sort of timed "finite limit" are quite different things. There is no finite limit on what we produce; we continue to do so as long as we are alive. Also, there is no basis for concluding that older people, any more than younger people, do not fully digest what they eat, regardless of whether or not the food is cooked. As for the conservation of digestive enzymes, it offers no support whatsoever for there being a timed limit on the amount of digestive enzymes we produce, or more generally, for the notion that eating raw food increases one's life span. Presuming that it offers evidence for such ideas does a disservice to a serious idea and the research that supports it.

THEORY #3: INSUFFICIENT DIGESTIVE ENZYMES LEAD TO POOR HEALTH, CHRONIC DISEASE, AND PREMATURE DEATH.

Howell alleged that every time you eat cooked food, your internal production of digestive enzymes escalates and your enzyme bank is depleted. When your enzyme potential drops too low, your health fails and you develop chronic degenerative diseases. When your enzyme potential is completely used up, you die. Two research projects are often cited as providing powerful evidence for the immense value of raw food and food enzymes for health and longevity. The first, conducted by Francis Pottenger, is known as "Pottenger's cats," and the second, by Paul Kouchakoff, is known as "digestive leukocytosis." We will briefly examine the claims of Howell and explore the research of Pottenger and Kouchakoff.

SCIENTIFIC FINDINGS

Howell's Theory

Although it would be difficult to test Howell's theory in a clinical study, a reasonable alternative would be to examine the diets of the world's healthiest, longest-living populations. One would expect that if food enzymes were critical to health and longevity, populations eating the highest proportion of raw food would live the longest, while those eating the highest proportion of cooked food would perish most rapidly.

There are a number of reports of extraordinary health and longevity in populations throughout the world. Among the most fascinating are the longevity articles in *National Geographic* and John Robbins extraordinary book *Healthy at 100*. In November 2005, *National Geographic*'s cover photo was that of an eighty-four-year-old Okinawan man doing a headstand on a beach. The feature article, "The Secrets of Living Longer," examined the lives of Okinawans, Sardians, and the Seventh-day Adventists from Loma Linda, California. Robbins' book gives a more detailed account of four of the healthiest, longest-living populations in the world: the Abkhasians from Russia, the Vilcabambans from South America, the Hunzans from Central Asia, and the Okinawans from Japan.

When we look at the diets of all of these long-lived peoples, we notice three common denominators immediately: they are largely plant-based, they include primarily unprocessed foods, and they provide moderate calories. Fresh fruits and vegetables from home gardens are staples in many of these diets, and consumption of raw food appears greater than it is in conventional Western diets. However, there are significant differences between the groups. For example, the Hunzans eat many of their foods raw—up to 80 percent raw in the summer—while the Okinawans eat the greater majority of their foods cooked. This difference is not reflected in their longevity, although there may be other factors at play. It is possible that some of the health habits of Okinawans are superior to those of the Hunzans, and if Okinawans ate more of their food raw, their lives would be further extended. However, there is no evidence to suggest that this is the case.

The fact that all of these long-lived populations have moderate caloric intakes could be regarded as proof that conserving enzymes lengthens lifespan. If we really have an enzyme bank, eating less would seem the perfect way to stretch our enzyme budget. On the other hand, no energy-restriction research has ever linked enzyme conservation to this phenomenon. It is generally thought that calorie restriction increases longevity because it lowers body weight, cholesterol, blood pressure, insulin resistance, inflammation, and numerous chronic degenerative diseases. It has also been shown to produce favorable metabolic changes, including better elimination of toxins from the body.[7, 8] Once again, this does not prove that enzymes could not be of some consequence in this regard; the evidence is simply lacking.

Stephen Rothman also weighed in on this question with the following response:

> I do not believe that eating raw food, animal or vegetable, extends your life or makes you healthier. Humans probably started cooking food to soften hard-to-chew food and to kill parasites. The softening that takes place includes the unraveling, or denaturation, of proteins, making them easier to digest (not harder). If we could remove the pancreas and all other sources of digestive enzymes in the gut (salivary glands, stomach, and small intestine) and depended solely on the enzymes in raw food, we would starve to death in short order.

Pottenger's Cats

Physician Francis M. Pottenger Jr. conducted a series of studies in California over a ten-year period from 1932–1942. In these studies, Pottenger examined the consequences of feeding raw versus cooked food to more than nine hundred cats.[9, 10] The raw diet, which contained raw meat and raw milk, produced excellent health in these animals, while the cooked-meat diet caused skin and bone disorders, allergies, infections, degenerative diseases, and adverse personality changes. By the fourth generation, the cats eating the all-cooked-meat diet had completely died out. Pottenger concluded that something in raw food helps to support the growth and development of cats, and whatever it is, it is destroyed by the cooking process. Many people cite these experiments as proof that raw food is healthful and cooked food is toxic. Some people attribute the differences in the health of the cats to the fact that raw food contains enzymes, or "vital life force," while cooked food is devoid of enzymes and therefore "dead."

The Pottenger experiments taught us far more about cat nutrition than about human nutrition. Carnivores, such as cats, have very different nutritional requirements than people. They require more protein and fat and far less carbohydrate. They produce their own vitamin C, while humans do not. (We have to get it from food.) So why would cats do so much better on raw meat than cooked meat? As Pottenger noted, something necessary for cat health was likely destroyed by the cooking process. In the mid '70s, decades after Pottenger's research was conducted, the mystery began to unfold. It was at this time that researchers discovered that an amino acid called taurine is an essential nutrient for cats. (It is not essential for humans, as we manufacture it.)[11–14] In the 1980s, studies showed remarkable similarities between taurine-deficient cats and the cats in Pottenger's study.[15–17] Finally, beginning in the 1990s, studies demonstrated the degradation of taurine by various cooking methods.[18–20] While there may have been other nutrients or beneficial dietary components missing from the cooked-meat diet, the lack of taurine was most likely the primary reason for the ill health of these animals.

With the research that currently exists on the essentiality of taurine in cat nutrition, it is surprising that Pottenger's work is still being cited as evidence for the food-enzyme theory. It also seems rather ironic that a study of carnivorous cats and their consumption of raw meat (the flesh of dead animals) would substantiate what humans should eat for good health and be considered solid evidence of the "vital life force" in raw plant foods.

Digestive Leukocytosis

Digestive leukocystosis is a condition in which there is rise in white blood cell (leukocyte) count following a meal. The condition was described by physiologist Jacob Moleschott in 1854 and was a hot topic among medical researchers at that time. While some were convinced that digestive leukocytosis was a proven fact, there were plenty of dissenters. Dozens of studies reported vastly different findings: some noted leukocyte changes throughout the day, regardless of whether a meal was consumed, others noted a response only when participants were standing rather than lying down. Some found high-protein foods (such as meat and fish) produced a significant response, while high-carbohydrate foods (such as bread and cake) did not.[21–23] In the early 1930s, Paul Kouchakoff, a researcher with the Institute of Clinical Chemistry in Lausanne, Switzerland, reported that the condition did not occur with the consumption of raw food. Kouchakoff found increases in white blood cell counts following the consumption of processed food or food cooked at temperatures of 189 degrees F (87 degrees C) or higher. (Critical temperatures were not the same for all foods.) From the point of view of the immune system, he said that whenever cooked food is eaten, the body reacts as though it is being invaded by a foreign or toxic substance. According to Kouchakoff, the phenomenon is worse when foods are pressure cooked, and still more severe when man-made processed foods are eaten. He maintained that eating cooked, smoked, or salted animal foods brings on violent leukocytosis consistent with ingesting poison.[24, 25]

While Kouchakoff's findings are fascinating, his results have not been reproduced in the eight decades since their original publication. This does not mean the results are invalid, but it would add considerable strength to the theory if the findings could be replicated by other research teams.

Raw-food proponents use Kouchakoff's work as evidence that raw foods are healthful and cooked foods are not. However, Kouchakoff suggested that, based on his findings, leukocytosis could be avoided by eating 10 percent of our food at a meal in its raw form or by heating foods below their critical temperature for less than thirty minutes. In his 1937 paper, he went into considerable detail regarding specific foods that should be eaten or avoided to minimize the risk of leukocytosis.[25] Foods that he suggested could be used without risk of leukocytosis included raw milk; yogurt; tea and coffee with lemon juice, water, cream, or raw milk added; whole-grain bread with butter; fresh or soft-boiled eggs; butter; cheese; raw or rare meats; fruits; vegetables (served with mayonnaise); cold-pressed vegetable oils; salt; pepper; and other condiments. He also recommended that boiled, braised, or grilled meats be served with a mixed salad or mixed vegetables to reduce leukocytosis. He recommended replacing sugar with honey, and if sugar is used, that it be balanced with at least two raw foods. Peanut oil and vinegar were cautioned against.

The scientific validity of Kouchakoff's theory is questionable. Using his theory as evidence for raw vegan diets ignores the author's findings and conclusions.

THEORY #4: COOKING DESTROYS ENZYMES IN FOOD.

The food-enzyme theory purports that heating food at temperatures reaching 118 degrees F (48 degrees C) or higher denatures food enzymes. All cooking temperatures exceed this limit. Even steaming or boiling a food will produce temperatures up to 212 degrees F (100 degrees C).

SCIENTIFIC FINDINGS

There is no question that heat denatures enzymes. It appears as though optimal food enzyme action (maximum reaction rate) occurs at around 104 degrees F (40 degrees C). However, even slightly higher temperatures can negatively affect enzyme activity. At first, the enzyme begins to unfold and the shape of the active site changes. The substrate may still attach, but not as strongly as it otherwise would. This slows down the reaction time. When the temperature reaches about 113 degrees F (45 degrees C), enzyme function can be more seriously compromised. By the time the temperature reaches 135–140 degrees F (57–60 degrees C), food enzymes are generally completely denatured. The longer the heat is maintained above 113 degrees F (45 degrees C), the more enzyme activity is lost. The whole process is quite gradual, and at certain stages, it is even reversible. However, once the enzyme is completely denatured, the process is usually irreversible. The magic number (118 degrees F/48 degrees C) offered by proponents of the food-enzyme theory is certainly consistent with scientific findings. However, while some imagine enzyme activity as going from 100 percent at temperatures under 118 degrees F (48 degrees C) to 0 percent over this temperature, the process is in fact very gradual.[26, 27]

THEORY #5: FOOD ENZYMES ARE VITAL FOR OPTIMAL HUMAN DIGESTION.

Proponents of the food-enzyme theory contend that food enzymes are not only vital to optimal human digestion, but also that enzymes in raw food actually take priority over digestive enzymes secreted by the body. Howell's explanation of the role of food enzymes in human digestion is as follows: Food enzymes become active the moment the plant cell wall is ruptured by chewing. As the food goes down the esophagus, it drops into the upper part of the stomach. The lower part of the stomach remains flat and closed while food sits in the upper part for thirty to forty-five minutes. During this phase of predigestion, minimal acid and enzymes are secreted by the body, and food enzymes continue to work on the food ingested. The greater the amount of food enzymes present during the predigestion phase, the less work the body has to do later. When the bottom section of the stomach opens up and this mass of food moves down, the body starts secreting acid and protein enzymes called pepsin. (Howell believed these enzymes could survive the acid of the stomach.) Even at this point, food enzymes continue to work unless they are either denatured or temporarily inactivated by the acid of the stomach. According to Howell, some enzymes survive to the small intestine; some can be reactivated and continue to assist with digestion in the small intestine.[28]

Many advocates also believe that food enzymes can then get through the small intestine to the bloodstream in their intact form and have healing effects on the body. Some advocates suggest that inhibition or destruction of food enzymes significantly decreases or even eliminates the total nutritive value of foods consumed. They add that food enzymes prime the digestive process so that the digestive enzymes can more effectively do their jobs. According to the food-enzyme concept, it is best to eat at least 75 percent of our food raw, and that if we eat cooked food, oral enzymes should be taken along with them.

SCIENTIFIC FINDINGS

The fundamental issue is whether or not food enzymes are vital for human digestion and health. In our effort to address all of the previous points, we will answer five critical questions.

Question 1: *Is Dr. Howell's description of digestion correct?*

Howell was quite accurate in his description of the physiology of the stomach. The stomach is divided into two compartments—the proximal stomach (upper part) and the distal stomach (lower part). The upper part of the stomach acts as a reservoir for food. Contractions in this part of the stomach are rare.[29] The time that solid food is held in this part of the stomach (lag time) ranges from twenty to sixty minutes, averaging about forty minutes.[30–32] The function of the distal stomach is to mix and grind food, turning it into a paste called chyme. Chyme is then dispensed into the small intestine at a very controlled rate of 1–5 milliliters (5 milliliters equals 1 teaspoon) about twice a minute. Food particles generally must be less than 3 millimeters in diameter to pass into the small intestine. If they're larger, they are generally returned to the stomach for further mastication.

Question 2: *Can food enzymes survive the harsh pH of the stomach or be reactivated once they arrive?*

Mainstream medical thinking on food enzymes is that they are completely broken down in the acidic environment of the stomach and therefore have no activity in the small intestine, where most digestive enzyme action occurs. This makes perfect sense. The pH of the empty stomach is generally between 1.3 and 2.5. After we eat, the stomach becomes less acidic, and the pH can rise to between 4.5 and 5.8. Within an hour after we eat, the pH falls to less than 3.1.[29] Food enzymes are largely denatured at a pH of less than 3.1[33, 34] so the logical assumption is that food enzymes could not survive past the stomach. Some people argue that food enzymes can survive acid with a pH as low as 2; however, there is only one study we could find that supported this claim. This study looked at a highly stable cysteine protease isolated from the latex of *Ervatamia coronaria*, a medicinal flowering plant that is native to India. The authors of this study stated that the cysteine protease from *Ervatamia coronaria* survives within a very broad pH range of 2–12, which, to their knowledge, is unique.[35]

While the mainstream view of food enzymes is theoretically accurate, there are many factors that could alter the typical scenario. For example, if hydrochloric acid secretion is low, antacids are consumed, food particles are not sufficiently reduced in size, or the stomach empties more quickly than usual, food enzymes could potentially survive into the small intestine. In some cases, food enzymes may begin to unravel somewhat but not become completely denatured, and they may become reactivated in the small intestine. Research has demonstrated some survival of salivary amylase into the small intestine. Salivary amylase, like food enzymes, is easily degraded at a pH of less than 4.[34, 36]

Based on the knowledge that the pH of a full stomach can rise to 4.5–5.8 for up to an hour after we have eaten, that food stays in the upper portion of the stomach for an average of forty minutes, and that the main function of this part of the stomach is as a reservoir, we can expect that the enzymes naturally present in raw food would survive and be active during this time. In addition, food preparation techniques (such as chopping, blending, and puréeing) and chewing release or activate some of the enzymes present within the plant cell walls. When food is pushed down to the lower part of the stomach, where the pH is below 3.1, and is ground into small particles, we can expect that most food enzymes will be deactivated or completely denatured by stomach acid. To summarize, food enzymes have some action before food is ingested (for example, when food is cut, blended, or processed) and in the upper part of the stomach after ingestion. However, they appear to have limited activity by the time they reach the small intestine. The more pressing question is: what is the significance of this predigestive action to the entire digestive process?

Question 3: *Are there enough enzymes in raw plant foods to contribute significantly to human digestion and human health?*

As we stated earlier, enzymes in plants are specifically designed to protect and propagate the plant. Digestive enzymes produced in the human body are designed specifically to break down the foods that we consume. While food enzymes can provide some of the initial digestion of protein, fat, and carbohydrate, the quantity of enzymes in food is small relative to the enzyme production that takes place in the pancreas and gastrointestinal tract. For this reason, most experts contend that food enzymes play a relatively minor role in human digestion. Unfortunately, research assessing the enzyme content of plant foods is scarce. Hallelujah Acres' researcher Michael Donaldson measured the amylase in carrot juice.[37] Amylase activity was only 20–30 units per liter of juice. Salivary amylase excretions have about 200 units of amylase per milliliter unstimulated (that is, without our having eaten beforehand).[38] Donaldson concludes:

> Overall, I think the quantity of digestive enzymes present in raw fruits and vegetables is going to be found to be rather small, especially when compared to the amount secreted by the pancreas.

According to enzyme researcher Stephen Rothman:

> I am unaware of any evidence that suggests that enzymes in raw vegetables or fruits, at quantities normally eaten, can substitute for our digestive enzymes or provide substantial assistance in the digestive process. Nor am I aware of any evidence that they pass safely through the acid environment of the stomach or are not rapidly degraded when they reach the intestines. Unless we eat large quantities of raw pancreas, the food we eat does not contain substantial quantities of enzymes to digest it, and those that it does contain are mostly denatured in the stomach before digestion occurs in the intestines.

One study reported that the effects of predigestion were minimal, even with oral enzymes, which are much more concentrated than enzymes in food.[39] Patients with cystic fibrosis (a disease that includes pancreatic insufficiency and minimal pancreatic enzyme secretion) were given either enterically coated enzymes (that is, enzymes in a capsule with a coating that protects the enzymes from stomach acid so they can survive into the small intestine) or enterically coated enzymes plus uncoated enzymes. All of these enzymes were derived from animal tissues. The patients receiving both forms of enzymes did not have a significant improvement in their digestion of food compared to the patients taking only the coated enzymes. This would suggest that predigestion had minimal effect on overall digestion and absorption. Some may argue that the animal enzymes function over a much narrower pH and that plant enzymes would have had a greater impact. While this may be a valid criticism, we would still expect significant action in the upper part of the stomach if this stage of digestion were as critical as some purport it to be.

It is important to note that there are enzymes in plants—apart from those that break down protein, carbohydrate, and fat—that are of value to human health in a very different way. These enzymes, myrosinase and alliinase, help to change phytochemicals in plants to active metabolites with anticancer properties (see page 51 for more information).

Question 4. *Do live food enzymes get absorbed into the bloodstream and have a healing effect on the body?*

Proponents of the food-enzyme theory believe that live enzymes in raw plant foods are able to cross the gastrointestinal tract intact and have a healing effect on the body. The most important scientific evidence for this, they say, comes from a research paper by Michael Gardner at the school of Biomedical Sciences in England titled "Gastrointestinal Absorption of Intact Proteins."[40] In this paper, Gardner concludes: "The concordance between results obtained by independent workers using different experimental approaches is now so strong that we cannot fail to accept that intact proteins and high-molecular fragments thereof do cross the gastrointestinal tract in humans and animals (both neonates and adults)."

We asked Michael Gardner if his research provides evidence of the value of food enzymes to human health. We also asked him if his research proves that enzymes in food pass through the stomach intact and provide subsequent health benefits. He replied as follows:

> There is plenty of sound evidence that small quantities of intact proteins, including enzymes, can be absorbed in their intact form across the gastrointestinal tract. However, this must *not* be interpreted as showing that absorbed enzymes have medicinal benefits. The evidence for this is weak and inconclusive. It is plausible that, in some individuals, some enzymes are absorbed in great enough quantity to have a systemic effect, but I am not aware of good proof of this— certainly not proof that would meet scientific rigor or the various regulatory bodies if such enzymes were being regarded as medicinal products. It is possible or plausible that some food enzymes might have benefit, but proof is lacking.
>
> Even if they do have benefit (I have not studied these claims, which would need to be supported by rigorous objective measurements), any benefit might arise from other constituents. My research has never measured any effects of absorbed enzymes on health. Some of my research, with collaborators, did show a strong indication that absorbed peptides from certain proteins (especially gluten and casein) were likely to have adverse effects on mental health, especially autism and probably schizophrenia. My research and my analysis of a wide range of literature from other scientists does not prove or disprove whether intact proteins in general can pass down through the stomach and into the small intestine

in their intact form; further, the extent of this will depend on the protein, the state of the person's gastric acidity, and the speed of gastric emptying. It would be most foolish to try to generalize on this. Certainly, if it is desired to administer small proteins, *such as insulin*, orally, protection from gastric digestion (mainly by pepsins) is essential. While I am sure that the food-enzyme claims are made in a bona fide way, objective evidence to support the powerful assertion that live foods are incredible life-giving and healing foods is not produced.

Question 5: *Are food enzymes necessary for optimal digestion?*

Many raw-food proponents believe that food enzymes survive the acid environment of the stomach, make it into the small intestine, and play a key role in digestion at this stage. Two reports that specifically address this issue were based on a medical hypothesis written by American biochemists L. J. Prochaska and W. V. Piekutowski in 1994 and 2000.[41, 42] Their enzyme-synergy hypothesis promotes the idea of a synergistic effect of enzymes in food with enzymes in the human body. It is important to recognize that a medical hypothesis does not prove cause and effect, but rather it is an idea that has yet to be conclusively proved.

The basis of the Prochaska and Piekutowski enzyme-synergy hypothesis is as follows: "Enzymes that occur naturally in foodstuffs can act synergistically with those in the human digestive tract to release the maximum amount of thermodynamic free energy from the food. This hypothesis predicts, and in fact, requires that endogenous enzymes in foodstuffs survive digestion until the bolus of food reaches the small intestine. The surviving enzyme molecules in foodstuffs are thought to be required for maximum thermodynamic energy release from consumed foods and that processes such as heating, hydrogenation, and the addition of preservatives into food may denature or inhibit the endogenous enzymes' activities. In this hypothesis, inhibition or destruction of these enzymes is thought to decrease or eliminate the total nutritive value of the ingested foodstuffs. These endogenous enzymes in food then play a central role in the digestion of foodstuffs and are thought to prime the digestive process so that the digestive enzymes can maximally release the thermodynamic energy of ingested food."[41, 42]

The contention that digestion absolutely requires that food enzymes survive the acid of the stomach to the small intestine is not one that is widely held. In fact, if this were true, cooked food would be very poorly digested. Numerous studies have shown that not only is cooked food digestible, sometimes it is more digestible than uncooked food.

The suggestion that cooking completely eliminates the nutritive value of ingested foods is also contentious, as carbohydrates, proteins, fats, vitamins, and minerals are well absorbed from foods whether they are cooked or not. If we could not digest and absorb nutrients from cooked food, people consuming primarily cooked food (which is virtually everyone eating the standard Western diet) would be underweight (due to a lack of available calories from food) and would suffer from multiple vitamin and mineral deficiencies. With over 65 percent of the American population being overweight or obese, we can safely surmise that most people have no problem digesting and absorbing carbohydrates, protein, and fat from cooked food.

However, Prochaska and Piekutowski's hypothesis puts forth some compelling evidence regarding the survival of food enzymes into the small intestine. The authors suggest that enzymes in dairy products, whole grains, and legumes can survive into the small intestine and enhance the digestibility of food. Here is a brief summary of the evidence they provide:

Dairy products. According to the enzyme-synergy hypothesis, dairy yogurt provides the most salient example of enzyme survival through the stomach. Yogurt contains about the same amount of a milk sugar called lactose as fluid milk. In order to digest this sugar, it must be split into glucose and galactose by an enzyme called beta-galactosidase. Yogurt has been shown to be more digestible for people with lactase deficiency (lactase is one member of the family of beta-galactosidases) than other dairy products. This is because the friendly bacteria in yogurt contain beta-galactosidase, which breaks down the lactose (milk sugar) in the small intestine.[43, 44] Beta-galactosidase survives the acid pH of the stomach because these enzymes are packaged within living microorganisms that are able to withstand the acid pH of the stomach to a much greater extent than they could otherwise.[45] These conclusions have been corroborated by other researchers[44, 46] and provide evidence that fermented foods, or foods containing viable microorganisms, improve the survival of enzymes within living microorganisms through the acidity of the stomach.

A similar phenomenon has been reported with fungal enzymes. An interesting report comes from the National Enzyme Company (NEC) of Forsyth, Missouri, an enzyme-manufacturing company, and TNO Nutrition and Food Research in Zeist, Netherlands.[47] The objective of their research was to determine the efficacy of an NEC fungal digestive-enzyme supplement on the digestibility of proteins and carbohydrates. A controlled dynamic gastrointestinal model was used to test the supplements, simulating both healthy human digestion and impaired digestion. The researchers conclude that "NEC fungal enzymes not only survive the acidity of the stomach, but also are active in that harsh environment where most other types of enzymes are inactivated." They add that NEC fungal enzymes should not be enterically coated to protect against stomach acid, because that would serve only to prevent them from working in the stomach. It appears as though these fungal enzymes are afforded protection that is similar to that of beta-galactosidase in yogurt and are better able to withstand stomach acid than food enzymes that are not associated with living microorganisms.

Grains. Prochaska and Piekutowski suggest that cooking impairs the digestibility of phytate (the storage form of phosphorus in plants) because phytase enzymes (the enzymes that break down phytate) are destroyed by the heat. They cite findings from a Swedish research team led by Ann-Sofie Sandberg on phytase activity in ileostomy patients (people who have had surgery to remove the large intestine, with digestion ending at the terminal part of their small intestine).[48] This research demonstrated that phytates are not digestible when heat-treated cereals are consumed but are quite digestible from unheated cereals. The authors of this study suggested that phytase activity may have been lost in the cooked product but not in the raw product. A 1987 study on ileostomy patients by the same team was also cited.[49] In this study, raw wheat bran was compared to heat-treated wheat bran. The authors reported that 95 percent of the phytate in the heat-treated bran was retained compared to only 40 percent in the raw-bran group. The conclusion in this study was also that dietary phytase was likely responsible. While Prochaska and Piekutowski suggest that these studies prove that phytase survives through the stomach, it may be that the phytase activity occurred in the upper part of the stomach. A 1996 study by the same group of Swedish researchers reported that the optimum pH for wheat phytase has been shown to be 5.15, and that wheat phytase activity decreases rapidly when the pH varies from this optimal level.[50] They add that plant phytase is inactivated when the pH is reduced to 2–3. We asked Ann-Sofie Sandberg whether she thought that the phytase survived to the small intestine, and she replied that on the basis of other work their team has completed, phytate is primarily degraded in the stomach, which offers the best conditions for phytate solubility and phytase activity (besides being degraded by enzymes secreted from the microorganisms of the large colon). Recall that the pH of the stomach after we eat can rise to between 4.5 and 5.8. (The optimal pH for phytase activity falls perfectly within this range.) Sandberg adds that phytases are generally poorly active at the intestinal pH, which is too alkaline for phytase activity. On the other hand, microbial phytases are active over a much wider pH range than plant phytases and have been shown to survive at pH levels as low as 1–3 (similar to the pH level of the stomach one hour after we have eaten). This may help to explain why studies using supplemental microbial phytases show their survival into the small intestine.[51] It is important to remember that the most effective way to reduce phytates in grains is to ferment them with phytase-producing microorganisms or to soak and sprout them so that naturally occurring phytases will break down the phytates. [50] For recipe examples, see Herbed Almond Cheese, page 270, and Sprouted Whole-Grain Cereal, page 261.

Legumes. According to the enzyme-synergy hypothesis, legumes provide the strongest evidence that endogenous proteins in food survive the digestive process in humans. Prochaska and Piekutowski contend that beans contain antinutrient proteins, such as protease inhibitors (compounds that block the action of protease enzymes), and lectins that survive stomach acid, so we can expect that the enzymes in beans will also survive. The authors overlook research showing that enzyme inhibitors have a more stable structure than enzymes and are often able to survive the acid pH of the stomach.[52]

The whole question of legumes being a source of enzymes is only relevant for raw or sprouted products, as cooking can deactivate both enzymes and enzyme inhibitors. For the majority of the world's population, legumes are consumed cooked. Sprouting would seem to be an excellent alternative to cooking, as it can deactivate enzyme inhibitors while significantly increasing enzymes. These enzymes degrade enzyme inhibitors and also may be useful for predigestion in the upper part of the stomach, although it is unlikely that most enzymes would survive the acid pH of the stomach after being mixed with

What We Know about Food Enzymes

1. Food enzymes are released when food is chewed or otherwise ground up. The activity of these enzymes is greatest in three locations: before we actually begin eating (for example, while a fruit smoothie is still in the blender or glass), in the mouth, and in the upper part of the stomach.

2. Food is held in the upper part of the stomach for twenty to sixty minutes, averaging about forty minutes. This part of the stomach serves primarily as a reservoir, without the release of hydrochloric acid and with little churning taking place during this time. We do not know precisely how significant this stage of pre-digestion is to the entire digestive process. However, we do know that the chemical breakdown of food occurs mainly in the small intestine. This leads us to the conclusion that food enzymes play a relatively minor role in human digestion.

3. Once food descends to the lower part of the stomach, the pH of the stomach drops from as much as 4.5–5.8 down to 1.3–2.5 and food enzymes are largely denatured or inactivated. Consequently, few food enzymes survive into the small intestine, although this is variable, depending on many circumstances.

4. Food enzymes that are found within viable organisms, such as friendly bacteria in yogurt and microbial or fungal enzymes, appear to have a much greater chance of surviving the acid of the stomach and functioning within the small intestine.

5. Some enzymes, such as myrosinase and allii-nase, help to convert phytochemicals into their active metabolites. These enzymes are degraded by cooking, so selecting raw sources of these enzymes (for example, cruciferous and *Allium* vegetables) may provide a health advantage (see page 51).

gastric juices. However, the use of sprouted legumes is often limited among raw-food practitioners. Some people find sprouted legumes unpalatable or difficult to digest, with the possible exceptions of lentils, chickpeas, mung beans, and peas. In addition, certain legumes, such as soybeans and chickpeas, are relatively high in enzyme inhibitors, even after sprouting (see pages 227–231).

In short, the medical hypothesis offered by Prochaska and Piekutowski provides strong evidence that beta-galactosidase enzymes in cultured dairy products survive stomach acid. The arguments for grains and legumes are less convincing. It would appear as though enzyme action from these foods likely occurs in the upper part of the stomach. Some studies have used supplemental microbial enzymes, and these have been shown to survive over a much broader pH range.

CONCLUSION: Edward Howell was a health pioneer who had tremendous insights about digestion in the early 1900s, when many vitamins had not yet even been discovered and phytochemicals were unheard of. Some of his theories have stood the test of time; others have long since been disproved. Raw food offers many advantages, and food enzymes are among them. There is good evidence that food enzymes play a positive role in health and digestion, although the role appears somewhat different, and less critical, than what proponents of the food-enzyme theory have suggested.

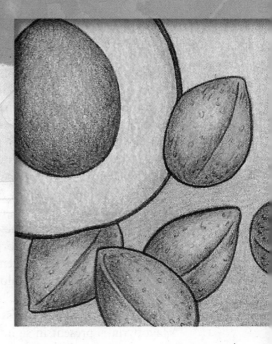

CHAPTER 11

Food Safety: Raw Case Files

You might imagine that edible plants are completely safe. Nature is rarely that simple. While the effects of plants on human health are overwhelmingly positive, there are three things that can turn plants from health heroes into potential villains:

1. Plants often have complex defense systems designed to protect them from predators, and these systems can include toxic chemicals. The same chemicals can be harmful to people too.

2. Whether they grow in the ocean or land, plants can be contaminated with environmental pollutants, such as heavy metals, dioxins, or PCBs.

3. Disease-causing bacteria that originate in the intestines of humans or animals can make their way onto plants.

This chapter provides a glimpse into the world of food safety, selecting six controversial issues of special interest to raw foodists. You will notice the framework for this chapter is based on criminal rap sheets. For each suspect, a charge is laid, evidence is summarized, and a verdict read. Please note that the charges are not statements of fact but rather common accusations made against that suspect food—you will discover whether the accusations are true or false after examining the evidence.

Suspect 001: Buckwheat Greens

Charge: Buckwheat greens (mature shoots with green leaves) contain a toxic compound called fagopyrin and should generally be minimized or avoided in the diet.

Evidence: Fagopyrism is a condition triggered in cattle and sheep by the ingestion of buckwheat greens. It creates a sensitivity to light that causes swelling and irritation of the skin. While fagopyrism has long been recognized in animals, it's a rather recent phenomenon in humans. With it, people (especially those with light-colored skin) experience extreme sensitivity to sunlight, skin irritation, and itching. Affected individuals also report tingling in the hands and face and an increased sensitivity to cold. While buckwheat greens are not traditionally consumed by humans, they have gained popularity as juicing greens by some health advocates.

The most comprehensive examination of fagopyrism in humans was published online by Gilles Arbour, a Canadian man who was affected by the condition after consuming raw juices containing buckwheat greens for an extended period of time.[1] The condition was said to be common among the staff and guests at Ann Wigmore's retreat where buckwheat greens were juiced.[1] Fagopyrin is a red fluorescent pigment in buckwheat. It is most concentrated in the buckwheat flowers, followed by the leaves. Little or no fagopyrin is present in other parts of the plant.[2]

Among the most pressing questions for raw-food adherents is whether fagopyrin is present in significant quantities in buckwheat sprouts (very young shoots before green leaves have developed). This gluten-free food is a popular base for crackers and cereals and is used extensively in raw vegan cuisine. One Korean study reported almost no fagopyrin present in buckwheat sprouts with up to eight days of sprouting.[3] In Korea, where buckwheat sprouts are commonly consumed, it is well known that buckwheat should only be sprouted in the dark. This is because exposure to light causes greening of the plant and an increase in the fagopyrin content. It is said that fagopyrin can be minimized by rinsing the buckwheat three to four times a day, as the fagopyrin will be lost in the pinkish rinse liquid. As buckwheat is normally soaked for twenty minutes, then sprouted for about a day (with regular rinsing), we would expect the fagopyrin to be negligible. Physician and raw-food advocate Gabriel Cousens described two individuals who developed symptoms after eating large quantities of buckwheat sprouts (an amount equal to 20 percent of their total food intake) for six months. No symptoms appeared with lesser intakes by these individuals.[4]

Verdict: Guilty as charged.

Although occasionally consuming fresh juices that include buckwheat greens is unlikely to produce adverse effects, regular consumption of buckwheat greens is ill advised. Buckwheat groats and seeds contain only trace amounts of fagopyrin and don't generally pose a risk. Buckwheat is often sprouted for only a day, but even with longer sprouting times, fagopyrin content appears minimal. However, eating very large amounts of sprouted buckwheat over a long period of time may produce symptoms in some individuals.

Suspect 002: Alfalfa Sprouts

Charge: Alfalfa sprouts contain a toxic compound called L-canavanine (LCN) and should be completely avoided.

Evidence: L-canavanine is a nonprotein amino acid that is structurally similar to the amino acid L-arginine. With regular, high consumption of alfalfa sprouts, L-canavanine can be inadvertently used in place of L-arginine to manufacture proteins in the body. Proteins containing L-canavanine instead of L-arginine cannot perform their usual assigned tasks in the body. These structurally aberrant molecules can disrupt both enzyme activity and metabolism.[5]

There is some evidence that L-canavanine can stimulate or exacerbate symptoms of systemic lupus erythematosus (SLE) and possibly other inflammatory diseases.[5] In 1981, a clinical trial using alfalfa seeds for cholesterol reduction resulted in enlargement of the spleen and reductions in various blood cells in one of the study participants.[6] In 1983, two lupus patients in remission experienced reactivation of their symptoms while taking alfalfa tablets.[7] Four healthy individuals were reported to have developed lupuslike symptoms while consuming twelve to twenty-four alfalfa tablets per day for three weeks to seven months.[8] In the Baltimore Lupus Environmental Study, a significant association between alfalfa consumption and the development of lupus was reported.[9] However, no such association was found in a Swedish study that reported similar alfalfa-sprout intakes in cases and controls.[10]

While it was once thought that germination reduces the content of L-canavanine in alfalfa sprouts, it is now known that L-canavinine increases slightly during germination, regardless of whether it is grown in a dark or light environment.[11]

Verdict: Guilty on a lesser charge.
L-canavanine is a toxic compound and can be dangerous when consumed in high amounts. However, the L-canavanine content of alfalfa sprouts is low and will not generally trigger negative health consequences in healthy individuals. Nevertheless, eating large portions (several cups) of alfalfa sprouts on a daily basis or juicing similar amounts of alfalfa sprouts is not advised. In addition, L-canavanine may be problematic for people with systemic lupus erythematosus, and until evidence to the contrary is available, it would be best for those individuals to minimize or avoid its consumption.

Suspect 003: Sprouted Legumes

Charge: Legumes are high in antinutrients (substances that block the absorption of nutrients), such as hemagglutinins and trypsin inhibitors. Cooking is the only preparation method that breaks down these compounds, so legumes should be avoided in raw vegan diets.

Evidence: To understand antinutrients in legumes and other seeds, it is helpful to explore the seed itself. A legume is the seed or small embryo of a plant, surrounded by a protective covering called a seed coat. Inside the seed coat is stored food (protein, carbohydrates, fat, vitamins, and minerals) along with substances that protect the seed from predators, such as microorganisms, insects, birds,

and animals. Not surprisingly, many of these substances work as antinutrients in human nutrition. These antinutrients include hemagglutinins as well as
compounds that inhibit the action of enzymes such as amylase (which breaks
down starches) and trypsin (which breaks down protein). When a legume is
germinated, enzymes are released to break down these antinutrients so that the
stored starch and protein become available for plant growth. When animals
eat ungerminated legumes, these antinutritional factors can adversely affect
the digestibility of the nutrients that are present. Some of these compounds are
actually toxic. For this reason, there has been considerable research examining
how best to rid plants of these compounds before they are consumed. Most of
this research has been conducted on animals and in test tubes.

Hemagglutinins are proteins that bind to sugar molecules. In excess, they
cause red blood cells to clump together, increase cell division, and interfere with
the transport of nutrients across intestinal-cell membranes. Hemagglutinins are
present in many foods but are most concentrated in legumes, particularly red
kidney beans and small red beans. Approximately one to three hours after a
person consumes raw or undercooked red kidney beans, three to four hours
of debilitating nausea, vomiting, and diarrhea ensue. Hemagglutinins are completely destroyed by conventional cooking practices. Boiling presoaked beans
for thirty minutes or simmering them at 176 degrees F (80 degrees C) for two
hours completely destroys this toxin, as does pressure cooking unsoaked beans
at 250 degrees F (121 degrees C) for fifteen minutes.[12] Germination can reduce
hemagglutinin by 75–100 percent,[13–16] although some studies have shown even
smaller reductions.[17] Despite the fact that the types of hemagglutinins in beans
are toxic, there is some evidence that those in lentils and peas are not.[18]

Trypsin is an enzyme that breaks protein into its component parts (amino
acids) so they can be absorbed into the bloodstream. Trypsin inhibitors are
proteins that block the action of trypsin, thereby reducing protein digestibility
from the food. There are two main families of trypsin inhibitors in legumes: the
Bowman-Birk type (found in most legume species, including soybeans) and the
Kunitz type (found mainly in soybeans). Soybeans are the most concentrated
sources of trypsin inhibitors; amounts in other legumes average only 15–40 percent of the quantity in soybeans.[19] Peas are low in trypsin inhibitors (less than
2–13 percent), while chickpeas and lima beans contain more than most other legumes, about 66 and 77 percent of the levels found in soy, respectively.[20] Studies
have shown that in soybeans, the Kunitz-type inhibitors are completely inactivated by the human gastric juices of the stomach, while the Bowman-Birk-type
inhibitors are impervious to these acidic conditions. As a result, Bowman-Birk-
type inhibitors generally arrive undamaged in the small intestine, decreasing the
digestibility of the protein in the food eaten.[18] When trypsin inhibitors block the
action of trypsin, the pancreas is stimulated to produce more of this enzyme.
This can drain the body's supply of sulfur-containing amino acids that are used
in making trypsin.[21–23] Legumes are already low in sulfur-containing amino acids, so when beans high in trypsin inhibitors are consumed, protein nutrition
could be compromised, especially when protein intakes are marginal.

In some small animals, particularly those fed an experimental diet of raw soybeans or that are injected with pure trypsin inhibitor, this continued stress damages the pancreas, causing the cells that produce digestive enzymes to increase in both size and number.[21, 24] It has been suggested by some raw foodists that trypsin inhibitors would cause similar damage to the pancreas in humans; however, evidence does not support this theory. In larger animals, such as pigs, dogs, cows, and monkeys, the pancreas appears completely unaffected by trypsin inhibitors.[24] Whether or not trypsin inhibitors cause damage to the pancreas seems to depend on the size of the pancreas relative to the total body weight of the animal. Therefore, scientists believe that it is highly unlikely that trypsin inhibitors would cause pancreatic damage in humans.[20] Numerous studies, as shown in table 11.1, below, demonstrate how different food-preparation methods reduce the amount of trypsin inhibitors in various legumes.

Generally, the quantity of trypsin inhibitors in germinated legumes decreases the longer the legumes are sprouted, as the seed slowly releases its store of nutrients until the plant is viable on its own. One study found that inhibitors in lentils were reduced by only 18 percent after six days but were reduced by 45 percent after ten days.[19] Another found that the trypsin inhibitors in soy continued to decline during germination until they were completely gone after thirteen days.[25]

Fermentation appears to produce even greater reductions in trypsin inhibitors than germination. One study tested six different legumes and found 38–47 percent reductions with fermentation.[26] A second study subjected lentils to natural fermentation for four days at 86 degrees F (30 degrees C) and reported a 50–82 percent drop in trypsin-inhibitor activity.[27] Another research team found that fermentation by fungi or bacteria eliminated 97–100 percent of the trypsin inhibitors in cowpeas within thirty-six hours.[28]

Most experts agree that the quantity of trypsin inhibitors that remains when using standard cooking methods does not present a risk to human health.[20, 23] There's evidence that Bowman-Birk inhibitors have both anticancer and anti-

TABLE 11.1 A comparison of preparation methods that reduce trypsin inhibitors in legumes

Preparation method	Percentage of reduction
Boiling[13, 14, 23, 26, 28, 32]	80%–100%
Soaking (at least 16 hours)[14, 27, 28, 33]	10%–20%
Soaking plus dissolved baking soda[28]	24%
Germination[13, 19, 27, 28, 32–40]	15%–65% (average of 30%)*

*The more commonly consumed sprouted legumes tended to fall at the lower end of this range (chickpeas, 34%;[13] mung beans, 22%;[14] and lentils 18–28%[19, 27]).

inflammatory actions,[23, 29] so eating small amounts of this inhibitor over time could offer some protection. However, considerably more trypsin inhibitor remains after germination than after cooking, so its potential negative effect on the digestion of protein may be of greater concern in raw vegan diets compared to mixed vegan diets containing both raw and cooked foods. Test-tube studies examining protein digestibility and protein quality have reported mixed results, with most studies finding little difference in the digestibility of boiled and germinated legumes.[13, 30] This may be because germination reduces phytates (which inhibit protein metabolism) even more than cooking does. At this point, we are uncertain about the health consequences of the increased intakes of trypsin inhibitors associated with raw vegan diets that include sprouted legumes.

Evidence suggests that the total trypsin produced by the average person in a day would be completely inhibited by the trypsin inhibitors contained in 100 grams of raw soybeans (just over one-half cup (125 milliliters).[18] We know that chickpeas contain about 66 percent of the trypsin inhibitors found in soy, while mung beans have about 37 percent and lentils about 25 percent. Using these figures, we can calculate the reduction of trypsin inhibitor that would be experienced by an individual consuming one cup (250 milliliters) of sprouted mung beans, lentils, or chickpeas, as shown in table 11.2, below.

While the significance of these figures is uncertain, the reduction in trypsin caused by eating mung bean or lentil sprouts is not significantly different from what would be produced by eating lightly boiled soybeans. (Approximately 14 percent of trypsin inhibitors remain after soaking and then boiling soybeans for twenty minutes.)[31] Using this very conservative estimate (longer cooking periods would result in greater reduction), if you eat one cup of these lightly cooked soybeans, the trypsin activity in your body would be reduced by approximately 9 percent. This decrease has not been shown to have negative consequences for human health. The much higher levels of inhibitors expected from sprouted chickpeas (compared with sprouted lentils or mung beans) may

TABLE 11.2 Estimated reduction in trypsin activity with the consumption of sprouted legumes

Legume	Reduction in trypsin activity*
1 cup sprouted chickpeas	21%
1 cup sprouted lentils	6%
1 cup sprouted mung beans**	5%

*The reduction in trypsin activity is the amount of trypsin that would essentially be disabled by the trypsin inhibitors contained in the sprouted legumes.

**While mung beans have higher trypsin inhibitors than lentils per 100 grams of unsprouted seed, the effect of one cup of sprouts is lower because mung beans produce a greater volume of sprouts.

be more of a concern, particularly if raw sprouted chickpeas are dietary staples and intakes of the sulfur-containing amino acids are borderline.[1]

Verdict: Mixed.

Many legumes are high in antinutritional factors, such as hemagglutinins and trypsin inhibitors, and these factors are most effectively reduced by cooking. While soaking and sprouting also reduce these factors significantly, about 70 percent of the trypsin inhibitors and up to 25 percent of the hemagglutinins remain. The significance of these findings for human health is not known. It would seem reasonable to limit sprouted legumes that provide high amounts of trypsin inhibitors, such as chickpeas. If using sprouted legumes, lentils and mung beans would appear to be better choices. It is worth noting that when consumed in small quantities as part of a health-promoting diet, many so-called antinutrients have been shown to provide health benefits.

Suspect 004: Mushrooms

Charge: Common edible mushrooms, such as button, crimini (brown), portobello, and shiitake, contain compounds called hydrazines, which are toxic to the liver and are carcinogenic. Shiitake mushrooms contain varying amounts of formaldehyde. Ingestion of shiitake mushrooms may cause dermatitis and photosensitivity in some people. They have also been linked to abdominal distress and abnormal blood counts in some individuals. Cooking mushrooms reduces or eliminates these toxic compounds, whereas raw mushrooms generally contain significant amounts. For this reason, raw mushrooms are best avoided.

Evidence: Common cultivated mushrooms, including button, crimini (brown), and portobello, contain hydrazines, which have been shown to be both carcinogenic and mutagenic in animals and in laboratory tests.[41, 42] Although they are suspected to be human carcinogens, more evidence would be required for definitive proof.[43-45] A Swedish research group estimated the carcinogenicity of a hydrazine in mushrooms called agaritine by figuring that the consumption of an average of 4 grams (1 tablespoon) of mushrooms per day would contribute to a lifetime cumulative cancer risk of about two cases per 100,000 lives.[46] It's important to recognize that while hydrazines appear carcinogenic, there are also studies suggesting that extracts of cooked white button mushrooms could be protective against breast cancer and prostate cancer.[47-49] These studies suggest that certain fatty acids and phytochemicals in mushrooms depress the activity of the enzyme aromatase, which is required for estrogen synthesis. A study following over 2,000 Chinese women reported a 64 percent reduction of breast cancer risk in those women who ate one-third of an ounce or more of mushrooms every day compared to those who did not eat mushrooms.[50]

Most methods of food preparation decrease the content of agaritine in mushrooms. Simply storing mushrooms in the refrigerator reduced agaritine by 25 percent in six days and 50 percent in fourteen days. Boiling mushrooms reduced agaritine up to 88 percent, one minute of microwaving decreased agaritine by about 65 percent, and frying resulted in about a 50 percent reduction. Dry baking was not as effective, with only a 23 percent reduction in ten minutes of baking time.[42] Canned mushrooms retain little agaritine, about 90 percent less than fresh mushrooms.[41] Dehydrating mushrooms at 77 degrees F (25 degrees C) for twenty-four hours resulted in an 18 percent reduction, while dehydrating them at 122 degrees C (50 degrees C) for seven to eight hours resulted in a 24 percent reduction.[42]

To our knowledge, no studies have examined whether marinating mushrooms affects their agaritine content. However, one study found that when agaritine (isolated from mushrooms) was kept in an open container with tap water, it was completely degraded within 48 hours. In closed containers, just under 50 percent of the agaritine remained after 120 hours. These findings show that agaritine breakdown is accelerated with exposure to oxygen. Temperatures ranging from 40 to 72 degrees F (4 to 22 degrees C) did not significantly affect agaritine levels, while a more acid pH resulted in significantly greater reductions than a more neutral pH.[51] It's possible that marinating mushrooms in lemon juice or vinegar for several hours may produce significant reductions in agaritine but, unfortunately, no studies have yet been done to confirm this hypothesis.

Fruits and vegetables, along with other living organisms, contain naturally occurring formaldehyde in the range of 2–60 milligrams per kilogram. While these levels are thought to pose little threat to health, higher amounts (100–406 milligrams per kilogram) have been reported in dried shiitake mushrooms.[52] One study suggests that the levels of formaldehyde detected in shiitake mushrooms exceeds safe limits.[31] Another study found that cooking shiitake mushrooms for six minutes produces significant reduction in formaldehyde levels, whereas storage for up to ten days had no effect on formaldehyde levels. (Interestingly, the authors of this study did not agree that the usual levels of formaldehyde in shiitake mushrooms were likely to pose an appreciable health risk.)[53]

Studies have also noted that shiitake mushrooms can cause dermatitis and photosensitivity in some individuals;[54, 55] however, this effect is not seen when the mushrooms are thoroughly cooked.[55] Finally, daily consumption of 4 grams (1 tablespoon) of shiitake mushroom powder (sixteen capsules, or the equivalent of four medium-sized dried mushrooms) for up to ten weeks resulted in abdominal discomfort and abnormal blood counts in seventeen of forty-nine patients in a cholesterol-lowering study and five out of ten patients in a study designed to investigate these effects.[56] Some experts suggest that shiitake mushrooms should be thoroughly cooked prior to consumption.[57–59] On the other hand, one of the key active compounds in shiitake mushrooms, lentinan, has been shown to have immune-regulating, antiviral, and anticancer activities.[60–62] Lentinan has been approved for use as a drug in Japan (generally as an adjunct to chemotherapy).[63]

Verdict: Mixed.

Hydrazines, such as agaritine, are considered probable human carcinogens. However, there is insufficient evidence to demonstrate beyond a reasonable doubt that human consumption of button, crimini (brown), and portobello mushrooms poses a serious threat to health. Conversely, while eating raw mushrooms is a common practice, it may not be risk free. It's worth noting that most of the favorable reports on mushrooms have been based on the cooked product. It seems reasonable to limit our exposure to hydrazines when possible, so limiting the amount of raw mushrooms we eat seems well advised. We know that dehydrating mushrooms results in small reductions in agaritine; however, reductions are less than what is achieved in cooking. There is a possibility that marinating mushrooms, particularly using an acidic medium, such as lemon juice or vinegar, is as effective at reducing agaritine as cooking, although further research is needed before we can be assured of this. Raw foodists who wish to eat raw mushrooms may be wise to marinate them overnight prior to their use. It is advisable to cook shiitake mushrooms prior to consumption. Finally, it's common knowledge that collecting wild mushrooms is risky business and is best done only by those who have the necessary expertise. (Most wild edible mushrooms are also safer when cooked.)

Suspect 005: Sea Vegetables

Charge: Sea vegetables are sources of heavy metals, particularly arsenic. Hijiki contains unsafe levels of inorganic arsenic and should be avoided.

Evidence: Sea vegetables have long been prized for their ability to behave like sponges, accumulating a rich supply of the ocean's minerals. Unfortunately, these nutritionally unique plants are also notorious for soaking up heavy metals, especially arsenic, from polluted waters. Generally, the type of arsenic that accumulates in sea vegetables is the less toxic form called organic arsenic. Exposure to organic arsenic has not been associated with adverse health consequences. However, inorganic arsenic is toxic. According to a 1981 World Health Organization (WHO) report, an ingested dose of 70–180 milligrams (70,000–180,000 micrograms) of arsenic (III) oxide (an inorganic form of arsenic) can prove fatal in humans.[64] Acute toxicity causes fever, vomiting, and diarrhea, and in severe cases, multiorgan failure. Chronic toxicity has been linked to nerve damage, respiratory disorders, skin lesions, and cancer. The Joint FAO/WHO Expert Committee on Food Additives set a provisional tolerable weekly intake for inorganic arsenic at 15 micrograms per kilogram of body weight.[65] For a person weighing 150 pounds (70 kilograms), this would amount to an upper limit of approximately 1 milligram (1,000 micrograms) per week.

Analyses done by governments in Canada, the United Kingdom, Hong Kong, and New Zealand have found high levels of inorganic arsenic in hijiki. In 2001, the Canadian Food Inspection Agency (CFIA) put out an advisory for consumers to avoid consuming hijiki. By 2005, health protection agencies in the United Kingdom, Hong Kong, Australia, and New Zealand had followed suit.[66-69] Government findings were later confirmed by independent research teams, as shown in table 11.3, page 234.

TABLE 11.3 Arsenic amounts in hijiki and other sea vegetables per kilogram (2.2 pounds) dry weight

Sea vegetables	Total arsenic (dry weight) mg/kg	Inorganic arsenic (dry weight) mg/kg
Hijiki[73]	68–149	42–117
Hijiki[74]	124	67–96
Hijiki[70]	92–132	65–105
Other sea vegetables[73]	4.1–116	0.14–1.44

Given the ranges of inorganic arsenic reported in hijiki (an average of 83 milligrams per kilogram/2.2 pounds), consumption of 7–15 grams (0.25–0.50 ounces) dry weight of hijiki could exceed the recommended upper limit of 1 milligram (1,000 micrograms) per week. (One-half cup/125 milliliters of dried hijiki weighs about 10 grams, or one-third ounce.) It's important to note that these figures are for dried sea vegetables, and most people soak and drain sea vegetables prior to consumption. Studies suggest that approximately 50 percent of the arsenic is lost with recommended soaking procedures. Cooking further reduces the initial concentrations to about 10 percent of the original levels.[70] There is some suggestion that the alginates in sea vegetables actually bind with heavy metals, rendering them indigestible and causing them to be quickly eliminated from the body. However, most of the evidence for this has been based on animal studies. In order to clarify the metabolism of arsenic from hijiki in humans, a research team from Japan investigated the fate of arsenic in a healthy volunteer who consumed 330 grams of a processed hijiki food (hijiki-bean combination) containing 0.869 milligrams (869 micrograms) of inorganic arsenic and 1.253 milligrams (1,253 micrograms) total arsenic, which is approximately the recommended upper limit. The researchers noted that the volunteer's urinary excretion of arsenic was comparable to that of someone with arsenic poisoning.[71]

A report of arsenic toxicity from kelp supplements led to an evaluation of arsenic in commercial kelp supplements. Of nine samples tested, eight showed levels higher than that deemed acceptable by the U.S. Food and Drug Administration.[72]

Verdict: Guilty on a lesser charge.
Although eating an occasional small serving of hijiki at your favorite restaurant may not be harmful, regular consumption of larger quantities seems ill advised, at least until evidence suggests otherwise. Intakes of inorganic arsenic from hijiki are generally overestimated, as losses of approximately 50 percent are incurred with soaking. However, the risk is greater for consumers of raw

hijiki, as they don't benefit from the reductions in arsenic that occur with heating. If you use kelp supplements, be sure that they're tested for heavy metals, and don't exceed intakes suggested on the label. While other sea vegetables have not been found to have high levels of inorganic arsenic, sea vegetables are known to absorb other heavy metals, such as cadmium and lead, and should be consumed in moderation.[73]

Suspect 006: Sprouts

Charge: Raw sprouts are a potential source of pathogenic bacteria and are best avoided.

Evidence: The three most prominent outbreaks of foodborne illness in the United States in 2008 were traced to hot peppers (chiles) and tomatoes (imported from Mexico), cantaloupes (imported from Honduras), and domestic peanuts. While most people associate food pathogens with animal products, such as fish, raw eggs, and undercooked hamburger or chicken, becoming a raw-food vegan is no guarantee you'll avoid food poisoning.

Food pathogens include a variety of organisms that contaminate food and make people sick. Symptoms of infection range from diarrhea, fever, vomiting, abdominal cramps, and dehydration to multiple organ failure and death.[75] The vast majority of cases go unreported, although the U.S. Centers for Disease Control and Prevention estimates that every year approximately 76 million people are infected and 5,000 die.[76, 77]

Most pathogenic bacteria originate in the intestines of animals or people. They usually make their way from animal or human intestines to our produce through the "back door." Fruits and vegetables may be grown in fresh manure and irrigated or washed with water that is contaminated by manure. Pathogens can be introduced from infected workers who handle the food in the field, in packing houses, or at the point of purchase. They can be transferred from a contaminated food to a clean food by a knife or other utensil, or through contact with a contaminated cutting board. Improper storage or holding conditions can also support bacterial growth. In the majority of cases, the original source of contamination can be traced back to concentrated animal-feeding operations (also known as factory farms). Livestock in the United States produce more than thirteen times the excrement of the entire American population, and unlike human waste, it goes largely untreated. Man-made lagoons on factory farms hold millions of gallons of pathogen-laden waste, which commonly seeps into waterways. This water may then be used for crop irrigation, resulting in pathogens being sprayed directly on our food.[78] This applies both to conventional and organic crops.

Heating food to an internal temperature above 160 degrees F (78 degrees C) effectively wipes out most pathogenic bacteria.[79] Animal products, such as meat, poultry, fish, and eggs, are almost always cooked prior to consumption. Food safety guidelines suggest very specific internal temperatures should be reached to ensure that pathogenic bacteria is destroyed. Dairy products are generally pasteurized to eliminate dangerous bacteria. Fruits, vegetables, and sprouts are less frequently cooked, and in raw diets they are rarely, if ever, cooked. Storing perishable foods at 40 degrees F (4.5 degrees C) helps to reduce the growth of bacteria. Washing produce can reduce contamination, but it does not always eliminate it.[80]

Alfalfa sprouts and other raw sprouts pose a unique challenge, as pathogens lurk in the tiny cracks and crevices of seeds. Even miniscule numbers of pathogens can multiply to millions during the sprouting process. This is because the best condition for growing sprouts is also the ideal medium for breeding bacteria. The pathogens most commonly associated with sprouts are *Salmonella* and *Escherichia coli* O157:H7, or *E. coli* (the leading cause of kidney failure in children). From 1990 to 2005, sprouts caused thirty-three outbreaks in North America: twenty-eight from alfalfa sprouts, four from mung bean sprouts, and one from clover sprouts. In a 2007 public meeting conducted by the FDA, an official of the Centers for Disease Control (CDC) reported that sprouts were implicated in 20 out of 168 outbreaks of all produce-related single food outbreaks between 1998 and 2004.[81] As a result, health authorities in the United States and Canada have issued warnings about the consumption of raw sprouts and advise high-risk groups (the elderly, young children, pregnant women, and people with weakened immune systems) to avoid eating raw sprouts altogether.[82, 83]

While the evidence against sprouts looks rather incriminating, it's important to remember that it's not sprouts or sprout seeds that are at the root of the problem; rather, it is manure from the concentrated livestock operations on factory farms. The first critical step to ensuring sprout safety is to begin with clean seeds. There is considerable debate as to how to best accomplish this task. For commercial sprouting, the U.S. Food and Drug Administration (FDA) currently recommends that seeds be treated with 20,000 ppm calcium hypochlorite (bleaching powder) prior to germination, and that sprouts and spent irrigation water samples be periodically tested for pathogens;[84, 85] however, organic sprout growers would lose their organic status if they used this method.[86] One solution would be for the FDA to endorse a more eco-friendly method for disinfecting sprouts. A simple alternative would be the use of dry heat. A study out of Cornell University in New York found that exposing mung beans and alfalfa seeds to 131 degrees F (55 degrees C) in an incubator for at least four days effectively eliminated *E. coli* and *Salmonella* pathogens without affecting germination rate.[87]

For home sprouting, consumers need to acquire sprouting seeds from a reputable dealer and disinfect them at home prior to sprouting. A researcher from Japan subjected seeds to a ninety-second hot-water bath (194 degrees F/90 degrees C), followed by immersion in chilled water for thirty seconds. No viable pathogens remained in the seeds, none were detected during the sprouting process, and germination was not significantly affected.[88] The findings of a microbiologist from Norringham University in the UK show exceptional results using hot water alone.[89] Finally, the University of California at Davis provides a handout on safe sprouting at home. They suggest heating the seeds on a stovetop for five minutes in a 3 percent hydrogen peroxide solution preheated to 140 degrees F (60 degrees C), followed by a cold rinse.[90]

Verdict: Not guilty.

While there is no doubt that sprouts can be contaminated with dangerous pathogenic bacteria, this does not mean that you must forever forgo this popular raw food. You can purchase sprouting seeds from reputable suppliers and further disinfect sprout seeds at home prior to sprouting them. If you purchase sprouts from a store, get to know your growers and find out what procedures they follow to ensure safe sprouts. Be selective at the supermarket, carefully checking to make sure the sprouts look fresh; keep them refrigerated and wash them thoroughly under cold running water before consuming them.

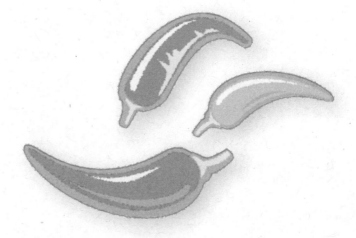

CHAPTER 12

Nutrition Guidelines and Menus

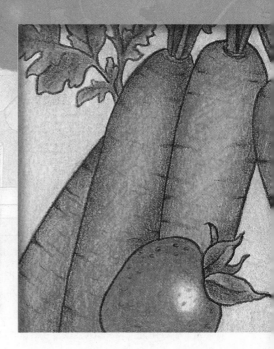

Creating a daily menu for raw vegan diets that includes all of the necessary vitamins, minerals, protein, and essential fats can be a bit of a challenge. The standard national food pyramids and food guides are not very helpful, since meat, milk, and grains form the majority of the food groups. In this chapter we provide guidelines and tips for raw meals and menus to make it easy for you to meet your optimum nutrition needs.

As in earlier chapters, we use as standards the Dietary Reference Intakes (DRIs), which have been developed by nutritional scientists. Although these were not developed specifically for people on raw vegan diets (unfortunately, such standards do not exist), the DRIs are based on an immense body of research about human requirements. DRIs are sometimes discounted as possible guidelines for raw menus, in part because it is believed that these standards cannot be met, especially for minerals and protein. However, in this chapter we illustrate how raw vegan diets can meet the DRIs for every nutrient.

There are numerous and diverse ways to accomplish this. At one end of the spectrum are the fruit-centered diets that include greens, seeds, and nuts. At another end are diets that include plenty of sprouted and fermented, or living, foods. You may wish to include sprouted or cooked legumes or sprouted grains in an otherwise raw diet. Your chosen way of eating can be entirely raw or high-raw, or you may just want to increase the proportion of raw food in your diet. You can enjoy elegant meals and wow your friends with fancy recipes, or you can eat very simply and keep preparation to a minimum. With well-planned menus, any of these approaches can keep you in excellent health.

In this chapter, we use as a standard the recommended nutrient intakes of healthy adults, apart from those who are pregnant and lactating. We do not include raw menus that meet the needs of infants, children, or teens. These topics

Top Ten Tips for Optimum Health on a Raw Vegan Diet

1. **Variety.** Include an assortment of raw plant foods: fruits, greens, peas and other vegetables, seeds, and nuts. Consider also incorporating sprouted grains and sprouted lentils and mung beans for additional calories and nutrients. If the diet is not 100 percent raw, cooked legumes, grains, and starchy vegetables can also make valuable contributions to overall nutrient intake.

2. **Greens.** Make the calcium-rich, low-oxalate greens (such as broccoli, bok choy, dandelion greens, kale, mustard greens, napa cabbage, turnip greens, and watercress) the backbone of every day's menus. It is wise to include greens at least twice a day in your meals or snacks, using a total of about 1⅓ pounds (600 grams) of greens on most days.

3. **Other vegetables.** Enjoy an assortment of vegetables in the full spectrum of colors. Vegetables are more nutrient dense than any other food.

4. **Fruits.** Fruits are a sweet, delicious, and vitamin-rich part of raw vegan diets. Their high sugar content can affect your dental health, so be sure to brush your teeth regularly and balance your menus with the other food groups that are higher in protein and minerals and lower in sugar.

5. **Seeds and nuts.** For protein and minerals, it's a good idea to include at least ½–⅔ cup (125–185 milliliters) of seeds and nuts each day in your menus. Include in this mix at least 2 teaspoons (10 milliliters) of ground flaxseeds, 2 tablespoons (30 milliliters) of walnuts, or 1 teaspoon (5 milliliters) of flaxseed oil, as these will top up your day's supply of essential omega-3 fatty acids. A little more may be necessary to get a good balance of omega-3 and omega-6 fatty acids (see page 122). When it comes to minerals and protein, seeds tend to be even more nutritious than nuts. The fat in seeds and nuts helps with the absorption of minerals and provides protective phytochemicals.

6. **Sprouted or cooked legumes.** Sprouted lentils and mung beans will help keep your blood sugar level between meals. If you include some cooked food in your menus, cooked legumes (such as a bowl of beans from a salad bar, or lentils, peas, or beans in a warm soup) would be a wise choice because they provide protein, iron, and zinc and contain very little fat.

7. **Sprouted grains.** Some people include sprouted grains (such as kamut and rye) or foods that are used as grains (such as buckwheat and quinoa) in the form of raw or dehydrated cereals and crackers. Another option, though it is not raw, is bloomed wild rice (see page 295). These carbohydrate- and protein-rich foods can help maintain your energy levels.

8. **Vitamin B_{12}.** Be certain to include a daily or weekly vitamin B_{12} supplement or use Red Star Vegetarian Support Formula nutritional yeast or other foods fortified with vitamin B_{12} as your source of this essential nutrient. (For more details, see page 166.)

9. **Vitamin D.** Make sure you have a source of vitamin D in the form of sunlight or a supplement. (For more details, see page 151.)

10. **Iodine.** Use a little kelp, iodized table salt, or a supplement that includes iodine for an intake of this mineral that meets recommended levels. When you eat significant amounts of cruciferous vegetables, such as broccoli, cabbage, and kale, or ground flaxseeds, it is especially important to maintain an adequate intake of iodine. (For more details, see page 187.)

are beyond the scope of this book and, at this time, there is insufficient research to establish safe guidelines that are based on a substantial body of evidence.

Supplements as a Safety Measure

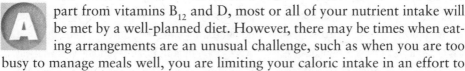

part from vitamins B_{12} and D, most or all of your nutrient intake will be met by a well-planned diet. However, there may be times when eating arrangements are an unusual challenge, such as when you are too busy to manage meals well, you are limiting your caloric intake in an effort to lose weight, you are traveling or are in other circumstances that restrict your food intake, or you are uncertain that you are meeting optimal nutrient intakes with diet alone. In such situations, a multivitamin-mineral supplement that has a wide range of minerals and vitamins (including vitamins B_{12} and D) at recommended levels can be a wise and reassuring choice. (See table 8.2, page 154, and table 9.2, page 185, for the adult DRIs for vitamins and minerals.)

Typical multivitamin-mineral supplements are low in calcium compared to the DRIs; otherwise, the pill would be too large to swallow. Therefore, in order to get significant amounts of calcium (preferably accompanied by vitamin D), you will need to take a separate calcium supplement, although it can be taken at the same time as your vitamin-mineral supplement.

Many brands of multivitamin-mineral supplements advise taking several tablets to meet the DRI or daily value (DV). Since most of what you need will come from your diet, you likely will do well with just one multivitamin-mineral supplement plus one calcium tablet per day or every few days. Aside from vitamin B_{12} (which can be taken either alone or as part of a multivitamin supplement), single-nutrient supplements are generally not the best choice, in part because the nutrients so often work as teams, and also because high intakes of one mineral (such as zinc) can interfere with absorption of another (such as copper).

Weight Management

ell-designed raw vegan diets are a powerful and effective choice for healthful weight loss. In addition to following a well-planned diet, make regular exercise part of your regimen for good health. If your weight drops to unhealthy levels or you suspect nutritional deficiencies, modify your diet to meet recommended intakes, making sure you obtain sufficient calories and protein. If necessary, enlist the support of a qualified health professional.

Menus for Excellent Health

n the pages that follow, you will find six raw vegan menus that meet the DRIs, providing that you include supplementary vitamin B_{12} (see page 166), a source of vitamin D (see page 151), and a little kelp or

Food Combining Theory and Fact

Food combining, a concept used in planning some raw diets, originates from a 1911 theory developed by New York physician Howard Hay. Hay took an interest in the research of 1904 Nobel Prize–winner Ivan Pavlov on the digestive process of dogs. Hay concluded that digestion is easier if we don't simultaneously eat foods that require different amounts of time to break down. Experimenting with his own diet during a time of ill health, Hay changed from a pattern of large meals that regularly featured meat with potatoes and white bread to a diet of whole foods with a much greater emphasis on plant foods. He eliminated cigarette smoking, lost weight, and regained his health. Hay's guidelines became the foundation for a system of food combining. The guidelines for this way of eating stated, for example, that "proteins" (meaning the food group that includes meat, poultry, fish, nuts, and legumes) interfere with good digestion when combined with starchy vegetables (such as potatoes), grains, or sweet fruit, but that "proteins" could be eaten with green leafy vegetables.

Since these origins, various proponents have adapted the food-combining principles by classifying foods into four to nine categories. The foods in each category are said to combine well or poorly with foods in other categories. For instance, it is said that fats do not combine well with fruits or starches; protein does not combine well with starches, fruits do not combine well with anything other than leafy greens, and melons do not combine well with any other foods. Food-combining rules can be complicated, and the permissible combinations differ depending on the presenter's interpretation, personal experience, and preferences. We now recognize that that food-combining theories have significant limitations and drawbacks. At the same time, we can learn from them.

LIMITATIONS

- Food combining was based on a belief that if a protein and a starch are eaten together, the body will wear itself out by producing both alkaline and acidic digestive juices, which nullify each other and impair digestion. This is simply not true. Since this theory was first developed, physiologists have learned that the stomach is always acidic and the small intestine is always alkaline, no matter what foods are eaten. When a plant food that contains

iodized salt for sodium and iodine (see page 187). Water or herbal tea can be added as desired. Each menu is presented at three different calorie levels:

- a basic 2,000-calorie menu
- a 2,500-calorie, higher-protein version of this menu, with a few added items
- a 1,600–1,700-calorie variation of the basic menu

The higher-calorie version is suitable for someone who is larger or more active. Athletes may further increase their calorie, protein, and iron intakes by increasing portion sizes or including more foods. The lower-calorie menu is designed for someone who is smaller, less active, or trying to lose weight. In a few cases where noted, the DRIs are not met for every nutrient. The recipes on pages 256–301 are used in the menus.

mostly carbohydrate is consumed, digestion starts with the salivary amylase in the mouth, then moves on to the acidic environment of the stomach, and continues in the small intestine. When a food high in protein is eaten, major steps in the digestive process take place in the stomach, due to the acidity there. These are followed by enzymatic actions that occur in the alkaline environment of the small intestine.

- Every whole plant food, without exception, contains protein, fat, *and* carbohydrate. The body is well adapted to digest these natural combinations.

- Scientific evidence to support the food-combining theories is lacking.

- Some combinations that break food-combining rules can be helpful to the body. For example, the vitamin C in many of the fruits listed in table 8.2 (page 154) can help to increase the absorption of iron from the iron-rich plant foods listed in table 9.4 (page 198). Also, the fat in foods such as seeds and avocados assists our absorption of minerals, fat-soluble vitamins, and phytochemicals from greens and other foods eaten at the same time.

POSITIVE INSIGHTS

- The century after Hay's theory was proposed was also the century in which the science of nutrition was born. Our understanding of digestion has evolved from where it was in 1911, yet Western science can learn from Eastern concepts of nutrition and from cultures such as Japan that place a greater emphasis on digestive health. A gap remains between Western scientific concepts and the subjective observations about digestion that form the core of food combining.

- Taking an interest in food combining can help people to simplify their meals and improve digestion. For example, some raw foodists have discovered that it works well for them to eat fresh fruit early in the day, and to wait a while before rounding out the menu with other foods.

- Indigestion may be improved by avoiding certain food combinations. If you experience bloating, gas, or indigestion, keep a journal of your eating habits and symptoms. This can help to determine whether certain foods or combinations cause difficulty. (Other factors, such as stress and uncomfortable emotions, can affect digestion too.)

Two menus have the option of either sprouted or cooked legumes and sprouted grains, buckwheat, or quinoa (menus 1 and 2). Two of the menus are centered on fruit, with added greens, seeds, and nuts (menus 3 and 4). Menu 4 is presented in terms of the weights of the different food groups for a day, rather than meals. Menu 5 requires little preparation apart from washing the produce. Menu 6 is a more gourmet approach, with a lovely dinner that is suitable for a celebration.

In practice, you may vary these menus; they are intended to illustrate how raw foods can be used to meet scientific recommendations. You might replace a lunch item with a Thai Spring Roll with Spicy Pecan Sauce (page 292). You may dine on Spicy Mexican Salad (page 288), Avocado Dip (page 269), and Salsa Flax Crackers (page 266), or set out a Whole Meal Salad Bar (page 296) in place of the supper listed. You don't need to meet the DRI for every nutrient every day, but aim to meet these as average intakes over time.

Menu 1

LIGHT AND NUTRITIOUS

This menu provides adequate protein, calcium, iron, zinc, other minerals, and vitamins, and is moderately low in fat. To maintain energy through the morning, some people like to have the juice first and the smoothie as a midmorning break. The ground flaxseeds, which provide omega-3 fatty acids, can be sprinkled on one of the other menu items if you prefer. The salad bar choices may be mixed into a salad or arranged on a plate.

BREAKFAST AND THROUGH THE MORNING

2 cups (500 ml) Green Giant Juice (page 259)

Blueberry-Kale Smoothie (page 258)

LUNCH

Whole Meal Salad Bar (page 296) choices: 4 cups (1 L) romaine lettuce, 1 cup (250 ml) kale, 1 tomato, ½ red sweet pepper, ¼ cucumber, 1 rib celery, 1 sheet nori, 1 cup (250 ml) sprouted mung beans (page 282)

¼ cup (60 ml) Avocado Dip or Spread (page 269), thinned with a little lime juice, lemon juice, or Nama Shoyu and used as dressing

SUPPER

2¼ cups (560 ml) Sprouted Quinoa Tabouli (page 290)

1¼ cups (310 ml) V-8 Vegetable Soup (page 274)

SNACKS OR DESSERTS

¼ cup (60 ml) pumpkin seeds

4 medjool dates, or 4 Coconut Macaroons (page 298)

2 pieces fresh fruit (such as 1 mango and 1 apple)

Nutritional analysis for menu: calories: 2005, protein: 59 g, fat: 60 g, carbohydrate: 364 g (198 g from sugar), dietary fiber: 71 g, calcium: 1132 mg, copper: 3850 mcg, iron: 33 mg, magnesium: 821 mg, phosphorus: 1553 mg, potassium: 8424 mg, sodium: 1245 mg, zinc: 12 mg, thiamin: 2.4 mg, riboflavin: 2.6 mg, niacin: 32 mg, vitamin B_6: 4 mg, folate: 1031 mcg, pantothenic acid: 6.8 mg, vitamin B_{12}: 1.0 mcg, vitamin A: 3036 mcg, vitamin C: 915 mg, vitamin E: 16 mg, vitamin K: 3399 mcg, omega-6 fatty acids: 14 g, omega-3 fatty acids: 4 g

Percentage of calories from: protein 11%, fat 24%, carbohydrate 65%

Note: About 85 percent of the sugar in this menu comes from fruit; the remainder comes from other vegetables and whole plant foods. The vitamin B_{12} comes from Vegetarian Support Formula nutritional yeast.

For a 2,500-calorie menu: For supper, increase the amount of Sprouted Quinoa Tabouli to 4½ cups (1,120 ml). For snacks, include both the 4 dates and 4 Coconut Macaroons and add 1 tablespoon (15 ml) of nuts or seeds or an extra piece of fruit.

For a 1,600–1,700-calorie menu: Omit the pumpkin seeds as a snack in the 2,000-calorie menu and have just 2 dates or 2 Coconut Macaroons.

Menu 2

ENJOYING NATURE'S BOUNTY

In this menu, lunch includes a choice of sprouted or cooked legumes. Unlike nuts and seeds, legumes allow menus to have higher protein, iron, and zinc, while contributing less fat. Items listed for breakfast, lunch, supper, or snacks may be interchanged.

BREAKFAST

2 cups (500 ml) Sprouted Whole-Grain Cereal (page 261)

³/4 cup (185 ml) Sunflower-Hemp Milk (page 260)

LUNCH

5 cups (1,250 ml) Build-Your-Bones Salad (page 278)

¹/2 cup (125 ml) sprouted lentils (see sidebar, page 289) or cooked beans

3 tablespoons (45 ml) Lemon-Tahini Dressing (page 275)

SUPPER

2 cups (500 ml) Garden Blend Soup (page 273)

¹/4 cup (60 ml) Pumpkin Seed Pâté (page 268)

4 Sunny Rye Crackers (page 265)

1 large tomato

SNACKS OR DESSERTS

2 oranges or other fruit

1 cup (250 ml) blueberries

1 cup (250 ml) Tutti-Frutti Ice Cream (page 301)

Nutritional analysis for menu: calories: 2015, protein: 79 g, fat: 80g, carbohydrate: 301 g (112 g from sugar), dietary fiber: 65 g, calcium: 1026 mg, copper: 4650 mcg, iron: 29 mg, magnesium: 869 mg, phosphorus: 1914 mg, potassium: 6141 mg, sodium: 1180 mg, zinc: 19 mg, thiamin: 5.4 mg, riboflavin: 3.6 mg, niacin: 45 mg, vitamin B$_6$: 5.4 mg, folate: 977 mcg, pantothenic acid: 10 mg, vitamin B$_{12}$: 1.4 mcg, vitamin A: 2833 mcg, vitamin C: 1000 mg, vitamin E: 37 mg, vitamin K: 2630 mcg, omega-6 fatty acids: 36 g, omega-3 fatty acids: 9 g

Percentage of calories from: protein 14%, fat 32%, carbohydrate 54%

For a 2,500-calorie menu: For breakfast, increase the Sunflower-Hemp Milk to 1½ cups (375 ml) and top the cereal with ¼ cup (60 ml) Crunchy Granola (page 262). For lunch, increase the Lemon-Tahini Dressing to 6 tablespoons (90 ml). Include an additional snack or dessert of a Chocolate-Cranberry Nut Ball (page 299) or a small piece of fruit.

For a 1,600–1,700-calorie menu: For breakfast, decrease the Sunflower-Hemp Milk to ½ cup (125 ml). For supper, omit the Pumpkin Seed Pâté. For snacks or dessert, omit either the Tutti-Frutti Ice Cream or the 2 pieces of fruit and berries. In this menu, the calcium drops to 940 milligrams.

Menu 3

FRUIT, GREENS, SEEDS, AND NUTS

For a mainly fruit menu to meet the DRIs, plenty of fruit is needed. Here we have 5 pounds (2.3 kilograms) of fruit that were chosen for their mineral contributions. The greens, nuts, and seeds add protein, essential fats, and other minerals—otherwise, this would be "the sugar diet." The large green salad takes a while to chew; in choosing this way of eating, you will need to make time for leisurely meals! The dressing provides omega-3 fatty acids. The breakfast items can be blended together to form a smoothie, or they can be served as a fruit salad or fruit platter on or beside the lettuce. Also, you may replace the strawberries and peaches with other berries and seasonal fruit. Menu 4 (page 247) is a more general version of this menu, providing weights instead of quantities to allow for easy shopping.

BREAKFAST AND THROUGH THE MORNING

2 cups (500 ml) strawberries, 2 peaches, 2 oranges, 2 cups (500 ml) romaine lettuce

LUNCH

4 cups (1 L) Three Melon Salad (page 291)

SUPPER

Whole Meal Salad Bar (page 296) choices: 4 cups (1 L) romaine lettuce, 3 cups (750 ml) napa cabbage, 2 cups (500 ml) kale

3 cups Raw Veggies (see sidebar, page 286)

¼ cup (60 ml) Liquid Gold Dressing (page 276)

SNACKS OR DESSERTS

⅓ cup (85 ml) currants, or 4 dried figs

¼ cup (60 ml) Nama Shoyu Sunflower Seeds, Pumpkin Seeds, or Almonds (page 297) or plain almonds and sunflower or pumpkin seeds

1 pound (454 g) fruit (such as 2 cups/500 ml berries, 1 banana, and 2 apricots)

Nutritional analysis for menu: calories: 1975, protein: 53 g, fat: 61 g, carbohydrate: 359 g (183 g from sugar), dietary fiber: 74 g, calcium: 1009 mg, copper: 3510 mcg, iron: 23 mg, magnesium: 618 mg, phosphorus: 1236 mg, potassium: 8240 mg, sodium: 1010 mg, zinc: 24 mg, thiamin: 5.5 mg, riboflavin: 4.9 mg, niacin: 47 mg, vitamin B_6: 6.2 mg, folate: 1260 mcg, pantothenic acid: 9.4 mg, vitamin B_{12}: 2.4 mcg, vitamin A: 1959 mcg, vitamin C: 958 mg, vitamin E: 24 mg, vitamin K: 1344 mcg, omega-6 fatty acids: 19 g, omega-3 fatty acids: 11 g

Percentage of calories from: protein 10%, fat 25%, carbohydrate 65%

For a 2,500-calorie menu: For supper, increase the Liquid Gold Dressing to 6 tablespoons (90 ml) and add another 1½ pounds (680 g) of berries and other fruit for snacks or desserts.

For a 1,600–1,700-calorie menu: Adjust the snacks or desserts in the 2,000-calorie menu by omitting the currants and the seeds or almonds or by omitting the pound of fruit. With these changes, the calcium in this menu drops to about 930 milligrams.

Menu 4

FRUIT, GREENS, NUTS, AND SEEDS (BY WEIGHT)

This fruit-based plan meets the DRIs, providing that you add sources of vitamins B$_{12}$ and D and a sprinkle of kelp for iodine and sodium. Along with a wide variety of fruits, it includes low-oxalate green veggies plus nuts and seeds. The nutritional analysis that follows includes a cross section of the foods mentioned. The specific items chosen could vary from day to day and include others that are not listed. Kale can be added to smoothies, thinly sliced for use in salads, or enjoyed in one of the delicious recipes in chapter 13.

FRUIT (ABOUT 5 POUNDS/2.25 KILOGRAMS), SUCH AS:

4 cups (1 L), 1½ pounds (680 g) melons: cantaloupe, honeydew, and/or watermelon

4 cups (1 L), 1¼ pounds (600 g) berries (such as blackberries or raspberries)

4 citrus fruits (14 oz/400 g) (such as oranges or tangerines)

3 whole fruits (12 oz/350 g) (such as apricots, bananas, or mangoes)

2 cups (250 g) cherries or chopped fruit (such as apples, durians, or peaches)

GREENS (ABOUT 1.32 POUNDS/600 GRAMS), SUCH AS:

5 cups (145 g) chopped lettuce or other leafy greens

3 cups (260 g) broccoli florets and stalks

3 cups (200 g) kale or broccoli leaves, thinly sliced or in smoothies

NUTS AND SEEDS (0.2 POUNDS/90 GRAMS), SUCH AS:

¼ cup (35 g) almonds

¼ cup (35 g) seeds (such as pumpkin or sunflower)

3 tablespoons (16 g) ground flaxseeds

1 Brazil nut

Nutritional analysis for menu: calories: 1995, protein: 60 g, fat: 64 g, carbohydrate: 350 g (178 g from sugar), dietary fiber: 84 g, calcium: 1070 mg, copper: 3920 mcg, iron: 23 mg, magnesium: 896 mg, phosphorus: 1532 mg, potassium: 7525 mg, sodium: 311 mg, zinc: 12 mg, thiamin: 2.4 mg, riboflavin: 2.1 mg, niacin: 29 mg, vitamin B$_6$: 3.5 mg, folate: 789 mcg, pantothenic acid: 7 mg, vitamin B$_{12}$: 0 mcg, vitamin A: 3041 mcg, vitamin C: 1067 mg, vitamin E: 23 mg, vitamin K: 2069 mcg, omega-6 fatty acids: 16 g, omega-3 fatty acids: 8 g

Percentage of calories from: protein 11%, fat 26%, carbohydrate 63%

For a 2,500-calorie menu: Increase the total weight of the fruits and nuts and seeds by 25–30 percent.

For a 1,600–1,700-calorie menu: Adjust the 2,000-calorie menu by decreasing the watermelon, bananas, and mango by about 1 pound (.45 kilogram), while retaining 4 pounds (1.75 kilograms) of the fruits, such as berries and apricots, which are more mineral-rich, and keeping the amounts of greens, nuts, and seeds the same.

Menu 5

NO-FUSS, RAW-FOOD FUN

This menu is helpful when you need to cut preparation to a minimum, such as when you are traveling or are away from home for the day. The tahini and juice from an orange can be stirred or shaken together in a little jar. A mini blender can be useful while traveling, as it will allow you to create smoothies, raw soups, and dressings or dips for veggies. Figs, oranges, tahini, and greens (lettuce, snow peas, and broccoli) are rich in calcium.

BREAKFAST

2 cups (500 ml) raspberries

3 fresh or dried figs

4 cups (1 L) romaine lettuce

ALTERNATIVE BREAKFAST

1 serving Blue Crush (page 257)

LUNCH AND SNACKS THROUGHOUT THE DAY

2½ cups (400 grams) snow peas

4 oranges

3 ripe bananas

1 cup (250 ml) cherry tomatoes

Trail mix: ⅓ cup (80 ml) walnuts,
1 Brazil nut, ¼ cup (60 ml) currants

SUPPER

Corn from 2 cobs

1 cup (250 ml) broccoli florets

1 cup (250 ml) carrot strips

1 cup (250 ml) sliced zucchini

Vegetable dip: ¼ cup (60 ml) sesame tahini mixed with ¼ cup (60 ml) orange juice

News Flash!

Every day innovative, high-quality raw products are finding their way into the marketplace. These products provide a convenient way to boost the nutritional value of meals, snacks, and smoothies. See page 346 for a brief list of recommended products and sources.

Nutritional analysis for menu: calories: 2057, protein: 60 g, fat: 64 g, carbohydrate: 361 g (167 g from sugar), dietary fiber: 78 g, calcium: 1025 mg, copper: 3430 mcg, iron: 21 mg, magnesium: 676 mg, phosphorus: 1613 mg, potassium: 7087 mg, sodium: 262 mg, zinc: 11 mg, thiamin: 3.3 mg, riboflavin: 2.0 mg, niacin: 32 mg, vitamin B$_6$: 3.8 mg, folate: 1108 mcg, pantothenic acid: 11 mg, vitamin B$_{12}$: 0 mcg, vitamin A: 1874 mcg, vitamin C: 838 mg, vitamin E: 10 mg, vitamin K: 374 mcg, omega-6 fatty acids: 30 g, omega-3 fatty acids: 4.3 g

Percentage of calories from: protein 11%, fat 25%, carbohydrate 64%

Note: This menu is a little low in vitamin E and in its ratio of omega 3 to omega-6 fatty acids. Vitamin E and balance can be restored on another day with flaxseed oil (for example, in a dressing as in menu 3).

For a 2,500-calorie menu: Increase the fruits, nuts, and vegetables throughout the day by 25 percent, according to your preferences.

For a 1,600–1,700-calorie menu: Adjust the 2,000-calorie menu by omitting the currants, 1 banana, and 1 cob of corn.

Menu 6

RAW GOES GOURMET

This menu is a pleasure when you want to impress guests with the delights of raw cuisine. The food is delicious!

BREAKFAST AND THROUGH THE MORNING

1½ cups (375 ml) Pink Cadillac Smoothie (page 256)

2 large fresh or dried figs

LUNCH

1 serving Celeriac Linguine with Bolognese Sauce and Hemp Parmesan (page 280)

3 cups (750 ml) Raw Veggies (see sidebar, page 286) served on 3 inner leaves of romaine lettuce

SUPPER

2½ cups (625 ml) Creamy Zucchini Soup (page 272)

2½ cups (625 ml) Kale Salad with Orange-Ginger Dressing (page 287)

1 serving Mango Pie with Coconut Crust (page 300)

SNACK OR DESSERT

1 cup (250 ml) grapes

Nutritional analysis for menu: calories: 2022, protein: 57 g, fat: 95 g, carbohydrate: 283 g (162 g from sugar), dietary fiber: 56 g, calcium: 821 mg, copper: 4260 mcg, iron: 25 mg, magnesium: 657 mg, phosphorus: 1585 mg, potassium: 6508 mg, sodium: 2982 mg, zinc: 12 mg, thiamin: 5.8 mg, riboflavin: 5.1 mg, niacin: 47 mg, vitamin B_6: 6.6 mg, folate: 726 mcg, pantothenic acid: 7.8 mg, vitamin B_{12}: 2.6 mcg, vitamin A: 1771 mcg, vitamin C: 886 mg, vitamin E: 19 mg, vitamin K: 962 mcg, omega-6 fatty acids: 31 g, omega-3 fatty acids: 6 g

Percentage of calories from: protein 10%, fat 39%, carbohydrate 51%

Note: This menu and its variations are higher in fat, omega-6 fatty acids, and sodium, and lower in calcium than menus 1 through 5.

For a 2,500-calorie menu: For breakfast, replace the figs with a hearty serving of Marvelous Muesli (page 264) plus ½ cup of Sunflower-Hemp Milk (page 260) or fruit juice.

For a 1,600–1,700-calorie menu: Adjust the 2,000-calorie menu by omitting the pie. Another option is to replace the Celeriac Linguine with Bolognese Sauce and Hemp Parmesan with V-8 Vegetable Soup (page 274) at lunch and to enjoy the whole dinner, including the pie.

For excellent information about shopping, foods to keep on hand, care and storage of produce, equipment (such as essential kitchen tools, juicers, food processors, blenders, and dehydrators), eating raw while traveling, weight management, and enjoying raw meals in cold weather, see *The Raw Food Revolution Diet* by Cherie Soria, Brenda Davis, and Vesanto Melina.

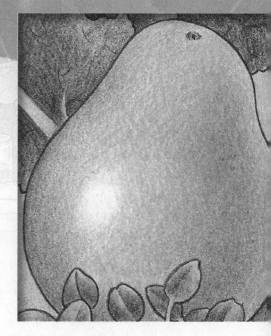

CHAPTER 13

Recipes

Welcome to this special collection of recipes that represents a cross section of raw eating styles. Many of these recipes require only the most basic equipment—a knife and a cutting board. We recommend that your first investment be a good chef's knife, if you do not already have one. For other recipes, you may need a blender, a food processor, a dehydrator, or a juicer. A more detailed discussion related to this equipment is included in chapter 4 of *The Raw Food Revolution Diet* by Cherie Soria, Brenda Davis, and Vesanto Melina. There you will find additional outstanding recipes.

How to Approach the Recipes

✔ Read each recipe through before you start. This will help ensure that it turns out successfully.

✔ Make the recipe exactly as it is written the first time you try it. After that, use your creativity to adapt it to your taste.

✔ Look for ingredients that are listed in **bold type**. This means a step needs to be completed before you start, such as soaking the ingredient.

✔ Look at the variations listed below many recipes, as you may find a version you prefer.

✔ Replace raw ingredients with the conventional form if necessary. Some raw ingredients—such as almond butter, tahini, oat groats, and rolled oats—may be a challenge to find. The conventional (not raw) versions may be substituted measure for measure.

✔ Select the ingredient options that you prefer or that are most readily available. Some recipes list two options for an ingredient—for example, one raw (such as Nama Shoyu) and one that was exposed to heat during processing (such as tamari). Either one may be used.

✔ Adjust the number of servings to suit your needs. Serving sizes are suggested for each recipe (in the yield or at the beginning of the nutritional analysis). However, we recognize that appetites vary immensely, and what could typically be enough to serve several people might be a single serving for one hungry, high-energy person.

The following recipes were developed and selected because of their nutritional value, simplicity, and flavor. We hope that they will get you off to a great start and add a little excitement to your current recipe repertoire. May these offerings be a blessing to your body and soul.

BEVERAGES

CEREALS AND CRACKERS

SPREADS, DIPS, AND CHEESES

SOUPS

SALAD DRESSINGS

MAIN DISHES AND SALADS

SNACKS AND SWEETS

NOTES ON THE NUTRITIONAL ANALYSES

- The nutritional analysis provided for each recipe does not include optional ingredients.
- Where two or more choices are given for an ingredient, the analysis is based on the first choice unless otherwise stated.
- Where there is a range in the amount of an ingredient, the smaller amount is used for the analysis.
- Metric measures were used for the analyses.
- Certain nutrients, such as choline, chromium, manganese, molybdenum, and selenium, are not included due to insufficient data.
- Although we list a specific amount of each nutrient per serving of a recipe, the actual amount will vary due to genetic differences in plant varieties, growing conditions, and farming practices.
- We used tamari rather than Nama Shoyu for the nutritional analyses because of the data available for it.
- We did not include whole flaxseeds in the analyses other than their fiber contribution because whole flaxseeds tend to pass through the gastrointestinal tract undigested.
- Most of the values for sugar in the nutritional analyses reflect naturally occurring sugars in fruits and vegetables. Added sugars, such as those from maple syrup, also are included in this figure.
- The value for niacin is represented by "mg NE" (milligrams of niacin equivalents).
- The value for folate is represented by "mcg DFE" (micrograms of dietary folate equivalents), which is the form found in food.
- The value for vitamin A is represented by "mcg RAE" (micrograms of retinol activity equivalents).

CALCULATING THE FAT IN RECIPES

The amounts of protein, fat, and carbohydrate are listed in grams in the nutritional analyses. Then at the bottom of the analysis is the percentage of calories that comes from protein, fat, and carbohydrate. Note that 45 percent or less calories from fat is very different from 45 percent or less of the food's *weight* coming from fat. From three energy-giving nutrients (protein, carbohydrate, and fat), protein and carbohydrate yield *approximately* 4 grams per calorie and fat yields *approximately* 9 grams per calorie. (These numbers are not exact and can vary slightly from one food to another.) Food weight includes water, which is calorie free, so when a food contains 15 percent fat by weight, depending on the water content, the percent of calories from fat could be a much higher number. For example, a California avocado can be 15 percent fat by weight, with about 30 grams of fat in a 200-gram avocado. Thirty grams of fat at 9 calories per gram equals 270 calories; this means that 270 of the total 336 calories in the avocado are from fat. As a result, approximately 80 percent of the avocado's calories are derived from fat.

PERCENTAGES OF PROTEIN, FAT, AND CARBOHYDRATES

You may recall the recommendation that a minimum of 10 percent of the calories in your overall diet should be derived from protein (page 93). Carbohydrates should make up approximately 45–75 percent of calories, while fat will generally range from 15 to 45 percent of calories for a healthy adult following a raw diet. (For more on this, see chapters 5, 6, and 7.) Though similar, the recommended range for fat extends slightly beyond the range advised by the World Health Organization and the Institute of Medicine's Acceptable Macronutrient Distribution Range (AMDR), allowing for a wider variety of healthful raw eating patterns (see chapters 5, 6, and 7). For individuals with chronic diseases, such as coronary artery disease, and who are on therapeutic diets aimed at disease reversal, recommended fat intakes may drop to 10 percent of calories from fat.

While we suggest upper and lower limits of protein, fat, and carbohydrates in raw vegan diets, the amounts in individual recipes will not necessarily fit neatly into these ranges. Some recipes will fall above or below these guidelines. For example, Tutti-Frutti Ice Cream (page 301) and Three-Melon Salad (page 291) provide fewer than 10 percent of calories from protein. This need be not a concern, as the 10 percent minimum refers to the average of all foods that are consumed during the day. The low percent of calories from protein in fruits can be boosted by adding seeds, nuts, and plenty of greens to the diet. A salad with dressing can be low in carbohydrates and typically provide more than the maximum 45 percent of calories from fat that is recommended for the whole diet. These percentages will be balanced by other plant foods in a varied raw diet. High intakes of fat can be offset by choosing more fruits, vegetables, grains, and legumes, because most of these foods provide 10 percent or less of their calories from fat. (See table 5.3, page 80.)

Smoothies

Smoothies have a lot going for them: vibrant colors, fruity aromas, and readily available and easily absorbed vitamins and protective phytochemicals. They are the ultimate healthful fast food—a smoothie can be prepared in minutes by almost anyone and can be made with fresh or frozen fruit. Don't have time for breakfast? Make a smoothie and take it with you!

Develop your own favorite combinations and, in doing so, consider the hues of the ingredients. Although blueberries, kale, and mango are a nutritious combo, they create a less-than-appealing brown when blended, whereas foods that are closer on the color spectrum can be gorgeous together.

This beautifully colored smoothie is a wonderful pick-me-up and a great vitamin C booster, with about double your daily requirement per serving. It provides potent antioxidants and anticancer agents.

Pink Cadillac **SMOOTHIE**

MAKES 3 CUPS (750 ML); 2 SERVINGS

Frozen Bananas

Use frozen bananas to make thick smoothies or Tutti-Frutti Ice Cream (page 301). Select ripe bananas, as they are much sweeter and have a less-starchy aftertaste. Peel the bananas and leave them whole or break them into chunks. A squeeze of lemon juice sprinkled over the fruit will keep it from turning brown. Put the bananas in zipper-lock freezer bags or airtight containers and freeze them. Frozen bananas will keep for several weeks, depending on their ripeness and the temperature of your freezer.

1 ½ cups (375 ml) **freshly squeezed orange juice**

1 cup (250 ml) **fresh or frozen sliced mango**

1 cup (250 ml) **fresh or frozen strawberries**

Combine all of the ingredients in a blender. Process until smooth.

Per 1½ cups (375 ml): calories: 169, protein: 2 g, fat: 1 g, carbohydrate: 41 g (33 g from sugar), dietary fiber: 3 g, calcium: 43 mg, copper: 220 mcg, iron: 1 mg, magnesium: 39 mg, phosphorus: 61 mg, potassium: 645 mg, sodium: 4 mg, zinc: 0.2 mg, thiamin: 0.2 mg, riboflavin: 0.1 mg, niacin: 1.9 mg, pyridoxine: 0.2 mg, folate: 89 mcg, pantothenic acid: 0.6 mg, vitamin B$_{12}$: 0 mcg, vitamin A: 54 mcg, vitamin C: 167 mg, vitamin E: 1 mg, omega-6 fatty acids: 0.1 g, omega-3 fatty acids: 0.1 g

Percentage of calories from: protein 5%, fat 4%, carbohydrate 91%

This meal-in-a-glass makes an excellent breakfast, snack, or emergency meal. This is a tasty way to boost your intake of vitamins, minerals, fiber, protein, and omega-3 fatty acids. If you like, toss in a supplement, such as calcium with vitamin D, a multivitamin, or a vitamin B_{12} tablet. Although you can use seeds and nuts that are not presoaked, soaking will increase their nutrient availability. If you prefer, remove the skins from the almonds (see sidebar, page 271). Smoothies that contain flaxseeds are best served immediately; if they stand for a while, the soluble fiber from the flaxseeds will make them gummy.

Blue CRUSH

MAKES 4 CUPS (1 L); 2 SERVINGS

1½ cups (375 ml) water

¼ cup (60 ml) **almonds, soaked in ½ cup (125 ml) water for 8–12 hours, drained and rinsed,** or 2 tablespoons (30 ml) raw almond butter (see sidebar, page 263)

2 tablespoons (30 ml) **sunflower seeds, soaked in ¼ cup** (60 ml) **water for 4–12 hours, drained, and rinsed,** or 2 tablespoons (30 ml) hempseeds

2 cups (500 ml) fresh or frozen blueberries

1½ cups (375 ml) chopped kale, romaine lettuce, or other greens

1 large fresh or frozen ripe banana (see sidebar, page 256)

1 tablespoon (15 ml) ground flaxseeds (optional)

Combine the water, almonds, and sunflower seeds in a blender. Process until smooth. Add the blueberries, kale, and banana. Process until smooth and creamy. Add the optional flaxseeds. Blend for a few more seconds. If you prefer, thin with a little water or juice. Serve immediately.

Creamy Blue Crush: For a creamier beverage, replace the water with Sunflower-Hemp Milk (page 260) or another nondairy milk, or add one-quarter to one-half of a ripe avocado.

Strawberry-Orange Crush: Omit the kale and replace the water with freshly squeezed orange juice. Substitute strawberries for the blueberries and add one-quarter to one-half of a ripe avocado, if desired.

Sweet Blue Crush: For a sweeter beverage, replace the water with fresh fruit juice.

Per 2 cups (500 ml): calories: 333, protein: 10 g, fat: 15 g, carbohydrate: 49 g (25 g from sugar), dietary fiber: 10 g, calcium: 144 mg, copper: 670 mcg, iron: 2.9 mg, magnesium: 130 mg, phosphorus: 214 mg, potassium: 796 mg, sodium: 29 mg, zinc: 1.7 mg, thiamin: 0.4 mg, riboflavin: 0.4 mg, niacin: 4.7 mg, vitamin B_6: 0.6 mg, folate: 60 mcg, pantothenic acid: 1.2 mg, vitamin B_{12}: 0 mcg, vitamin A : 415 mcg, vitamin C: 85 mg, vitamin E : 9.3 mg, vitamin K: 465 mcg, omega-6 fatty acids: 5.4 g, omega-3 fatty acids: 0.3 g (with hempseeds and flaxseeds: omega-6 fatty acids: 4.1 g, omega-3 fatty acids: 2.6)

Percentage of calories from: protein 11%, fat 36%, carbohydrate 53%

Made with the most nutritious ingredients you can find, this thick smoothie is a winner. It is low in fat and a rich source of calcium and omega-3 fatty acids. If you do not plan to drink it all immediately, omit the flaxseeds, as otherwise it will thicken over time.

Blueberry-Kale SMOOTHIE

MAKES 2½ CUPS (625 ML); 1 SERVING

2 cups (500 ml) coarsely torn kale

1¼ cups (310 ml) blueberries

1 fresh or frozen ripe banana (see sidebar, page 256)

1 orange, peeled

¾ cup (185 ml) water

1 tablespoon (15 ml) ground flaxseeds

Put the kale, blueberries, banana, orange, and water in a blender. Process until smooth and creamy. Add the flaxseeds. Blend for a few more seconds. If you prefer, thin with a little water or orange juice. Serve immediately.

Per whole recipe: calories: 199, protein: 5 g, fat: 3 g, carbohydrate: 45 g (24 g from sugar), dietary fiber: 8 g, calcium: 138 mg, copper: 390 mcg, iron: 2 mg, magnesium: 70 mg, phosphorus: 99 mg, potassium: 766 mg, sodium: 33 mg, zinc: 1 mg, thiamin: 0.2 mg, riboflavin: 0.2 mg, niacin: 2.7 mg , vitamin B_6: 0.5 mg, folate: 62 mcg, pantothenic acid: 0.6 mg, vitamin B_{12}: 0 mcg, vitamin A: 520 mcg, vitamin C: 130 mg, vitamin E: 1.3 mg, vitamin K: 566 mcg, omega-6 fatty acids: 0.5 g, omega-3 fatty acids: 1.1 g

Percentage of calories from: protein 9%, fat 11%, carbohydrate 80%

This juice is rich in superstars from the bone-building team. The greens in this recipe supply plenty of calcium, vitamin A (beta-carotene), vitamin K, and folate. As a bonus, the calcium from kale is about twice as available to the body as the calcium from cow's milk.

Green Giant JUICE

MAKES 3 CUPS (750 ML); 2 SERVINGS

1 **bunch** (about 8 ounces/220 g) **kale, including stems**

½ head romaine lettuce

1 cucumber, quartered lengthwise

1 apple, cored and quartered

4 ribs celery

1 lemon, peeled and quartered

1 **piece** (1 in/3 cm) **ginger** (optional)

Juice all of the ingredients. Serve immediately.

Juicing Kale with Different Juicers

Centrifugal juicer. Centrifugal juicers are not efficient at juicing greens and are not recommended.

Champion Juicer. If you use a Champion Juicer, roll the kale leaves tightly and feed them through the chute in small quantities. To maximize the yield, put the pulp through the juicer a second time.

Green Power Juicer. If you use a Green Power or Green Star Juicer, feed the stem end of the leaves in first and allow the twin gears to pull the leaves through the gears. You do not need to chop or roll the leaves.

Per 1½ cups (375 ml): calories: 57, protein: 5 g, fat: 0.4 g, carbohydrate: 8 g, dietary fiber: 3 g, calcium: 155 mg, copper: 110 mcg, iron: 1.4 mg, magnesium: 48 mg, phosphorus: 119 mg, potassium: 835 mg, sodium: 111 mg, zinc: 0.6 mg, vitamin C: 16 mg, vitamin E: 1.5 mg, omega-6 fatty acids: 0.1 g, omega-3 fatty acids: 0.2 g

Percentage of calories from: protein 36%, fat 7%, carbohydrate 58%

While almond milk is a favorite of raw-food adherents, it requires several steps, including squeezing the milk through a porous bag to remove the almond pulp. This recipe provides a quick and easy alternative. If you prefer a thick, creamy milk, use the smaller amount of water; for a thinner milk, use the larger amount. Unlike most commercial nondairy milks, which are white, Sunflower-Hemp Milk is creamy beige, though the color is not noticeable in smoothies or when poured over cereal. You can make this milk with seeds that are not presoaked; however, soaking starts the germination process, which reduces phytates, thereby increasing mineral availability.

Sunflower-Hemp **MILK**

MAKES 4 TO 5 CUPS (1 TO 1.25 L)

3 to 4 cups (750 ml to 1 L) water

½ cup (125 ml) **sunflower seeds, soaked in 1 cup** (250 ml) **water for 4–12 hours, drained, and rinsed**

¼ cup (60 ml) **hempseeds**

¼ teaspoon (1 ml) **vanilla extract** (optional)

Pinch **salt** (optional)

1 ripe **banana**

Put 1 cup (250 ml) of the water and all of the sunflower seeds, hempseeds, vanilla extract, and optional salt in a blender. Process on high speed until thick and creamy. Add the remaining 2 to 3 cups of water and the banana. Process until smooth. Refrigerate until thoroughly chilled. Serve cold. Sunflower-Hemp Milk does not keep well, so it is best to make just what you can use within 24 hours.

VARIATION: For longer storage, replace the banana with 3 pitted dates or 2 teaspoons (10 ml) of maple syrup or other sweetener, and use 3 cups (750 ml) of water. Process as directed. Store in a glass jar in the refrigerator for 3 to 4 days.

Per cup (250 ml): calories: 168, protein: 6 g, fat: 11 g, carbohydrate: 13 g (4 g from sugar), dietary fiber: 5 g, calcium: 32 mg, copper: 400 mcg, iron: 1.7 mg, magnesium: 73 mg, phosphorus: 133 mg, potassium: 230 mg, sodium: 5 mg, zinc: 1 mg, thiamin: 0.4 mg, riboflavin: 0.1 mg, niacin: 1 mg, pyridoxine: 0.2 mg, folate: 47 mcg, pantothenic acid: mg, vitamin B$_{12}$: 0 mcg, vitamin A: 1 mcg, vitamin C: 3 mg, vitamin E: 6.2 mg, vitamin K: 0.6 mcg, omega-6 fatty acids: 6.4 g, omega-3 fatty acids: 1.4 g

Percentage of calories from: protein 14%, fat 58%, carbohydrate 29%

Note: Vitamin values and most mineral values for hempseeds are not available; therefore, most of the values provided in the nutritional analysis below are actually lower than they would be if this data were available.

This whole-grain cereal is a far cry from the flaked or puffed boxed cereals many of us grew up on. If whole-grain cereals were placed in a hierarchy of healthfulness, this one would sit unrivaled at the top. Serve Sprouted Whole-Grain Cereal with Sunflower-Hemp Milk (page 260) or other nondairy milk, and top it with Crunchy Granola (page 262), if desired.

Sprouted Whole-Grain CEREAL

MAKES ABOUT 4 CUPS (1 LITER); 2 SERVINGS

3 cups (750 ml) chopped fresh or thawed frozen fruit and/or berries

½ cup (125 ml) **sprouted grains** (see sidebar)

3 tablespoons (45 ml) **nuts and seeds, soaked for 4–12 hours, drained, and rinsed**

1 tablespoon (15 ml) ground flaxseeds

Combine all of the ingredients in a medium bowl. Serve immediately.

TIP: Be creative with your fruit combinations and use locally grown organic produce, if possible. Freezing fresh fruits and berries will allow you to enjoy them during winter, when they are out of season. The liquid from thawed frozen fruits, especially berries, makes a lovely addition to this cereal.

Per one-half recipe (2 cups/500 ml): calories 242, protein: 8 g, fat: 9 g, carbohydrate: 37 g (9 g from sugar), dietary fiber: 15 g, calcium: 94 mg, copper: 420 mcg, iron: 2.6 mg, magnesium: 112 mg, phosphorus: 191 mg, potassium: 446 mg, sodium: 8 mg, zinc: 1.8 mg, thiamin: 0.2 mg, riboflavin: 0.2 mg, niacin: 3.6 mg, pyridoxine: 0.2 mg, folate: 42 mcg, pantothenic acid: 1 mg, vitamin B$_{12}$: 0 mcg, vitamin A: 3 mcg, vitamin C: 49 mg, vitamin E: 4.8 mg, vitamin K: 15 mcg, omega-6 fatty acids: 2.2 g, omega-3 fatty acids: 1.2 g

Percentage of calories from: protein 12%, fat 32%, carbohydrate 56%

Note: Analysis was done using raspberries, sprouted wheat, and almonds.

Sprouted Grains

MAKES ABOUT 2 CUPS (500 ML)

Almost any whole grain can be sprouted. Try barley, kamut, rye, spelt, triticale, or wheat, or try a combination of whole grains.

½ cup (125 ml) whole grains

Put the grains in a quart (1 L) mason jar. Cover the grains with water and let soak at room temperature for 24 hours.

Put a sprouting lid on the jar or a piece of mesh or cheesecloth secured with a wide elastic band. Drain and rinse the grains a few times, or until the water is almost clear. (If you, like you can save the rinse water for your plants or garden.) Place the jar at a 45-degree angle over a saucer (to collect any water that may run off) or in a dish rack.

Rinse the grains several times a day. They will be ready to use when they have a small sprout, about ¼ inch (0.6 cm) or smaller. This will take a day or two, depending on the temperature and humidity of your kitchen. (If the sprouts get much longer, they will acquire a grassy taste. They will still be nutritious, just less palatable.) Once the sprouts have reached the desired length, they can be refrigerated to slow their growth so you can enjoy them for several days.

Reminiscent of traditional baked granola, which typically contains oil and sugar, our delicious raw version is moistened and sweetened with almond butter and dried fruit. Soak Crunchy Granola in Sunflower-Hemp Milk (page 260) just before serving to soften it, and top it with fresh fruit. Alternatively, try Crunchy Granola as a topping on Sprouted Whole-Grain Cereal (page 261) or as a snack when you go hiking.

Crunchy GRANOLA

MAKES 18 CUPS (4.5 L); 36 SERVINGS

3 cups (750 ml) dried fruit (one kind or a mixture)

1½ cups (375 ml) almost-boiling water

¾ cup (180 ml) raw almond butter (see sidebar, page 263)

2 apples, cored and quartered

2 ripe bananas

1 tablespoon (15 ml) ground cinnamon

1 teaspoon (5 ml) vanilla extract

10 cups (2.5 L) rolled oats (see sidebar, page 264)

1 cup (250 ml) whole or chopped almonds, soaked for 6 hours, drained, and rinsed

1 cup (250 ml) pumpkin seeds, soaked for 6 hours, drained, and rinsed

1 cup (250 ml) sunflower seeds, soaked for 6 hours, drained, and rinsed

1 cup (250 ml) unsweetened shredded dried coconut (optional)

1 cup (250 ml) walnuts, whole or coarsely chopped

½ cup (125 ml) flaxseeds, soaked for 10–30 minutes in 1 cup (250 ml) water (do not drain)

Soak the dried fruit in the almost-boiling water for about 30 minutes. Transfer the soaked fruit and its soaking water to a food processor. Process into a paste, stopping occasionally to scrape down the sides of the work bowl with a rubber spatula. Add the almond butter and process for a few more seconds. Add the apples, bananas, cinnamon, and vanilla extract. Process for a few more seconds, just until the mixture is fairly smooth, stopping as needed to scrape down the sides of the work bowl.

Combine the oats, almonds, pumpkin seeds, sunflower seeds, optional coconut, walnuts, and flaxseeds in a large bowl. Add the fruit mixture. Stir until well combined.

Spread the granola onto five 14-inch (35-cm) square dehydrator trays lined with nonstick sheets, or see the tip that follows. Dehydrate at 115 degrees F (46 degrees C) for about 24 hours, or until dry and crispy. Break the granola apart or crumble it into chunks. Stored in sealed glass jars, Crunchy Granola will keep for 1 month at room temperature or 3 months in the refrigerator.

TIP: If you use 9 dehydrator trays with 2 cups (500 ml) of the granola mix spread thinly on each tray, the granola will be easier to break apart than if it is spread over fewer trays.

Granola Cookie Chunks: Using a table knife, score each tray of the mix with 5 lines in both directions to make about 36 Granola Cookie Chunks per tray.

Per ½ cup (125 ml): calories: 287, protein: 9 g, fat: 15 g, carbohydrate: 33 g (11 g from sugar), dietary fiber: 6 g, calcium: 59 mg, copper: 360 mcg, iron: 2.5 mg, magnesium: 96 mg, phosphorus: 221 mg, potassium: 348 mg, sodium: 27 mg, zinc: 1.5 mg, thiamin: 0.3 mg, riboflavin: 0.1 mg, niacin: 1.9 mg, pyridoxine: 0.14 mg, folate: 30 mcg, pantothenic acid: 0.6 mg, vitamin B_{12}: 0 mcg, vitamin A: 1 mcg, vitamin C: 1 mg, vitamin E: 4.2 mg, vitamin K: 1 mcg, omega-6 fatty acids: 4 g, omega-3 fatty acids: 0.8 g

Percentage of calories from: protein 12%, fat 44%, carbohydrate 44%

How to Make Raw Almond Butter

MAKES 1¼ CUPS (10 OUNCES)

2 cups raw almonds

Instead of using commercial almond butter, which is available raw or roasted, you may choose to make your own. Pulverize the almonds into a paste in a food processor, stopping as needed to scrape down the sides of the work bowl with a rubber spatula. This will take about 10 minutes. Alternatively, process the almonds through a Green Star or Champion Juicer using the blank attachment. Stored in a sealed glass jar, Raw Almond Butter will keep for 1 month in the refrigerator.

Muesli is a favorite European breakfast cereal that was first developed around 1900 by Swiss physician Maximilian Bircher-Benner as a part of his therapy for his patients. Most granola is coated with oil and sugar and then baked, but muesli has no added fat or sugar. Traditional muesli consists of a combination of rolled oats, fruit, and nuts that is soaked overnight, making its wealth of minerals more available. A wonderful alternative to rolled oats is soaked oat groats.

Marvelous MUESLI

MAKES 5½ CUPS (1.38 L); 2 TO 3 HEARTY SERVINGS

1 cup (250 ml) rolled oats (see sidebar, below), or ¾ cup (185 ml) oat groats, soaked for at least 24 hours, drained, and rinsed

1 cup (250 ml) Sunflower-Hemp Milk (page 260) or other nondairy milk, plus more for serving

3 tablespoons (45 ml) raisins, currants, dried cranberries, or chopped dried fruit (such as apricots, peaches, or prunes)

2 tablespoons (30 ml) coarsely chopped nuts (see tips)

2 tablespoons (30 ml) seeds (see tips)

2 tablespoons (30 ml) unsweetened shredded dried coconut (optional)

3 cups (750 ml) chopped or sliced fresh fruit or berries

1 to 2 tablespoons (15 to 30 ml) ground flaxseeds

Per one-half recipe (2¾ cups/685 ml): calories: 509, protein: 15 g, fat: 20 g, carbohydrate: 76 g (28 g from sugar), dietary fiber: 14 g, calcium: 105 mg, copper: 700 mcg, iron: 5.0 mg, magnesium: 141 mg, phosphorus: 253 mg, potassium: 993 mg, sodium: 10 mg, zinc: 1.7 mg, thiamin: 0.8 mg, riboflavin: 0.2 mg, niacin: 4.5 mg, pyridoxine: 0.6 mg, folate: 109 mcg, pantothenic acid: 1.8 mg, vitamin B$_{12}$: 0 mcg, vitamin A: 5 mcg, vitamin C: 110 mg, vitamin E: 7 mg, vitamin K: 5 mcg, omega-6 fatty acids: 9.9 g, omega-3 fatty acids: 2.5 g

Percentage of calories from: protein 12%, fat 33%, carbohydrate 55%

Combine the oats, Sunflower-Hemp Milk, raisins, nuts, seeds, and optional coconut in a bowl or container that can be covered. Stir to mix. Cover and refrigerate for 8–12 hours.

Just before serving, stir in the fresh fruit and top with the ground flaxseeds. Serve with additional Sunflower-Hemp Milk, if desired.

TIPS

- The nuts and seeds can be soaked for 4–8 hours and then drained and rinsed, or they can be soaked and dehydrated prior to using them in this recipe.

- Use whole hempseeds, sunflower seeds, or flaxseeds in this recipe. If using whole flaxseeds, add them along with the fresh fruit, just before serving, to prevent the muesli from becoming gummy.

Oat groats are generally hulled and passed through a heat-and-moisture treatment (kilned) to stabilize them. (Once the hull is removed, the oat groat will become rancid within four days if it isn't stabilized.) An oat groat is not considered raw if it has been kilned, and it will not sprout. Hulless oats that have not been heat-treated will sprout, however they are not widely available.

Regular rolled oats are steamed during processing to soften them; therefore they are not a raw food. "Raw" rolled oats are available, but are often made by cold-pressing kilned oats, so they are not technically raw. Raw rolled oats can be prepared at home by using hulless oats that have not been heat-treated and a grain-roller mill (or another similar machine).

Rye is a rich and hearty-tasting grain that is especially delicious in crackers. These wonderful raw crackers are highly textured and packed with flavor and nutrition. Enjoy them spread with Herbed Almond Cheese (page 270), Pumpkin Seed Pâté (page 268), or Morocc-Un-Butter (page 267), along with a slice of avocado, a slice of tomato, and/or a few sprouts.

Sunny Rye CRACKERS

MAKES ABOUT 72 CRACKERS

2 cups (500 ml) **rye berries, soaked for 24 hours, sprouted for 2 days, and rinsed**

2 cups (500 ml) **sunflower seeds, soaked for 4–6 hours, drained, and rinsed**

1 cup (250 ml) ground flaxseeds

1 red or white onion, chopped

¼ cup (60 ml) water

¼ cup (60 ml) fresh herbs, or 4 teaspoons (20 ml) dried herbs (use basil, dill, oregano, or parsley, or a mix)

¼ cup (60 ml) black or white sesame seeds (optional)

2 cloves garlic, minced

1½ teaspoons (7 ml) salt

Combine all the ingredients in a food processor. Process for about 2 minutes to make a thick dough, stopping as needed to scrape down the sides of the work bowl with a rubber spatula.

Spread one-third of the dough about ¼ inch (.5 cm) thick on three 14-inch (36-cm) square dehydrator trays lined with a nonstick sheet or parchment paper. Dehydrate at 115 degrees F (46 degrees C) for about 3 hours. Remove from the dehydrator and score the cracker dough into 3-inch (8 cm) squares, rectangles, or diamonds (making about 24 crackers per tray). Return to the dehydrator and dehydrate for 5 hours longer.

Remove the trays from the dehydrator. Place a mesh dehydrator screen and tray over the cracker dough and flip the dough onto the screen. Remove the top dehydrator tray and peel off the nonstick sheet. Put the trays back in the dehydrator and dehydrate for 24 hours longer, or until the crackers are completely dry. Break the crackers along the score lines. Let cool completely. Stored in airtight containers, Sunny Rye Crackers will keep for 2 weeks at room temperature, 1 month in the refrigerator, or 3 months in the freezer.

Per 4 crackers: calories: 205, protein: 8 g, fat: 12 g, carbohydrate: 20 g (1 g from sugar), dietary fiber: 7 g, calcium: 48 mg, copper: 480 mcg, iron: 2.2 mg, magnesium: 113 mg, phosphorus: 242 mg, potassium: 242 mg, sodium: 188 mg, zinc: 1.9 mg, thiamin: 0.6 mg, riboflavin: 0.1 mg, niacin: 3.6 mg, pyridoxine: 0.2 mg, folate: 59 mcg, pantothenic acid: 1.5 mg, vitamin B$_{12}$: 0 mcg, vitamin A: 4 mcg, vitamin C: 2 mg, vitamin E: 6 mg, vitamin K: 16 mcg, omega-6 fatty acids: 6.1 g, omega-3 fatty acids: 1.7 g

Percentage of calories from: protein 15%, fat 49%, carbohydrate 36%

TIP: If you prefer a saltier-tasting cracker without adding extra sodium, reserve ½ teaspoon (2 ml) of the salt called for in this recipe and sprinkle it evenly over the rolled dough before placing it in the dehydrator. Alternatively, mix the reserved salt with ¼ cup (60 ml) of sesame seeds and sprinkle the mixture over the dough.

There are as many ways to make these crackers as there are salsa recipes—and there are a multitude of salsa recipes! Adapt the recipe to suit your taste by using whichever vegetables you like, as long as they total about four cups.

Salsa-Flax CRACKERS

MAKES 108 CRACKERS

1 cup (250 ml/20 grams) **sundried tomatoes, soaked for 1 hour in** ½ **cup** (125 ml) **very hot water** (do not drain)

2 cups (500 ml) chopped zucchini

1 cup (250 ml) chopped tomatoes

1 cup (250 ml) chopped red sweet pepper

½ (125 ml) red or white onion, chopped

1 small or large jalapeño chile, chopped

Zest of 1 lime (optional)

½ lime, juiced (optional)

2 teaspoons (10 ml) salt

1 teaspoon (5 ml) chili powder

1¼ cups (310 ml) ground flaxseeds

1 cup (250 ml) **whole flaxseeds, soaked for 8 hours in 2 cups water** (do not drain)

¼ cup (60 ml) finely chopped fresh parsley or cilantro

Put the sundried tomatoes and their soaking water in a food processor or blender. Add the zucchini, tomatoes, sweet pepper, onion, chile, optional lime zest, optional lime juice, salt, and chili powder. Process until smooth. If your blender or processor is large enough, add the ground flaxseeds and process until smooth. Then add the whole flaxseeds, the flaxseed soaking water, and the parsley. Pulse to combine. If your blender or processor is not very large, transfer the blended mixture to a large bowl and stir in the ground flaxseeds until well combined. Then add the whole flaxseeds, the flaxseed soaking water, and the parsley. Stir to combine.

Spread about 2⅓ cups (580 ml) of the batter onto each of three 14-inch (36-cm) square dehydrator trays lined with a nonstick sheet or parchment paper. Dehydrate at 105 degrees F (40 degrees C) for 2–3 hours.

Remove the trays from the dehydrator and score each sheet into 36 square crackers by making 5 cuts in each direction with a table knife. Alternatively, score them into other shapes, such as diamonds.

Return the trays to the dehydrator and dehydrate at 105 degrees F (40 degrees C) for 9–10 hours, or until the tops of the crackers are dry and crisp. If the score marks are barely visible, score the crackers again.

Place a mesh dehydrator screen and tray over the cracker dough and flip the dough onto the screen. Remove the top dehydrator tray and peel off the nonstick sheet. Put the trays back in the dehydrator and dehydrate for 8–12 hours longer, or until the crackers are completely dry. Break the crackers along the score lines and let cool completely. Stored in sealed containers, Salsa-Flax Crackers will keep for 3 months at room temperature or 6 months in the refrigerator or freezer.

Per 6 crackers: calories: 62, protein: 2 g, fat: 4 g, carbohydrate: 5 g (2 g from sugar), dietary fiber: 6 g, calcium: 32 mg, copper: 150 mcg, iron: 0.8 mg, magnesium: 45 mg, phosphorus: 77 mg, potassium: 210 mg, sodium: 292 mg, zinc: 0.5 mg, thiamin: 0.2 mg, riboflavin: 0.1 mg, niacin: 1.2 mg, pyridoxine: 0.1 mg, folate: 19 mcg, pantothenic acid: 0.2 mg, vitamin B$_{12}$: 0 mcg, vitamin A: 26 mcg, vitamin C: 23 mg, vitamin E: 0.3 mg, vitamin K: 17 mcg, omega-6 fatty acids: 0.6 g, omega-3 fatty acids: 2.2 g

Percentage of calories from: protein 14%, fat 55%, carbohydrate 31%

Based on sesame seeds, this spicy North African spread has far more nutritional value than butter or margarine and no cholesterol or trans-fatty acids. Feel free to play with the seasonings to create your own variation. Serve it with Sunny Rye Crackers (page 265) or your favorite raw vegetables.

Morocc-**UN-BUTTER**

MAKES ABOUT 1 CUP (250 ML)

¼ cup (60 ml) freshly squeezed lemon juice

½ cup (125 ml) tahini

¼ cup (60 ml) chopped fresh parsley or cilantro, plus additional for garnish

3 tablespoons (45 ml) chopped green onion (optional)

1 to 2 cloves garlic

1½ teaspoons (7 ml) ground cumin (optional)

1 teaspoon (5 ml) Nama Shoyu or tamari

½ teaspoon (2 ml) paprika

¼ teaspoon (1 ml) chili powder (optional)

Pour the lemon juice into a food processor. Add the tahini, parsley, optional green onion, garlic, cumin, Nama Shoyu, paprika, and optional chili powder. Process until smooth. If the mixture is too thick, add a small amount of water to achieve the desired consistency. Garnish with additional parsley just before serving. Stored in a sealed container in the refrigerator, Morocc-Un-Butter will keep for 5 days.

Per 2 tablespoons (30 ml): calories: 98, protein: 3 g, fat: 8 g, carbohydrate: 4 g (0.2 g from sugar), dietary fiber: 1 g, calcium: 27 mg, copper: 260 mcg, iron: 0.9 mg, magnesium: 17 mg, phosphorus: 129 mg, potassium: 99 mg, sodium: 49 mg, zinc: 0.8 mg, thiamin: 0.3 mg, riboflavin: 0 mg, niacin: 1 mg, pyridoxine: 0 mg, folate: 20 mcg, pantothenic acid: 0 mg, vitamin B$_{12}$: 0 mcg, vitamin A: 11 mcg, vitamin C: 7 mg, vitamin E: 0.4 mg, vitamin K: 32 mcg, omega-6 fatty acids: 3.6 g, omega-3 fatty acids: 0.1 g

Percentage of calories from: protein 11%, fat 72%, carbohydrate 17%

This pâté is simple to prepare, so don't be daunted by the number of ingredients. Enjoy it spread on crackers, rolled up in a green leaf, or scooped on a salad. A serving of pâté supplies 15 grams of protein, which is more than in a 2-ounce burger patty or veggie burger and is about one-quarter of your day's supply.

Pumpkin Seed PÂTÉ

MAKES 3 CUPS (750 ML); 6 SERVINGS

1 cup (250 ml) **pumpkin seeds, soaked for 4–6 hours, rinsed, and drained**

1 cup (250 ml) **walnuts, soaked for 4–6 hours, rinsed, and drained**

3 carrots, grated or coarsely chopped

3 green onions, sliced

2 ribs celery, coarsely chopped

3 tablespoons (45 ml) tahini

3 tablespoons (45 ml/18 g) nutritional yeast flakes

3 tablespoons (45 ml) freshly squeezed lemon juice

2 tablespoons (30 ml) Nama Shoyu or tamari

Freshly ground black pepper (optional)

½ cup (125 ml) chopped fresh parsley

Put the pumpkin seeds, walnuts, carrots, green onions, celery, tahini, nutritional yeast flakes, lemon juice, Nama Shoyu, and pepper in a food processor. Process for at least 3 minutes, or until all the ingredients are finely ground and well mixed, stopping as needed to scrape down the sides of the work bowl with a rubber spatula. Add the parsley. Process for 30–60 seconds longer, or until the parsley is evenly distributed. Stored in a sealed container in the refrigerator, Pumpkin Seed Pâté will keep for 3 days.

Per ½ cup (125 ml): calories: 386, protein: 15 g, fat: 32 g, carbohydrate: 14 g (3 g from sugar), dietary fiber: 5 g, calcium: 84 mg, copper: 520 mcg, iron: 4.2 mg, magnesium: 56 mg, phosphorus: 190 mg, potassium: 388 mg, sodium: 388 mg, zinc: 1.8 mg, thiamin: 2.2 mg, riboflavin: 2.1 mg, niacin: 13 mg, pyridoxine: 2.1 mg, folate: 46 mcg, pantothenic acid: 5 mg, vitamin B_{12}: 1.5 mcg, vitamin A: 286 mcg, vitamin C: 15 mg, vitamin E: 0.5 mg, vitamin K: 126 mcg, omega-6 fatty acids: 7.9 g, omega-3 fatty acids: 2 g

Percentage of calories from: protein 15%, fat 69%, carbohydrate 16%

Note: Analysis was done using Red Star Vegetarian Support Formula nutritional yeast flakes.

For a Mexican flair, serve this dip or spread with Salsa-Flax Crackers (page 266) and a raw soup. Avocados are celebrated for their healthful fat, but they also have other outstanding nutritional attributes (see page 135). If you use Red Star Vegetarian Support Formula nutritional yeast, you'll increase your intake of B vitamins, including vitamin B_{12}.

Avocado **DIP OR SPREAD**

MAKES ABOUT 1 CUP (250 ML)

1 large or 2 small ripe avocados

2 to 3 teaspoons (10 to 15 ml) **freshly squeezed lime juice**

2 teaspoons (10 ml/4 g) **nutritional yeast flakes**

½ to 1 teaspoon (2 to 5 ml) **Nama Shoyu or tamari**

¼ teaspoon (1 ml) **chili powder**

¼ teaspoon (1 ml) **garlic powder**

Pinch **ground black pepper**

2 teaspoons (10 ml) **chopped green onion**

2 teaspoons (10 ml) **chopped fresh parsley or cilantro** (optional)

Halve the avocado and remove the seed. Scoop the avocado flesh into a bowl and mash until smooth. Stir in the lime juice, nutritional yeast flakes, Nama Shoyu, chili powder, garlic powder, and pepper until well blended. Then stir in the green onion and optional parsley. If desired, adjust the seasonings to taste. Serve immediately.

Per ¼ cup (60 ml): calories: 104, protein: 2 g, fat: 9 g, carbohydrate: 5 g (0.7 g from sugar), dietary fiber: 3 g, calcium: 9 mg, copper: 170 mcg, iron: 0.7 mg, magnesium: 26 mg, phosphorus: 38 mg, potassium: 396 mg, sodium: 42 mg, zinc: 0.5 mg, thiamin: 0.7 mg, riboflavin: 0.7 mg, niacin: 5 mg, pyridoxine: 0.8 mg, folate: 54 mcg, pantothenic acid: 0.7 mg, vitamin B_{12}: 0.5 mcg, vitamin A: 42 mcg, vitamin C: 6 mg, vitamin E: 1 mg, vitamin K: 15 mcg, omega-6 fatty acids: 1.1 g, omega-3 fatty acids: 0.1 g

Percentage of calories from: protein 7%, fat 74%, carbohydrate 19%

Note: Analysis was done using Red Star Vegetarian Support Formula nutritional yeast flakes.

Nut cheeses are a wonderful way to add probiotics and vitamin E to your diet. This recipe is heavenly. Serve it on Salsa-Flax Crackers (page 266) or Sunny Rye Crackers (page 265), or use it as a topping for raw pizza.

Herbed Almond CHEESE

MAKES 2 CUPS (500 ML); 6 TO 8 SERVINGS

2 cups (500 ml) **almonds, soaked for 8–12 hours, drained, rinsed, and skinned** (see sidebar, page 271)

1 cup (250 ml) water

1 teaspoon (5 ml) light miso

½ teaspoon (2 ml) probiotic powder

1 teaspoon (5 ml) dried chives

1 teaspoon (5 ml) dried dill weed

1 teaspoon (5 ml) dried parsley

½ teaspoon (2 ml) salt

Put the almonds, water, miso, and probiotic powder in a high-powered blender. Process until smooth.

Line a large strainer or colander with cheesecloth, allowing several inches of the cloth to drape down around the sides. Set the strainer on top of a bowl. Pour the blended mixture into the cheesecloth (the bowl will catch the liquid as it drains; the solids will remain in the cloth to create the cheese). Fold the excess cheesecloth over the top of the cheese. Place a weight on top of the cheese to help press out more of the liquid. Let the cheese ferment in a warm (not hot) location for 12–24 hours (less fermentation time is required in warmer weather).

Once the cheese has fermented (see tips), stir in the chives, dill weed, parsley, and salt. Stored in a sealed container in the refrigerator, Herbed Almond Cheese will keep for 1 week.

Per ⅓ cup (80 ml): calories: 294, protein: 11 g, fat: 26 g, carbohydrate: 10 g (2 g from sugar), dietary fiber: 6 g, calcium: 131 mg, copper: 570 mcg, iron: 2.3 mg, magnesium: 140 mg, phosphorus: 242 mg, potassium: 378 mg, sodium: 195 mg, zinc: 1.7 mg, thiamin: 0.1 mg, riboflavin: 0.4 mg, niacin: 4.5 mg, pyridoxine: 0.1 mg, folate: 0.4 mcg, pantothenic acid: 0.2 mg, vitamin B$_{12}$: 0 mcg, vitamin A: 1.4 mcg, vitamin C: 0 mg, vitamin E: 13 mg, vitamin K: 1 mcg, omega-6 fatty acids: 6.2 g, omega-3 fatty acids: 0.2 g

Percentage of calories from: protein 14%, fat 73%, carbohydrate 13%

- A jar filled with water or grain (with the lid screwed on tightly) works well as a weight.

- It is not always easy to tell when nut cheese is adequately fermented. The best indicators are a bit of bubbling or rising and a change in aroma. Unfermented cheese does not have much aroma at all; properly fermented nut cheese will have a distinct, cheeselike smell.

VARIATIONS

- Spice up Herbed Almond Cheese with garlic, coarsely ground black pepper, and hot chiles.

- Replace the chives, dill weed, and parsley with dried basil, oregano, and thyme, or other fresh or dried herbs of your choice.

- Omit the herbs and use the plain Almond Cheese as you would plain cream cheese.

How to Skin Almonds

Soak raw almonds for 8–12 hours. Drain and rinse them. Transfer the almonds to a heatproof bowl and cover them with almost-boiling water. Let the almonds soak for 10 minutes, then drain. Remove the brown skins by squeezing the almonds between your fingers.

This soup always gets rave reviews.

Creamy Zucchini SOUP

MAKES 2½ CUPS (625 ML); 1 LARGE OR 2 SMALL SERVINGS

2 tablespoons (30 ml) **cashews, soaked in ¼ cup** (60 ml) **water for 1 hour** (do not drain)

1 cup (250 ml) chopped zucchini

1 rib celery, chopped

½ ripe avocado

½ cup (125 ml) cold or hot water

1 tablespoon (15 ml) tahini

1 tablespoon (15 ml) freshly squeezed lemon juice

1 teaspoon (5 ml/2 g) nutritional yeast flakes

1 teaspoon (5 ml) miso

1 clove garlic, minced

¼ teaspoon (1 ml) salt

Dash cayenne

1 tablespoon (15 ml) fresh dill, or ½ teaspoon (2 ml) dried dill weed

1 sprig dill, pine nuts, or Namu Shoyu Sunflower Seeds (page 297), for garnish

Put the cashews and their soaking water in a blender. Add the zucchini, celery, avocado, water, tahini, lemon juice, nutritional yeast flakes, miso, garlic, salt, and cayenne. Process until smooth. Add the dill. Blend briefly, just to mix.

For a warm soup, put in a dehydrator set at 115 degrees F (45 C) or warmer for about 30 minutes. For a chilled soup, refrigerate for at least 2 hours before serving. Garnish with the dill sprig just before serving.

Per 2½ cups (625 ml): calories: 410, protein: 12 g, fat: 32 g, carbohydrate: 28 g (6 g from sugar), dietary fiber: 9 g, calcium: 145 mg, copper: 1050 mcg, iron: 5 mg, magnesium: 154 mg, phosphorus: 377 mg, potassium: 1419 mg, sodium: 762 mg, zinc: 3.3 mg, thiamin: 1.8 mg, riboflavin: 1.7 mg, niacin: 11.4 mg, pyridoxine: 2 mg, folate: 75 mcg, pantothenic acid: 1.6 mg, vitamin B$_{12}$: 1 mcg, vitamin A: 32 mcg, vitamin C: 42 mg, vitamin E: 2.1 mg, vitamin K: 45 mcg, omega-6 fatty acids: 6.9 g, omega-3 fatty acids: 0.3 g

Percentage of calories from: protein 11%, fat 64%, carbohydrate 25%

Note: Analysis was done using Red Star Vegetarian Support Formula nutritional yeast flakes.

The vibrant green leaves of the kale plant impart an earthy flavor and offer more nutritional value per calorie than almost any other food. Vary the flavors of this soup to suit your taste; some people like it spicy, others like it sweet. In cool months, use very hot water for a warming soup.

Garden Blend SOUP

MAKES 2½ CUPS (625 ML); 1 TO 2 SERVINGS

¼ cup (60 ml) **freshly squeezed orange juice, or** ½ orange, peeled and coarsely chopped

1½ teaspoons (7 ml) **freshly squeezed lemon juice**

3 to 4 cups (750 ml to 1 L) **chopped kale leaves**

½ apple, cored and chopped, or ½ small cucumber, peeled and chopped

¼ cup (60 ml) **fresh herbs (such as basil, cilantro, dill, or parsley), packed**

1½ tablespoons (22 ml) **light miso**

½ green onion, coarsely sliced (optional)

¼ red jalapeño chile with seeds, or pinch cayenne

½ clove garlic

¾ cup (185 ml) **cold or hot water**

¼ **cup** (60 ml) **sunflower seeds, soaked for 1 hour, rinsed, and drained,** or ½ ripe avocado, coarsely chopped

¼ cup (60 ml) **mung bean sprouts or pumpkin seeds** (optional), **for garnish**

Put the orange juice and lemon juice in a blender. Add the kale, apple, fresh herbs, miso, optional green onion, chile, and garlic. Add the water and process until smooth. Add the sunflower seeds and process again until smooth. Garnish each serving with the mung bean sprouts. Serve immediately.

TIPS

- Use a variety of vegetables instead of or in addition to the kale, such as celery, cucumber, romaine lettuce, spinach, sweet pepper, tomato, or zucchini.
- The orange juice or orange gives sweetness to the soup. For a less sweet soup, reduce or eliminate the orange juice or orange and replace it with an additional ¼ cup (60 ml) of water or an additional ½ peeled cucumber, coarsely chopped.

Per 2½ cups (625 ml): calories: 399, protein: 17 g, fat: 20 g, carbohydrate: 48 g (15 g from sugar), dietary fiber: 10 g, calcium: 348 mg, copper: 1330 mcg, iron: 6.4 mg, magnesium: 216 mg, phosphorus: 399 mg, potassium: 1431 mg, sodium: 448 mg, zinc: 2.9 mg, thiamin: 1.2 mg, riboflavin: 0.4 mg, niacin: 7.6 mg, pyridoxine: 1 mg, folate: 168 mcg, pantothenic acid: 2.8 mg, vitamin B_{12}: 0 mcg, vitamin A: 14 mcg, vitamin C: 296 mg, vitamin E: 14 mg, vitamin K: 1740 mcg, omega-6 fatty acids: 12.3 g, omega-3 fatty acids: 0.4 g

Percentage of calories from: protein 15%, fat 41%, carbohydrate 43%

Smooth, flavorful, and nutritious, this soup is an everyday staple. The first time you make it, follow these directions exactly. Then feel free to adapt it according to your preferences or what you have on hand. Add fresh or dried herbs, such as basil or oregano, or spices, such as chili powder or cumin. You can easily double the recipe to make two servings.

V-8 Vegetable SOUP

MAKES 1⅓ CUPS (330 ML); 1 SERVING

1 cup (250 ml) torn lettuce leaves or spinach

⅓ cup (80 ml) chopped celery

⅓ cup (80 ml) chopped cucumber

⅓ cup (80 ml) chopped red sweet pepper

⅓ cup (80 ml) chopped tomato

¼ cup (60 ml) chopped fresh parsley, cilantro, arugula, or a combination

2 tablespoons (30 ml) water

1½ teaspoons (7 ml) miso

1 teaspoon (5 ml) freshly squeezed lemon juice

½ small clove garlic

¼ teaspoon (1 ml) grated fresh ginger

⅓ cup (80 ml) chopped avocado

Salt

Ground black pepper

½ cup (125 ml) mung bean or alfalfa sprouts, for garnish

Put the lettuce, celery, cucumber, red sweet pepper, tomato, parsley, water, miso, lemon juice, garlic, and ginger in a blender. Process until smooth, stopping as needed to scrape down the sides of the blender jar with a rubber spatula. Add the avocado. Process until smooth. Season with salt and pepper to taste. Transfer to a soup bowl. Garnish with the sprouts.

Per 1⅓ cups (330 ml): calories: 216, protein: 7 g, fat: 13 g, carbohydrate: 24 g (9 g from sugar), dietary fiber: 10 g, calcium: 126 mg, copper: 460 mcg, iron: 3.9 mg, magnesium: 85 mg, phosphorus: 151 mg, potassium: 1288 mg, sodium: 385 mg, zinc: 1.5 mg, thiamin: 0.3 mg, riboflavin: 0.4 mg, niacin: 4.9 mg, pyridoxine: 0.6 mg, folate: 101 mcg, pantothenic acid: 1.6 mg, vitamin B$_{12}$: 0 mcg, vitamin A: 185 mcg, vitamin C: 155 mg, vitamin E: 1.5 mg, vitamin K: 439 mcg, omega-6 fatty acids: 1.9 g, omega-3 fatty acids: 0.2 g

Percentage of calories from: protein 12%, fat 49%, carbohydrate 39%

This lovely, creamy dressing is a popular favorite. Enjoy it with Build-Your-Bones Salad (page 278), Brilliant Broccoli Salad (page 277), or Whole Meal Salad Bar (page 296).

Lemon-Tahini **DRESSING**

MAKES ABOUT 1³/₄ CUPS (435 ML)

½ cup (125 ml) water

⅓ cup (80 ml) freshly squeezed lemon juice

⅓ cup (80 ml) tahini

¼ cup (60 ml) flaxseed oil

3 tablespoons (45 ml) Nama Shoyu or tamari

2 tablespoons (30 ml/12 g) nutritional yeast flakes

2 tablespoons (30 ml) maple syrup or other sweetener

2 cloves garlic, minced

Salt

Ground black pepper

Combine all the ingredients in a blender. Process on high speed for a few seconds until well blended. Stored in a glass jar in the refrigerator, Lemon-Tahini Dressing will keep for 1 week.

VARIATION: For a lower-oil version of this recipe, reduce the oil to 2 tablespoons (30 ml). Add 1 cup (250 ml) chopped zucchini and omit the water. Blend until smooth.

Per 2 tablespoons (30 ml): calories: 81, protein: 2 g, fat: 7 g, carbohydrate: 4 g (2 g from sugar), dietary fiber: 1 g, calcium: 27 mg, copper: 110 mcg, iron: 0.3 mg, magnesium: 8 mg, phosphorus: 57 mg, potassium: 56 mg, sodium: 145 mg, zinc: 0.5 mg, thiamin: 0.6 mg, riboflavin: 0.6 mg, niacin: 4.1 mg, pyridoxine: 0.5 mg, folate: 20 mcg, pantothenic acid: 0.1 mg, vitamin B₁₂: 0.5 mcg, vitamin A: 0.1 mcg, vitamin C: 3 mg, vitamin E: 0.7 mg, vitamin K: 0 mcg, omega-6 fatty acids: 1.7 g, omega-3 fatty acids: 2.1 g

Percentage of calories from: protein 8%, fat 71%, carbohydrate 21%

Note: Analysis was done using Red Star Vegetarian Support Formula nutritional yeast flakes.

This is a tasty and nutritious dressing that is good to keep on hand. Two tablespoons provides your day's supply of omega-3 fatty acids, which can help balance your intake of omega-6 and omega-3 fatty acids for the day. When the dressing is made with Red Star Vegetarian Support Formula nutritional yeast, two tablespoons will provide half of the recommended daily intake of vitamin B_{12}, along with plenty of other B vitamins. Ground flaxseeds thicken the dressing; adjust the amount according to your preference.

Liquid Gold DRESSING

MAKES ABOUT 1³/₄ CUPS (435 ML)

½ cup (125 ml) flaxseed oil or hempseed oil

½ cup (125 ml) freshly squeezed lemon juice

½ cup (125 ml) water

⅓ cup (80 ml/34 g) nutritional yeast flakes

¼ cup (60 ml) Nama Shoyu or tamari

1 to 2 tablespoons (15 to 30 ml) ground flaxseeds

2 teaspoons (10 ml) Dijon mustard

4 teaspoons (20 ml) maple syrup or other sweetener (optional)

1 teaspoon (5 ml) ground cumin

Combine all the ingredients in a blender. Process until smooth. The dressing will thicken more as it rests. Stored in a glass jar in the refrigerator, Liquid Gold Dressing will keep for 2 weeks.

VARIATION: For a lower-oil version of this recipe, reduce the oil to 2 tablespoons (30 ml) and omit the water. Add 1 cup (250 ml) chopped zucchini and include the agave syrup. Blend until smooth.

Per 2 tablespoons (30 ml): calories: 91, protein: 2 g, fat: 9 g, carbohydrate: 2 g (0.3 g from sugar), dietary fiber: 1 g, calcium: 7 mg, copper: 40 mcg, iron: 0 mg, magnesium: 9 mg, phosphorus: 40 mg, potassium: 80 mg, sodium: 310 mg, zinc: 0.6 mg, thiamin: 1.5 mg, riboflavin: 1.5 mg, niacin: 9.3 mg, pyridoxine: 1.5 mg, folate: 39 mcg, pantothenic acid: 0.2 mg, vitamin B_{12}: 1.2 mcg, vitamin A: 0 mcg, vitamin C: 4 mg, vitamin E: 1.5 mg, vitamin K: 0 mcg, omega-6 fatty acids: 1.1 g, omega-3 fatty acids: 4.5 g

Percentage of calories from: protein 8%, fat 82%, carbohydrate 10%

Note: Analysis was done using Red Star Vegetarian Support Formula nutritional yeast flakes.

Broccoli is one of the most nutrient-packed foods available. It is brimming with vitamins A and C, calcium, and folic acid. It is also a source of fiber, providing the perfect balance of soluble and insoluble fibers. As a member of the cruciferous family, broccoli also boasts an abundance of phytochemicals. Broccoli contains an enzyme that helps convert certain phytochemicals to more active, cancer-fighting forms; because this enzyme is destroyed by heat, the enzyme activity is greatest when broccoli is eaten raw.

Brilliant Broccoli SALAD

MAKES 8 CUPS (2 L)

1 bunch broccoli

2 carrots, grated

½ small red onion, finely diced

¾ **cup** (185 ml) **Lemon-Tahini Dressing** (page 275)

Salt

½ cup (125 ml) dried cranberries, currants, or raisins, plus extra for garnish

¼ cup (60 ml) **Nama Shoyu Sunflower Seeds, Pumpkin Seeds, or Almonds** (page 297), plus extra for garnish

Wash the broccoli and remove the stems. Peel and grate the stems. Chop the broccoli tops into very small florets. Combine the broccoli (stems and florets), carrots, and onion in a large bowl. Add the dressing and stir well to coat the vegetables. Season with salt to taste.

Add the cranberries and sunflower seeds and toss briefly. Transfer the salad to a serving bowl and garnish with additional cranberries and the sunflower seeds. Serve immediately.

VARIATION: Replace the Lemon-Tahini Dressing with an equal amount of Liquid Gold Dressing (page 276) or Orange–Poppy Seed Dressing (page 283).

TIP: For some people, broccoli that is a little older is easier to digest after it has been immersed briefly in very hot water. Put the broccoli florets and the grated stem in a fine-mesh sieve and immerse the broccoli for about 1 minute in a bowl of very hot water. Drain well and proceed as directed.

Per 2 cups (500 ml): calories: 144, protein: 6 g, fat: 5 g, carbohydrate: 24 g (11 g from sugar), dietary fiber: 9 g, calcium: 86 mg, copper: 180 mcg, iron: 2.1 mg, magnesium: 56 mg, phosphorus: 137 mg, potassium: 620 mg, sodium: 77 mg, zinc: 0.9 mg, thiamin: 0.3 mg, riboflavin: 0.2 mg, niacin: 1.4 mg, pyridoxine: 0.3 mg, folate: 102 mcg, pantothenic acid: 1.1 mg, vitamin B$_{12}$: 0 mcg, vitamin A: 413 mcg, vitamin C: 112 mg, vitamin E: 3.5 mg, vitamin K: 4 mcg, omega-6 fatty acids: 2.2 g, omega-3 fatty acids: 0.2 g

Percentage of calories from: protein 14%, fat 26%, carbohydrate 60%

This can be a super meal for two or a number of smaller side salads. If you spend thirty minutes assembling it each week, it can be ready whenever you arrive home from work or need to quickly pack a lunch. This salad combines well with Lemon-Tahini Dressing (page 275), Liquid Gold Dressing (page 276), or Orange-Ginger Dressing (page 287).

Build-Your-Bones SALAD

MAKES 10 TO 14 CUPS (2.5 TO 3.5 L); 2 GENEROUS SERVINGS

2 to 3 cups (500 to 750 ml) thinly sliced kale or collard greens

2 to 3 cups (500 to 750 ml) romaine lettuce torn into bite-size pieces (see tips)

2 to 3 cups (500 to 750 ml) chopped napa cabbage

2 to 3 cups (500 to 750 ml) broccoli florets and peeled and grated stems

2 to 3 cups (500 to 750 ml) thinly sliced red cabbage

1 red sweet pepper, cut into thin strips

Combine all of the ingredients in a large bowl. Toss to mix well.

Full-Meal Salad: To increase the protein, add 2 cups (500 ml) of one or a combination of the following: sprouted lentils (see sidebar, page 289), sprouted mung beans (see sidebar, page 282), seeds, nuts, or cooked beans.

TIPS

- To keep Build-Your-Bones Salad for up to 5 days, omit the red sweet pepper and store the salad in a tightly sealed container in the refrigerator. Chop and add the red sweet pepper just before serving.

- You may prefer to tear lettuce into bite-size pieces rather than chopping it, especially if it will be stored. Cutting lettuce causes the edges to brown more quickly; it also releases more ascorbic acid oxidase (an oxidizing enzyme), which results in greater losses of vitamin C.

Per 5 cups (1.25 L): calories: 115, protein: 8 g, fat: 1 g, carbohydrate: 24 g (6 g from sugar), dietary fiber: 7 g, calcium: 213 mg, copper: 380 mcg, iron: 3.9 mg, magnesium: 76 mg, phosphorus: 160 mg, potassium: 1072 mg, sodium: 86 mg, zinc: 4.6 mg, thiamin: 0.2 mg, riboflavin: 0.3 mg, niacin: 3.8 mg, pyridoxine: 0.7 mg, folate: 661 mcg, pantothenic acid: 0.9 mg, vitamin B$_{12}$: 0 mcg, vitamin A: 948 mcg, vitamin C: 325 mg, vitamin E: 2 mg, vitamin K: 661 mcg, omega-6 fatty acids: 0.2 g, omega-3 fatty acids: 0.4 g

Percentage of calories from: protein 23%, fat 9%, carbohydrate 68%

This outstanding version of a familiar favorite is not only tasty but also nutritious; each serving is a powerhouse of B vitamins. Although romaine is the traditional choice for Caesar salad, feel free to use other types of lettuce. Instead of anchovies, nori offers a hint of the flavors of the sea.

Caesar's Better **SALAD**

MAKES ABOUT 24 CUPS (6 L); 4 LARGE SERVINGS

CAESAR DRESSING
MAKES ¾ CUP (185 ML)

⅓ cup (80 ml) water

¼ cup (60 ml/25 g) nutritional yeast flakes

3 tablespoons (45 ml) freshly squeezed lemon juice

1 tablespoon (15 ml) Dijon mustard

1 tablespoon (15 ml) tahini

1 tablespoon (15 ml) extra-virgin olive oil or flaxseed oil

1 tablespoon (15 ml) Nama Shoyu or tamari, or ½ teaspoon (2 ml) salt

2 cloves garlic, pressed or chopped

CAESAR SALAD
MAKES ABOUT 24 CUPS (6 L)

2 heads romaine lettuce, torn into bite-size pieces (see tips, page 278)

¼ cup (60 ml) julienne carrot

8 baby or cherry tomatoes, cut in half

12 pitted raw or kalamata olives, cut in half

¼ sheet nori, cut into matchsticks

To make the dressing, combine all the ingredients in a blender. Process on high speed for 1 minute, or until smooth, stopping as needed to scrape down the sides of the blender jar with a rubber spatula. For optimal flavor, chill the dressing in the refrigerator for at least 1 hour prior to serving. Stored in a glass jar in the refrigerator, Caesar Dressing will keep for 1 week.

To assemble the salad, put the lettuce in a large bowl. Add the dressing. Toss until all of the leaves are evenly coated. Scoop the salad onto 4 plates. Arrange 1 tablespoon (15 ml) of the carrot down center of each salad vertically. Arrange 4 tomato halves evenly around each plate. Garnish the top of each salad with the olives and nori.

Per one-quarter recipe (about 6 cups/1½ L): calories: 184, protein: 9 g, fat: 10 g, carbohydrate: 19 g (5 g from sugar), dietary fiber: 9 g, calcium: 130 mg, copper: 300 mcg, iron: 3.8 mg, magnesium: 62 mg, phosphorus: 219 mg, potassium: 1040 mg, sodium: 569 mg, zinc: 2.3 mg, thiamin: 4.3 mg, riboflavin: 4.2 mg, niacin: 26 mg, pyridoxine: 4.1 mg, folate: 514 mcg, pantothenic acid: 0.9 mg, vitamin B_{12}: 3.2 mcg, vitamin A: 989 mcg, vitamin C: 83 mg, vitamin E: 1.4 mg, vitamin K: 310 mcg, omega-6 fatty acids: 1.1 g, omega-3 fatty acids: 0.4 g (with flaxseed oil: omega-3 fatty acids: 2.2 g)

Percentage of calories from: protein 17%, fat 45%, carbohydrate 38%

Note: Analysis was done using Red Star Vegetarian Support Formula nutritional yeast flakes.

This elegant dish incorporates a novel vegetable called celeriac, also known as celery root; for this recipe you will need about two (depending on their size). Unlike other root vegetables, which are high in starch, celery root contains only about 5 percent starch by weight. It has a very mild celery flavor. Being a fairly firm vegetable, it spiralizes and juliennes beautifully. The Tomato Sauce can also be used on pizza, and the Seed Mix and Hemp Parmesan make nutritious additions to salads.

Celeriac Linguine
WITH BOLOGNESE SAUCE AND HEMP PARMESAN

MAKES 4 HEARTY SERVINGS

TOMATO SAUCE
MAKES ABOUT 4 CUPS (1 L)

20 sundried tomato halves or pieces, soaked for 6–24 hours in 1²/₃ cups (414 ml) water

5 pitted medjool dates, or 10 pitted regular dates, soaked for 6–24 hours in ¹/₃ cup (80 ml) water

¼ red onion, chopped

1 tablespoon (15 ml) dried oregano

1 clove garlic, minced

2 tomatoes, chopped

1 cup (250 ml) grated carrots

SEED MIX
MAKES ABOUT 2 CUPS (500 ML)

½ cup (125 ml) shredded carrot

½ cup (125 ml) chopped fresh parsley

½ cup (125 ml) sunflower seeds, soaked for 1 hour, drained, and rinsed

¼ cup (60 ml) pumpkin seeds, soaked for 1 hour, drained, and rinsed

2 to 4 tablespoons (30 to 60 ml) Nama Shoyu or tamari

2 tablespoons (30 ml) freshly squeezed lemon juice or apple cider vinegar

1 tablespoon (15 ml) miso

¼ cup (60 ml) sesame seeds, soaked for 1 hour, drained, and rinsed

¼ cup (60 ml) hempseeds

To make the Tomato Sauce, put the sundried tomatoes and their soaking water in a food processor or blender. Add the dates and their soaking water. Then add the onion, oregano, and garlic. Process until smooth. Transfer to a bowl. Stir in the fresh tomatoes and carrots.

To make the Seed Mix, put the carrot, parsley, sunflower seeds, pumpkin seeds, Nama Shoyu, lemon juice, and miso in a food processor. Process until smooth. Add the sesame seeds and hempseeds. Pulse until evenly mixed. Stored in a sealed container in the refrigerator, Seed Mix will keep for 3 days.

Alternatively, spread the Seed Mix on a dehydrator tray with a nonstick sheet. Dehydrate at 115 degrees F (46 degrees C) for 3 hours. Crumble with your fingers. Serve warm or store in the refrigerator.

CELERIAC LINGUINE
MAKES 8 CUPS (2 L)

8 cups (2 L) shredded celeriac (spiralized, julienned with a mandolin, or grated)

2 tablespoons (30 ml) extra-virgin olive oil

Juice of 1/2 lemon

HEMP PARMESAN
MAKES: 1/4 CUP (60 ML)

2 tablespoons (30 ml) hempseeds

2 tablespoons (30 ml) nutritional yeast flakes

1/8 teaspoon (3/4 ml) salt

To make the Celeriac Linguine, combine all the ingredients in a large bowl. Toss until evenly mixed. Cover and refrigerate until serving time, up to 4 hours.

TIP: To keep the shredded celeriac moist while preparing the remainder of the recipe, sprinkle it with a little water so it does not dry out.

To make the Hemp Parmesan, combine all the ingredients in a small bowl. Stir until evenly mixed. Stored in a sealed container in the refrigerator, Hemp Parmesan will keep for 1 month.

Assemble the finished dish just before serving. For each serving, arrange 2 cups (500 ml) of the Celeriac Linguine on a plate. Combine the Tomato Sauce and the Seed Mix to create the Bolognese Sauce and stir gently. Top each serving with about 1 1/2 cups (375 ml) of the Bolognese Sauce. Sprinkle with about 1 tablespoon (15 ml) of the Hemp Parmesan.

VARIATIONS

- For Zucchini Linguine, replace the celeriac in the Celeriac Linguine with 8 cups of shredded zucchini (spiralized, julienned with a mandolin, or grated).

- For Sunflower Parmesan, grind 2 tablespoons of sunflower seeds (in a coffee grinder or hand grinder) until almost all of the seeds are broken into smaller pieces (do not process so long that the seeds become a paste). Use the sunflower seeds to replace the hempseeds in the Hemp Parmesan.

Per one-quarter recipe: calories: 568, protein: 21 g, fat: 32 g, carbohydrate: 59 g (25 g from sugar), dietary fiber: 17 g, calcium: 277 mg, copper: 1300 mcg, iron: 9 mg, magnesium: 242 mg, phosphorus: 629 mg, potassium: 1663 mg, sodium: 1171 mg, zinc: 4.3 mg, thiamin: 2.7 mg, riboflavin: 2.3 mg, niacin: 20.1 mg, pyridoxine: 2.6 mg, folate: 162 mcg, pantothenic acid: 2.7 mg, vitamin B$_{12}$: 1.6 mcg, vitamin A: 438 mcg, vitamin C: 45 mg, vitamin E: 7.8 mg, vitamin K: 154 mcg, omega-6 fatty acids: 13.6 g, omega-3 fatty acids: 1.1 g

Percentage of calories from: protein 14%, fat 47%, carbohydrate 39%

Note: Analysis was done using Red Star Vegetarian Support Formula nutritional yeast flakes.

To serve this nourishing salad, simply sprinkle on a little lemon juice and Nama Shoyu, or serve it with Lemon-Tahini Dressing (page 275), Liquid Gold Dressing (page 276), Orange-Ginger Dressing (page 287), or Orange–Poppy Seed Dressing (page 283) on the side.

CRUNCHY Sprouts and Veggies

MAKES ABOUT 6 CUPS (1.5 L); 2 LARGE SERVINGS OR 4 SMALLER SERVINGS

3 cups (750 ml) chopped napa cabbage

1 cup (250 ml) **mung bean sprouts** (see sidebar, page 282)

1 cup (250 ml) **lentil sprouts** (see sidebar, page 289)

½ red sweet pepper

½ rib celery, cut into matchsticks

15 snow peas, quartered

1 green onion, finely sliced

2 large leaves napa cabbage or lettuce

½ to 1 avocado, diced

½ cup (125 ml) alfalfa sprouts or other sprouts (optional)

Combine the chopped cabbage, mung bean sprouts, lentil sprouts, red sweet pepper, celery, snow peas, and green onion in a bowl. Toss until mixed. Put a whole cabbage leaf on each serving plate. Spoon the chopped cabbage mixture over the cabbage leaf. Top with the avocado and optional alfalfa sprouts.

How to Sprout Mung Beans

MAKES 3 TO 4 CUPS (750 ML TO 1 L) SPROUTS

¼ cup (60 ml) dried mung beans

2 cups (500 ml) water

Put the beans in a 1-quart (I-L) jar and cover them with the water. Put a sprouting lid on the jar or cover it with piece of mesh or cheesecloth secured with a wide elastic band. Let stand at room temperature for 12–24 hours. Drain the beans; then rinse them thoroughly with cool water and drain again.

Place the jar at a 45-degree angle over a saucer (to collect any water that may run off) or in a dish rack. Cover the jar with a tea towel or place the jar away from direct sunlight so the sprouts can grow in the dark.

Rinse and drain the beans 2 or 3 times a day for 3–5 days, until a short tail is visible. Store the well-drained sprouts in a sealed container in the refrigerator for up to 1 week.

Note: Homegrown mung bean sprouts will have much shorter tails than commercially grown sprouts. The tails become longer if mung beans are sprouted under a weight that exerts pressure on them. For information on how to do this, see Ann Wigmore's *The Sprouting Book.*

Per 3 cups (750 ml): calories: 404, protein: 21 g, fat: 17 g, carbohydrate: 56 g (16 g from sugar), dietary fiber: 18 g, calcium: 355 mg, copper: 850 mcg, iron: 7 mg, magnesium: 129 mg, phosphorus: 322 mg, potassium: 1420 mg, sodium: 91 mg, zinc: 2.7 mg, thiamin: 0.6 mg, riboflavin: 0.5 mg, niacin: 6.6 mg, pyridoxine: 0.9 mg, folate: 353 mcg, pantothenic acid: 2.8 mg, vitamin B_{12}: 0 mcg, vitamin A: 315 mcg, vitamin C: 300 mg, vitamin E: 2.9 mg, vitamin K: 122 mcg, omega-6 fatty acids: 2.2 g, omega-3 fatty acids: 0.2 g

Percentage of calories from: protein 18%, fat 33%, carbohydrate 49%

You can use leaf lettuce, spinach, or any combination of mixed greens in this light, uplifting salad.

Elegant Greens
WITH STRAWBERRIES, ALMONDS, AND ORANGE–POPPY SEED DRESSING

MAKES 16 CUPS (4 L); 4 LARGE SERVINGS

ORANGE–POPPY SEED DRESSING
MAKES ABOUT ½ CUP (125 ML)

3 tablespoons (45 ml) extra-virgin olive oil, flaxseed oil, or a combination

3 tablespoons (45 ml) freshly squeezed orange juice

2 tablespoons (30 ml) maple syrup or agave syrup

1 tablespoon (15 ml) chopped fresh dill, or 1 teaspoon (5 ml) dried dill weed

1 tablespoon (15 ml) Dijon mustard

2 teaspoons (10 ml) poppy seeds

GREENS, STRAWBERRIES, AND ALMONDS
MAKES 16 CUPS (4 L)

1 pound (454 g) leaf lettuce or other tender greens, torn or chopped (about 15 cups/3.75 L)

2 cups (500 ml) sliced strawberries

½ cup (125 ml) sliced almonds

To make the dressing, combine all the ingredients in a jar with a tight-fitting lid. Shake to mix well just before adding to the salad.

To make the salad, combine the lettuce, strawberries, and almonds in a large bowl. Add the dressing just before serving. Toss gently to distribute the dressing evenly.

Per 4 cups (1 L): calories: 297, protein: 7 g, fat: 22 g, carbohydrate: 25 g (16 g from sugar), dietary fiber: 6 g, calcium: 129 mg, copper: 320 mcg, iron: 2.4 mg, magnesium: 84 mg, phosphorus: 166 mg, potassium: 533 mg, sodium: 126 mg, zinc: 1.2 mg, thiamin: 0.2 mg, riboflavin: 0.3 mg, niacin: 2.9 mg, pyridoxine: 0.2 mg, folate: 74 mcg, pantothenic acid: 0.4 mg, vitamin B_{12}: 0 mcg, vitamin A: 422 mcg, vitamin C: 78 mg, vitamin E: 5.6 mg, vitamin K: 199 mcg, omega-6 fatty acids: 2.8 g, omega-3 fatty acids: 0.1 g (with flax oil, omega-3 fatty acids: 5.7 g)

Percentage of calories from: protein 8%, fat 61%, carbohydrate 31%

Use half of the crust squares to make this recipe and store the remaining squares to quickly make pizza at a later time. The squares can also be used as crackers. Try the scrumptious pesto in this recipe as a spread or dip or as a topping for raw zucchini or celeriac "pasta." (pages 280–281)

Pesto and Sundried Tomato
PIZZA WITH VEGGIES

MAKES 16 (3-INCH/8-CM) PIZZA SQUARES, PLUS 16 CRACKERS (FOR FUTURE PIZZAS)

PIZZA CRUST

MAKES 32 (3-INCH/8-CM) PIZZA CRUSTS
OR CRACKERS

1½ cups (375 ml) buckwheat groats, soaked for 4–6 hours, drained, and rinsed

¾ cup (185 ml) sunflower seeds, soaked for 4–6 hours, drained, and rinsed

1 carrot, shredded

2 teaspoons (10 ml) Italian seasoning

2 teaspoons (10 ml) salt

¼ cup (60 ml) ground flaxseeds

½ cup (125 ml) water

Per 3-inch (8-cm) pizza: calories: 137, protein: 5 g, fat: 3 g, carbohydrate: 14 g (3 g from sugar), dietary fiber: 4 g, calcium: 39 mg, copper: 320 mcg, iron: 1.4 mg, magnesium: 63 mg, phosphorus: 120 mg, potassium: 317 mg, sodium: 338 mg, zinc: 1 mg, thiamin: 0.9 mg, riboflavin: 0.9 mg, niacin: 6.6 mg, pyridoxine: 0.9 mg, folate: 52 mcg, pantothenic acid: 0.6 mg, vitamin B$_{12}$: 0.6 mcg, vitamin A: 67 mcg, vitamin C: 29 mg, vitamin E: 1.9 mg, vitamin K: 37 mcg, omega-6 fatty acids: 3.4 g, omega-3 fatty acids: 1.4 g

Percentage of calories from: protein 13%, fat 50%, carbohydrate 37%

Note: Analysis was done using Red Star Vegetarian Support Formula nutritional yeast flakes.

To make the pizza crust dough, combine the buckwheat groats, sunflower seeds, carrot, Italian seasoning, and salt in a food processor. Process until smooth, stopping as needed to scrape down the sides of the work bowl with a rubber spatula. Add the flaxseeds, then add the water. Process for a few more seconds until thoroughly blended.

Spread half the dough evenly over 2 dehydrator trays lined with nonstick sheets or parchment paper (about 1½ cups/375 ml of dough should be used for each tray). The dough will not completely cover the trays; simply spread it as thinly as possible, making sure there are no holes in it. Dehydrate at 125 degrees F (52 degrees C) for 2 hours.

Remove the trays from the dehydrator. Score the crust 3 times in each direction to make 16 (3-inch/8-cm) squares per tray. Flip each crust by placing another dehydrator tray lined with a nonstick sheet on top and turning them over in unison. Remove the nonstick sheet that had been below the crust by peeling it back. Alternatively, score the dough into rectangles or triangles. Put the trays back in the dehydrator and dehydrate at 115 degrees F (46 degrees C) for 12 hours, or until the crust is dry and crispy.

Stored in sealed containers, Pizza Crust will keep for 1 month in the refrigerator or 3 months in the freezer.

SUNDRIED TOMATO SAUCE

MAKES 1 1/4 CUPS (310 ML)

10 sundried tomatoes, soaked for 6–24 hours in 3/4 cup (185 ml) water

2 to 3 pitted medjool dates, or 5 pitted small dates, soaked for 6–24 hours in 3 tablespoons (45 ml) water

2 tablespoons (30 ml) chopped red onion

1 1/2 teaspoons (7 ml) miso

1 teaspoon (5 ml) dried oregano

PESTO-THE-BEST-OH!

MAKES ABOUT 1 CUP (250 ML)

3/4 cup (185 ml) walnuts, pine nuts, or hempseeds, or a mix

3 cups (750 ml) fresh basil leaves (about 3 ounces/85 g)

1 1/2 tablespoons (22 ml) flaxseed oil or extra-virgin olive oil

1 1/2 tablespoons (22 ml) freshly squeezed lemon juice

1 to 1 1/2 tablespoons (15 to 22 ml) Nama Shoyu or tamari

1 to 4 cloves garlic

1/8 teaspoon ground black pepper

3 tablespoons (45 ml/19 g) nutritional yeast flakes

To make the sauce, transfer the sundried tomatoes and their soaking water to a blender (for the smoothest results) or a food processor. Add the dates and their soaking water. Then add the onion, miso, and oregano. Process until well combined, stopping as needed to scrape down the sides of the work bowl or blender jar with a rubber spatula. Stored in a sealed container in the refrigerator, Sundried Tomato Sauce will keep for 1 week.

To make the pesto, process the walnuts in a food processor until finely ground. Add the basil, oil, lemon juice, Nama Shoyu, garlic, and pepper. Pulse until well combined. Add the nutritional yeast, and pulse a few times until it is incorporated. Stored in a sealed container, Pesto-the-Best-Oh! will keep for 4 days in the refrigerator or 3 months in the freezer.

See next page for veggie variations.

VEGGIES

MAKES 3 TO 3½ CUPS (750 TO 810 ML)

4 to 5 cups (1 to 1.25 L) seasonal vegetables (such as broccoli, sweet peppers, and/or zucchini), julienned or cut into bite-size pieces

¼ red onion, thinly sliced

2 tablespoons (30 ml) apple cider vinegar or freshly squeezed lemon juice

1 to 2 tablespoons (15 to 30 ml) Nama Shoyu or tamari

1 tablespoon (15 ml) extra-virgin olive oil

2 teaspoons (10 ml) Italian seasoning or other dried herbs

1 teaspoon (5 ml) paprika

To make the veggies, combine all of the ingredients in a large bowl and stir until evenly mixed. Marinate at room temperature for at least 30 minutes or in the refrigerator for up to 24 hours. Spread the vegetable mixture evenly on a dehydrator tray with a nonstick sheet. Dehydrate at 115 degrees F (46 degrees C) for 1 hour. Stored in a covered container in the refrigerator, Veggies will keep for 5 days.

To assemble the pizzas, spread 1 heaping tablespoon (20 ml) of Sundried Tomato Sauce on each pizza crust. Top with ¼ cup (60 ml) of Veggies and 1 tablespoon (15 ml) of Pesto-the-Best-Oh! Serve immediately or warm in a dehydrator at 115 degrees F (45 C) for 30 minutes.

Tomato Sauce and Almond Cheese Pizza: Spread 1 to 2 tablespoons (15 to 30 ml) plain or herbed Almond Cheese (page 270) and 1 to 2 tablespoons (15 to 30 ml) Sundried Tomato Sauce, with or without Veggies, on each 3-inch (8-cm) pizza crust.

TIP: Be creative with the vegetables you use— add asparagus tips, baby spinach, or pitted sundried olives, or explore more exotic choices, such as julienned golden beet or hokkaido pumpkin.

Raw Veggies

An assortment of raw veggies makes an excellent snack or addition to a meal. Two cups of these will provide, on average, 3 grams of protein, 61 grams of calcium, an entire day's supply of vitamins A and C, and plenty of protective phytochemicals—all with less than a gram of fat. Cut them into a variety of interesting shapes: cubes, strips, sticks, straight or diagonal slices, julienne, or spirals—let your creativity take over! Serve any combination of the following raw veggies on their own or with a dip, spread, or thick salad dressing.

asparagus tips	parsnips
bok choy	radishes (red, watermelon,
broccoli	or white)
carrots	snow peas
cauliflower	sweet peppers (orange, red,
celery	or yellow)
cucumbers	tomatoes
daikon	turnips (choose young ones)
green onions	yams
jicama	zucchini

Kale has gained fame as a source of calcium that is absorbed by our bodies about twice as well as the calcium from dairy products. It can be a rather tough green to eat raw, especially if large, older leaves are used. A trick to improve its appeal is to cut it matchstick thin and marinate it in a citrus-based dressing. For those who have never known what to do with kale, this recipe is an amazing initiation!

Kale Salad
WITH ORANGE-GINGER DRESSING

MAKES 10 CUPS (2 1/2 L)

KALE SALAD

MAKES 10 CUPS (2½ L)

1 bunch kale (275 to 300 g), stemmed and thinly sliced

1 to 2 carrots, grated or julienned

1 cup (250 ml) thinly sliced red cabbage

½ cup (125 ml) julienne daikon

1 red sweet pepper, thinly sliced

¼ cup (60 ml) chopped fresh parsley or cilantro

¼ cup (60 ml) chopped fresh mint

Dulse flakes (optional)

Sesame seeds (optional)

ORANGE-GINGER DRESSING

MAKES 1½ CUPS (375 ML)

4 pitted dates

1 cup (250 ml) freshly squeezed orange juice

2 tablespoons (30 ml) tahini

2 tablespoons (30 ml) chopped or grated fresh ginger

2 tablespoons (30 ml) miso

2 tablespoons (30 ml) cider vinegar or freshly squeezed lemon juice

2 tablespoons (30 ml) Nama Shoyu or tamari

2 teaspoons (10 ml) sesame oil (optional)

Pinch cayenne or ground black pepper

To make the salad, combine the kale, carrots, cabbage, daikon, red sweet pepper, parsley, and mint in a large bowl. Toss well. Sprinkle with the optional dulse flakes and sesame seeds if desired.

To make the dressing, soak the dates in ½ cup (125 ml) of the orange juice for 1 hour. Transfer the dates and their soaking liquid to a blender. Add the tahini, ginger, and miso. Process until smooth. Add remaining ½ cup (125 ml) of orange juice and all of the vinegar, Nama Shoyu, optional sesame oil, and cayenne. Process until smooth. Taste and adjust the seasonings if necessary.

To serve, add the dressing to the salad to taste and toss to combine. Let marinate for at least 20 minutes before serving. Stored in a sealed container in the refrigerator, Kale Salad with Orange-Ginger Dressing will keep for 1 day.

VARIATION: Add ¼ to ½ cup (60 to 125 ml) Namu Shoyu Sunflower Seeds, Pumpkins Seeds, or Almonds (page 297).

Per 2½ cups (625 ml), ¼ recipe: calories: 180, protein: 7 g, fat: 6 g, carbohydrate: 30 g (14 g from sugar), dietary fiber: 5 g, calcium: 155 mg, copper: 450 mcg, iron: 3 mg, magnesium: 62 mg, phosphorus: 167 mg, potassium: 782 mg, sodium: 889 mg, zinc: 1.2 mg, thiamin: 0.3 mg, riboflavin: 0.2 mg, niacin: 3.7 mg, pyridoxine: 0.4 mg, folate: 78 mcg, pantothenic acid: 0.5 mg, vitamin B_{12}: 0 mcg, vitamin A: 741 mcg, vitamin C: 194 mg, vitamin E: 1.7 mg, vitamin K: 638 mcg, omega-6 fatty acids: 2.1 g, omega-3 fatty acids: 0.2 g

Percentage of calories from: protein 15%, fat 25%, carbohydrate 60%

This salad is not only packed with nutrition but also offers a tantalizing variety of colors and textures. For a larger meal, serve this fabulous salad with a soup (see pages 272 to 274) and Salsa-Flax Crackers (page 266).

Spicy Mexican SALAD

MAKES 8 CUPS (2 L); 4 SERVINGS

SALAD
MAKES 8 CUPS (2 L)

3 tomatoes, chopped

2 ripe avocados, finely diced

2 cups (500 ml) fresh corn kernels or thawed frozen corn kernels

2 ribs celery, diced

1 large orange, red, or yellow sweet pepper, sliced into matchsticks

1 cup (250 ml) **sprouted lentils** (see sidebar, page 289) or cooked black beans

1 cup (250 ml) finely chopped fresh cilantro or parsley, packed

3 green onions, sliced

SPICY MEXICAN DRESSING
MAKES ⅔ CUP (165 ML)

¼ cup (60 ml) freshly squeezed lime juice

2 tablespoons (30 ml) extra-virgin olive oil

2 tablespoons (30 ml) flaxseed oil

2 tablespoon (30 ml) Nama Shoyu or tamari

1 tablespoon (15 ml) maple syrup, agave syrup, or other liquid sweetener

2 cloves garlic, minced

1 teaspoon (5 ml) minced red or green chile

½ **teaspoon** (2 ml) ground cumin (optional)

To make the salad, combine all the ingredients in a large bowl.

To make the dressing, combine all the ingredients in a jar or blender. Seal the jar and shake well, or process until well combined.

To serve, add the dressing to the salad and toss until evenly distributed. Serve at once or chill for up to 2 hours.

Per 2 cups (500 ml): calories: 428, protein: 9 g, fat: 31 g, carbohydrate: 40 g (11 g from sugar), dietary fiber: 10 g, calcium: 45 mg, copper: 500 mcg, iron: 3 mg, magnesium: 100 mg, phosphorus: 203 mg, potassium: 1272 mg, sodium: 543 mg, zinc: 1.5 mg, thiamin: 0.4 mg, riboflavin: 0.3 mg, niacin: 6.1 mg, pyridoxine: 0.6 mg, folate: 152 mcg, pantothenic acid: 2 mg, vitamin B$_{12}$: 0 mcg, vitamin A: 119 mcg, vitamin C: 115 mg, vitamin E: 4.9 mg, vitamin K: 59 mcg, omega-6 fatty acids: 4 g, omega-3 fatty acids: 3.9 g

Percentage of calories from: protein 8%, fat 58%, carbohydrate 34%

How to Sprout Lentils

½ cup (125 ml) dried lentils

2 cups (500 ml) water

Put the lentils in a 1-quart (1-L) sprouting jar and cover them with the water. Put a sprouting lid on the jar or cover it with piece of mesh or cheesecloth secured with a wide elastic band. Let stand at room temperature for 12–24 hours. Drain and rinse the lentils thoroughly with cool water.

Place the jar at a 45-degree angle over a saucer (to collect any water that may run off) or in a dish rack. Cover the jar with a tea towel or position the jar away from direct sunlight so the sprouts can grow in the dark.

Rinse and drain the lentils 2 or 3 times a day for 3–5 days, until a short tail is visible. Store the well-drained sprouts in a sealed container in the refrigerator for up to 1 week.

Raw-food enthusiasts will welcome a warm salad on chilly days. This easy-to-make salad is traditionally served warm, and it is bursting with health-building properties. The vegetables in the *Brassica* (cabbage) family contain valuable phytochemicals, which help protect us against cancer. Walnuts are rich in essential omega-3 fatty acids.

Warm Red Cabbage SALAD

MAKES 3 CUPS (750 ML); ABOUT 2 SERVINGS

4 cups (1 L) thinly sliced red cabbage

2 tablespoons (30 ml) water

1 to 2 teaspoons (5 to 10 ml) extra-virgin olive oil (optional)

1 teaspoon (5 ml) Nama Shoyu or tamari

2 tablespoons (30 ml) freshly squeezed lemon juice

¼ cup (60 ml) walnuts

Per 1½ cups (375 ml): calories: 132, protein: 4 g, fat: 8 g, carbohydrate: 14 g (6 g from sugar), dietary fiber: 4 g, calcium: 77 mg, copper: 230 mcg, iron: 1.6 mg, magnesium: 45 mg, phosphorus: 91 mg, potassium: 422 mg, sodium: 208 mg, zinc: 0.7 mg, thiamin: 0.1 mg, riboflavin: 0.1 mg, niacin: 1.5 mg, pyridoxine: 0.4 mg, folate: 40 mcg, pantothenic acid: 0.3 mg, vitamin B_{12}: 0 mcg, vitamin A: 79 mcg, vitamin C: 87 mg*, vitamin E: 0.3 mg, vitamin K: 54 mcg, omega-6 fatty acids: 4.9 g, omega-3 fatty acids: 1.2 g

Percentage of calories from: protein 12%, fat 52%, carbohydrate 37%

*Values for vitamin C are based on raw cabbage; some loss is expected during warming.

Put the cabbage in a wide, shallow dish or pie plate. Add the water, optional oil, and Nama Shoyu. Toss to distribute evenly. Put in a dehydrator at 110 degrees F (43 degrees C) for 30–60 minutes, or until the cabbage is wilted. Sprinkle with the lemon juice. Add the walnuts. Toss to distribute evenly. Serve immediately.

VARIATION: Replace the lemon juice with 1 tablespoon (15 ml) apple cider vinegar. Add it to the cabbage before it goes into the dehydrator rather than after.

TIP: If you are dehydrating other foods and your dehydrator is already set at a temperature slightly lower or higher than 110 degrees F (43 degrees C), it is fine to use that temperature instead.

Quinoa (pronounced keen-wah) is an ancient crop, native to the high Andes regions of South America. It often is called a superfood because of its excellent protein quality and content. Quinoa is a good source of fiber and is high in calcium, magnesium, phosphorous, potassium, iron, vitamin E, and several B vitamins. Quinoa is also gluten free and easy to digest.

Sprouted Quinoa **TABOULI**

MAKES 9 CUPS (2.25 L); 4 TO 5 SERVINGS

SPROUTED QUINOA TABOULI

MAKES ABOUT 9 CUPS (2.25 L)

3 cups (750 ml) finely chopped fresh parsley

2 cups (500 ml) sprouted quinoa (see sidebar, page 291)

1 cucumber, finely diced

3 tomatoes, finely diced

½ cup (125 ml) finely chopped fresh mint (about 1½ ounces/45 g), or 1 tablespoon (15 ml) dried

5 green onions, thinly sliced

LEMON DRESSING

MAKES ⅔ CUPS (185 ML)

⅓ cup (80 ml) freshly squeezed lemon juice

2 to 3 tablespoons (30 to 45 ml) extra virgin olive oil

1½ tablespoons (22 ml) Namu Shoyu or tamari

2 cloves garlic, finely minced

½ teaspoon (2 ml) psyllium powder, or 1 tablespoon (15 ml) ground flaxseeds

Pinch ground black pepper or cayenne

LETTUCE OR CABBAGE CUPS

4 to 5 large lettuce or cabbage leaves

SEED TOPPING (OPTIONAL)

1 cup (250 ml) Nama Shoyu Sunflower Seeds, Pumpkin Seeds, or Almonds (page 297) or plain sunflower or pumpkin seeds

To make the tabouli, combine all the ingredients in a large bowl. Toss to mix.

To make the dressing, combine all the ingredients in a blender. Process until smooth.

To assemble, pour the dressing over the tabouli. Toss gently with a fork to mix well. Put a lettuce leaf on each salad plate. Heap about 2 cups (500 ml) of the tabouli on each lettuce leaf. Sprinkle ¼ cup (60 ml) of the optional seed topping over each serving or serve it in a small side dish.

Per serving (about 2 cups/500 ml): calories: 302, protein: 11 g, fat: 10 g, carbohydrate: 46 g (6 g from sugar), dietary fiber: 8 g, calcium: 169 mg, copper: 580 mcg, iron: 9 mg, magnesium: 152 mg, phosphorus: 287 mg, potassium: 1150 mg, sodium: 423 mg, zinc: 2.6 mg, thiamin: 0.2 mg, riboflavin: 0.3 mg, niacin: 5.2 mg, pyridoxine: 0.3 mg, folate: 190 mcg, pantothenic acid: 1 mg, vitamin B_{12}: 0 mcg, vitamin A: 346 mcg, vitamin C: 109 mg, vitamin E: 4.8 mg, vitamin K: 871 mcg, omega-6 fatty acids: 1.8 g, omega-3 fatty acids: 0.2 g

Percentage of calories from: protein 13%, fat 29%, carbohydrate 58%

How to Sprout Quinoa

1 cup (250 ml) quinoa
2 cups (500 ml) water

Put the quinoa in a fine-mesh sieve. Rinse it well to remove any residue of saponin (a soapy-tasting compound that naturally coats the seeds). Transfer the quinoa to a 1-quart (1-L) sprouting jar and cover it with the water. Put a sprouting lid on the jar or cover it with a piece of mesh or cheesecloth secured with a wide elastic band. Let stand at room temperature for 4–6 hours.

Drain and rinse the quinoa thoroughly with cool water several times. Place the jar at a 45-degree angle over a saucer (to collect any water that may run off) or in a dish rack. Rinse and drain the quinoa every 8–12 hours for 1–2 days, until most of the seeds have sprouted tiny roots. Store the sprouts in a sealed container in the refrigerator. They will keep for 1 to 2 days.

This delectable salad makes a refreshing light meal and includes a variety of appealing textures and colors.

Three-Melon SALAD

MAKES 8 CUPS (2 L); 2 LARGE SALAD SERVINGS OR 8 DESSERT SERVINGS

MELON DRESSING

MAKES 1¼ CUPS (310 ML)

½ **cup** (125 ml) **cantaloupe chunks**

¼ **cup** (60 ml) **honeydew chunks**

¼ **cup** (60 ml) **watermelon chunks**

1 ripe banana

1 pitted medjool date, or 2 pitted regular or deglet noor dates

Juice of ½ lime

MELON SALAD

MAKES 8 CUPS (2 L)

½ **cantaloupe, peeled, seeded, and cut into chunks** (about 2 cups/500 ml)

¼ **honeydew melon, peeled, seeded, and cut into chunks** (about 2 cups/500 ml)

¼ **watermelon, peeled, seeded, and cut into chunks** (about 4 cups/1 L)

½ **cup** (125 ml) **pecans**

To make the dressing, combine all the ingredients in a blender. Process until smooth.

To make the salad, combine the cantaloupe, honeydew, and watermelon in a large bowl. Add the dressing and toss until evenly mixed. Garnish with the pecans.

Per one-half recipe (4 cups/1 L): calories: 519, protein: 8 g, fat: 22 g, carbohydrate: 85 g (50 g from sugar), dietary fiber: 8 g, calcium: 82 mg, copper: 680 mcg, iron: 2.6 mg, magnesium: 134 mg, phosphorus: 189 mg, potassium: 1792 mg, sodium: 74 mg, zinc: 2.3 mg, thiamin: 0.5 mg, riboflavin: 0.2 mg, niacin: 5.5 mg, pyridoxine: 0.8 mg, folate: 113 mcg, pantothenic acid: 1.8 mg, vitamin B_{12}: 0 mcg, vitamin A: 460 mcg, vitamin C: 150 mg, vitamin E: 1.4 mg, vitamin K: 12 mcg, omega-6 fatty acids: 6.2 g, omega-3 fatty acids: 0.5 g

Percentage of calories from: protein 6%, fat 34%, carbohydrate 60%

The sauce makes these spring rolls truly divine. Serve the rolls as a hearty appetizer, an entrée with soup, or a packed lunch.

Thai Spring Rolls
WITH SPICY PECAN SAUCE

MAKES 6 SPRING ROLLS; 2 SERVINGS OR 6 HORS D'OEUVRES

SPICY PECAN SAUCE
MAKES ⅜ CUP (48 ML) SAUCE

¾ cup (185 ml) pecans, or ¼ cup (60 ml) peanut butter

1 tablespoon (15 ml) freshly squeezed lime juice

1 tablespoon (15 ml) flaxseed oil

1 tablespoon (15 ml) maple syrup or agave syrup

1 teaspoon (5 ml) miso

1 teaspoon (5 ml) apple cider vinegar or additional lime juice

1 clove garlic, pressed

½ teaspoon (2 ml) grated fresh ginger

Dash chili powder or cayenne

To make the sauce, process the pecans in a blender until they form a paste. Add the lime juice, oil, maple syrup, miso, vinegar, garlic, ginger, and chili powder. Process into a smooth sauce. Stored in a sealed container in the refrigerator, Spicy Pecan Sauce will keep for 5 days.

To make the rolls, cut each collard leaf in half lengthwise (to make 6 pieces), slicing out the spine. Lay the leaves vertically in front of you. On each half leaf, spread about 1 tablespoon (15 ml) of the Spicy Pecan Sauce, covering the leaf to the edges. Layer one-sixth of the vegetables on each half leaf in this order: carrots, cucumber, mung bean sprouts, parsley, avocado, and alfalfa sprouts. Roll up each leaf tightly. If necessary, secure each roll with a toothpick to keep it closed.

Per one-half recipe: calories: 571, protein: 11 g, fat: 49 g, carbohydrate: 33 g (14 g from sugar), dietary fiber: 13 g, calcium: 184 mg, copper: 940 mcg, iron: 3.9 mg, magnesium: 121 mg, phosphorus: 246 mg, potassium: 1051 mg, sodium: 182 mg, zinc: 182 mg, thiamin: 0.5 mg, riboflavin: 0.4 mg, niacin: 5.9 mg, pyridoxine: 0.5 mg, folate: 215 mcg, pantothenic acid: 1.7 mg, vitamin B$_{12}$: 0 mcg, vitamin A: 563 mcg, vitamin C: 61 mg, vitamin E: 5.4 mg, vitamin K: 310 mcg, omega-6 fatty acids: 11.6 g, omega-3 fatty acids: 4.3 g

Percentage of calories from: protein 7%, fat 72%, carbohydrate 21%

THAI SPRING ROLLS
MAKES 6 ROLLS

3 large collard leaves

1 cup (250 ml) shredded carrots

1 (3-inch/8-cm) piece cucumber, peeled and julienned

1 cup (250 ml) mung bean sprouts (see sidebar, page 282)

½ cup (125 ml) chopped fresh parsley or cilantro

½ ripe avocado, sliced

1 cup (250 ml) alfalfa sprouts

Rice Paper and Lettuce Wraps: Replace the collard leaves with 6 rice paper sheets and 6 lettuce leaves. Immerse each rice paper sheet in warm water for a few seconds until it softens. Place it on a flat surface and lay a lettuce leaf on top. Spread about 1 tablespoon of the Spicy Pecan Sauce on the lettuce leaf. Layer the carrots, cucumber, mung bean sprouts, parsley, avocado, and alfalfa sprouts as directed for the collard leaves. Roll up the rice paper sheet and lettuce together over the filling, tucking in the ends as you go. (Although rice paper is not raw, it holds the wrap together very well.)

TIP: If the collard leaves are too stiff to roll, immerse them in almost-boiling water for 30 seconds to soften and wilt them.

Veggie Fillings: Create your own combination of vegetable fillings. Try grated zucchini, finely chopped broccoli, diced red sweet pepper, finely sliced celery, broccoli sprouts, finely chopped napa cabbage or lettuce, or other vegetables of your choice.

Napa Cabbage Wraps: Replace the collard leaves with 6 leaves of napa cabbage. Immerse the leaves in almost-boiling water for 30 seconds to soften and wilt them. Fill and roll as directed.

Wild rice is the seed of a grass that grows in shallow lake waters and slow-flowing streams. It is threshed into canoes by First Nations people and smoked according to traditional methods. As a result, it is not strictly a raw food. When placed in warm, wet conditions, it will "bloom" and soften to a fluffy texture. Wild rice is gluten free, and it is high in protein, including the amino acid lysine. It also provides B vitamins (niacin, riboflavin, and thiamin), calcium, and iron. This colorful dish is great for a summer picnic or a festive winter holiday meal, or even for breakfast. The rich, deep flavor of the wild rice is accentuated by the sweetness of the berries and the nip of fresh ginger.

Wild Rice Salad
WITH PECANS AND CRANBERRIES

MAKES 5½ CUPS (1375 ML)

SALAD
MAKES 5½ CUPS (1,375 ML)

1 cup (250 ml) **wild rice, bloomed**
(see sidebar, page 295)

½ cup (125 ml) red sweet pepper, diced

½ cup (125 ml) dried cranberries

½ cup (125 ml) chopped pecans

½ cup (125 ml) chopped green onion

CITRUS DRESSING
MAKES 6 TABLESPOONS (90 ML)

¼ cup (60 ml) freshly squeezed orange juice

2 tablespoons (30 ml) extra-virgin olive oil
(optional)

2 teaspoons (10 ml) minced fresh ginger

1 teaspoon (5 ml) salt

GARNISH
Lime wedges

To make the salad, combine all the ingredients in a large bowl.

To make the dressing, put all the ingredients in a jar or a small bowl. Seal the jar and shake well or whisk until well combined.

To assemble, pour the dressing over the salad and stir until well mixed. Garnish with lime wedges if desired.

Per one-quarter recipe: calories: 324, protein: 8 g, fat: 12 g, carbohydrate: 49 g (14 g from sugar), dietary fiber: 6 g, calcium: 33 mg, copper: 430 mcg, iron: 1.7 mg, magnesium: 100 mg, phosphorus: 238 mg, potassium: 348 mg, sodium: 595 mg, zinc: 3.3 mg, thiamin: 0.2 mg, riboflavin: 0.2 mg, niacin: 5.2 mg, pyridoxine: 0.3 mg, folate: 60 mcg, pantothenic acid: 0.7 mg, vitamin B$_{12}$: 0 mcg, vitamin A: 32 mcg, vitamin C: 39 mg, vitamin E: 1.2 mg, vitamin K: 29 mcg, omega-6 fatty acids: 3.4 g, omega-3 fatty acids: 0.3 g

Percentage of calories from: protein 10%, fat 32%, carbohydrate 58%

How to Bloom Wild Rice

Bloomed wild rice may be used in a salad or for a pilaf. Mix it with your choice of fruits and nuts, or take it in a savory direction by adding grated or chopped vegetables, seeds, and your choice of dressing.

1 cup (250 ml) wild rice

Put the wild rice in a 1-quart (1-L) jar. Fill the jar with water, close the lid, and put in a dehydrator set at 105 degrees F (40 degrees C) for about 24 hours, or until the rice has "bloomed" (that is, the rice kernels will have opened up and softened to a fluffy texture). The rice may require less time to bloom if the temperature of the dehydrator is set a little higher.

At earlier stages, it might appear as though the rice has bloomed because many of the kernels will have opened up. Look carefully at the jar. If you are unsure whether the rice is ready, open up the jar and look for unbloomed kernels. Taste one to see if it is still hard. If it is, you will need to let the rice soak in the dehydrator a little longer.

Once the rice has bloomed, drain it in a fine-mesh sieve. Stored in a sealed container in the refrigerator, bloomed wild rice will keep for 4 days.

This jewel-like salad is excellent tossed with Orange-Ginger Dressing (page 287) or Lemon-Tahini Dressing (page 275). For a different twist, try Orange–Poppy Seed Dressing (page 283) or Liquid Gold Dressing (page 276). Alternatively, offer several dressings at the table and let each guest choose his or her favorite.

Ruby Red SALAD

MAKES ABOUT 7 CUPS (1.75 L); 4 GENEROUS SERVINGS

3 cups (750 ml) grated carrots

2 cups (500 ml) grated beets

1 cup (250 ml) chopped fresh parsley

½ cup (125 ml) dried cranberries

½ cup (125 ml) coarsely chopped walnuts

2 tablespoons (30 ml) sliced fresh chives (optional)

Salad dressing of your choice

Salt

Ground black pepper

Seeds from ½ pomegranate (optional)

Combine the carrots, beets, parsley, cranberries, walnuts, and optional chives in a large bowl. Add the salad dressing to taste and stir until the vegetables are thoroughly coated. Season with salt and pepper to taste. Top with the optional pomegranate seeds if desired. Serve immediately.

VARIATION: Add 1 to 2 chopped red apples.

Per 1¾ cups (435 ml) without salad dressing: calories: 221, protein: 5 g, fat: 11 g, carbohydrate: 30 g (20 g from sugar), dietary fiber: 6 g, calcium: 78 mg, copper: 360 mcg, iron: 2.4 mg, magnesium: 59 mg, phosphorus: 122 mg, potassium: 669 mg, sodium: 124 mg, zinc: 1.1 mg, thiamin: 0.2 mg, riboflavin: 0.1 mg, niacin: 2.4 mg, pyridoxine: 0.3 mg, folate: 134 mcg, pantothenic acid: 0.5 mg, vitamin B_{12}: 0 mcg, vitamin A: 801 mcg, vitamin C: 30 mg, vitamin E: 1 mg, vitamin K: 277 mcg, omega-6 fatty acids: 6 g, omega-3 fatty acids: 1.4 g.

Percentage of calories from: protein 8%, fat 41%, carbohydrate 51%

The items listed here will allow you to make a wide range of salads, from simple to gourmet. Select one or two items from the various groups for each meal. Change the combinations from one meal to the next and introduce other choices to create an endless array of interesting salads. Place bowls of ingredients on the table and let diners select their favorites, or just toss everything together in a big salad bowl. Prepare the ingredients using a single technique, such as julienne, or get creative and give each ingredient a unique treatment or shape.

Whole-Meal SALAD BAR

DRESSINGS

Caesar Dressing, page 279

Citrus Dressing, page 294

Lemon Dressing, page 290

Lemon-Tahini Dressing, page 275

Liquid Gold Dressing, page 276

Orange-Ginger Dressing, page 287

Orange–Poppy Seed Dressing, page 283

Spicy Mexican Dressing, page 288

EDIBLE PODS AND PEAS

green peas

snow peas

sugar snap peas

FRUIT VEGETABLES

avocados

cucumbers

olives

peppers, sweet (orange, red, or yellow)

tomatoes

winter squash

zucchini or other summer squash

FLOWERING VEGETABLES

broccoli

broccoflower

broccolini

cauliflower

LEAFY VEGETABLES

arugula, dandelion greens, endive, radicchio, or watercress

cabbage (green or red)

collard greens or kale

lettuce (such as butterhead, leaf, or romaine)

napa cabbage

purslane

spinach

spring mix

NUTS AND SEEDS
(see table 4.3, page 58)

plain, or soaked and dehydrated

Nama Shoyu Sunflower Seeds, Pumpkin Seeds, or Almonds (page 297)

ONIONS

green onions

red or sweet white onion

ROOT VEGETABLES

carrots

beets

celeriac

daikon

radishes

rutabaga

turnips

SEA VEGETABLES

dulse

nori

SPROUTS

alfalfa, broccoli, radish, or sunflower

mung bean (see sidebar, page 282) or lentil (see sidebar, page 289)

quinoa (see sidebar, page 291)

STALK VEGETABLES

asparagus tips

celery

fennel

TUBERS

Jerusalem artichokes

jicama

Seeds provide us with a wealth of trace minerals, especially iron, magnesium, manganese, and zinc. Although presoaking is not essential, it increases the mineral availability, improves the balance of the amino acids of the protein, and creates a texture that is delightful to bite into. These tasty seeds and nuts are a valuable snack and a welcome addition to salad bars; they are also delightful on salads and soups.

Nama Shoyu
SUNFLOWER SEEDS, PUMPKIN SEEDS, OR ALMONDS

MAKES 2³/₄ CUPS (685 ML)

2 cups (500 ml) **sunflower seeds, pumpkin seeds, or almonds, or a mix, soaked for 4–6 hours, drained, and rinsed**

1 tablespoon (15 ml) Nama Shoyu or tamari

Put the seeds in a bowl. Sprinkle the Nama Shoyu over them and stir until it is evenly distributed. Spread the seeds on a 14-inch (36-cm) square dehydrator tray lined with mesh sheets. Dehydrate at 105 degrees F (40 degrees C) for about 12 hours, or until the seeds are crisp. Stored in an airtight container in the refrigerator or freezer, Nama Shoyu Sunflower Seeds, Pumpkin Seeds, or Almonds will keep for 6 months.

TIP: For crisp seeds or nuts without soaking, simply season them with the Nama Shoyu and dehydrate as directed for about 8 hours, or until crisp.

Per ¼ cup (60 ml): calories: 150, protein: 6 g, fat: 13 g, carbohydrate: 5 g (0.7 g from sugar), dietary fiber: 3 g, calcium: 31 mg, copper: 500 mcg, iron: 1.8 mg, magnesium: 93 mg, phosphorus: 187 mg, potassium: 184 mg, sodium: 94 mg, zinc: 1.3 mg, thiamin: 0.6 mg, riboflavin: 0.1 mg, niacin: 1.2 mg, pyridoxine: 0.2 mg, folate: 60 mcg, pantothenic acid: 1.8 mg, vitamin B$_{12}$: 0 mcg, vitamin A: 2 mcg, vitamin C: 0 mg, vitamin E: 9 mg, vitamin K: 1 mcg, omega-6 fatty acids: 8.5 g, omega-3 fatty acids: 0 g

Percentage of calories from: protein 15%, fat 72%, carbohydrate 12%

We were determined to create a recipe for delicious, raw vegan macaroons. These not only fill the bill, they are super simple to make. Try the variations too—they are outstanding.

Coconut MACAROONS

MAKES 48 COOKIES

1½ cups (375 ml) pitted soft dates (see tip)

1 cup (250 ml) cashew pieces, soaked for 4 hours, drained, and rinsed

1 teaspoon (5 ml) vanilla extract

1¼ cups (310 ml) **unsweetened shredded dried coconut**

Put the dates, cashews, and vanilla extract in a food processor. Process for about 3 minutes, or until smooth. Add the coconut. Pulse a few times, just until the coconut is evenly distributed.

Drop by tablespoons (15 ml) onto dehydrator trays with nonstick sheets. Dehydrate at 110 degrees F (43 degrees C) for about 4 hours. Transfer the cookies from the nonstick sheets to unlined trays. Dehydrate for 8 more hours. Stored in an airtight container, Coconut Macaroons will keep for 1 month in the refrigerator or 4 months in the freezer.

Apricot or Peach Macaroons: Replace half of the dates with unsulfured dried apricots or peaches. Proceed as directed.

Carob or Cacao Macaroons: Increase the dates to 2 cups (500 ml). Add 2 tablespoons (30 ml) of cacao or carob powder to the food processor along with the dates, cashews, and vanilla extract.

TIP: If the dates (or apricots or peaches, if you are making the variation) are hard, soak them in almost-boiling water for 30 minutes. Drain well. Proceed as directed.

Per cookie: calories: 43, protein: 1 g, fat: 3 g, carbohydrate: 5 g (3 g from sugar), dietary fiber: 1 g, calcium: 3 mg, copper: 90 mcg, iron: 0.3 mg, magnesium: 12 mg, phosphorus: 24 mg, potassium: 62 mg, sodium: 1 mg, zinc: 0.2 mg, thiamin: 0 mg, riboflavin: 0 mg, niacin: 0.1 mg, pyridoxine: 0 mg, folate: 2 mcg, pantothenic acid: 0.1 mg, vitamin B$_{12}$: 0 mcg, vitamin A: 0 mcg, vitamin C: 0 mg, vitamin E: 0 mg, vitamin K: 1 mcg, omega-6 fatty acids: 0.2 g, omega-3 fatty acids: 0 g

Percentage of calories from: protein 7%, fat 50%, carbohydrate 43%

How to Make Homemade Raw Nut Butter

YIELD: 1/3 TO 3/4 CUP (85 TO 185 ML)

The yield of homemade nut butter depends on the type of nut used. Softer, more oily nuts, such as pecans, will require more nuts to equal the same yield as harder nuts like almonds.

1 to 2 cups (250 to 500 ml) raw nuts (such as almonds, cashews, hazelnuts, pecans, or walnuts)

Pulverize the nuts into a paste in a food processor, stopping as needed to scrape down the sides of the work bowl with a rubber spatula. This can take up to 10 minutes. Stored in a sealed container in the refrigerator, homemade raw nut butter will keep for 1 month.

These balls are fun and easy to make. While they are a delicious treat, they provide far more nutritional value than the traditional cookies they replace.

Chocolate-Cranberry **NUT BALLS**

MAKES 36 BALLS

2 cups (500 ml) **dates** (see tip, page 298)

3/4 cup (185 ml) **raw nut butter** (see sidebar)

1/3 cup (80 ml) **raw carob or cacao powder**

1 teaspoon (5 ml) **vanilla extract**

1 cup (250 ml) **coarsely chopped walnuts or pecans**

1/2 cup (125 ml) **dried cranberries**

36 hazelnuts, or 18 brazil nuts

1/3 cup (80 ml) **unsweetened shredded dried coconut or sesame seeds**

Combine the dates, nut butter, carob powder, and vanilla extract in a food processor. Process for about 3 minutes, or until smooth. Add the walnuts and cranberries. Process for a few more seconds, just until evenly incorporated. Refrigerate the mixture for 2–3 hours.

Form the chilled mixture into 1-inch (2.5-cm) balls around 1 hazelnut or 1/2 brazil nut so that the nut is in the middle of the ball. Roll each ball in the coconut. Stored in a covered container, Chocolate-Cranberry Nut Balls will keep for 1 month in the refrigerator or 3 months in the freezer.

Chocolate-Cherry Nut Balls: Replace the cranberries with dried cherries.

Chocolate Fruit-and-Nut Balls: Replace up to 1/2 cup (125 ml) of the dates with dried apricots, peaches, or nectarines (see tip, page 298).

Per ball: calories: 85, protein: 1.5 g, fat: 5 g, carbohydrate: 10 g (8 g from sugar), dietary fiber: 2 g, calcium: 24 mg, copper: 100 mcg, iron: 0.4 mg, magnesium: 25 mg, phosphorus: 43 mg, potassium: 123 mg, sodium: 1 mg, zinc: 0.3 mg, thiamin: 0 mg, riboflavin: 0 mg, niacin: 1 mg, pyridoxine: 0 mg, folate: 8 mcg, pantothenic acid: 0.1 mg, vitamin B$_{12}$: 0 mcg, vitamin A: 0 mcg, vitamin C: 0 mg, vitamin E: 2 mg, vitamin K: 0 mcg, omega-6 fatty acids: 1 g, omega-3 fatty acids: 0.1 g

Percentage of calories from: protein 7%, fat 49%, carbohydrate 44%

This irresistible pie is quick to prepare because the nuts and dates in the crust are not presoaked. You will still need to plan ahead, however, because the finished pie must chill for at least three hours so the filling can firm up. If you prefer, make the recipe without the crust and serve the filling as a pudding topped with sliced strawberries or other fruit.

Mango Pie **WITH COCONUT CRUST**

MAKES 1 PIE; 8 SERVINGS

COCONUT CRUST

MAKES 1 (9-IN./23-CM) CRUST

1½ cups (375 ml) **unsweetened shredded dried coconut**

1½ cups (375 ml) **walnuts or macadamia nuts**

¼ teaspoon (1 ml) **salt**

½ cup pitted medjool or regular dates

MANGO FILLING

MAKES 2 TO 2½ CUPS (500 TO 575 ML)

3 cups (750 ml) chopped fresh mango

1 cup (250 ml) **chopped dried mango** (use scissors to cut it into pieces), **soaked for 10 minutes and drained well** (use your hands to press out the excess liquid)

1 cup (250 ml) or more sliced strawberries or other fruit

To make the crust, put the coconut, walnuts, and salt in a food processor. Process until coarsely ground. Add the dates. Process until the mixture resembles coarse crumbs and begins to stick together. Scoop the mixture into a 9-inch (23-cm) pie plate.

With your palm and fingers, distribute the crumbs evenly along the bottom and up the sides of the pan. There should be a 3/4-inch (2-cm) lip of crumbs along the sides. After the crumbs are evenly distributed, press the crust down on the bottom of the pan using your fingers and palm. Be sure to press especially firmly where the bottom of the pan joins the sides. Then press the crust against the pan's sides, shaping it so that the edges are flush with the rim. Put the crust in the freezer for 15 minutes.

To make the filling, put the fresh and well-drained dried mango in a blender. Process on high speed until smooth.

To assemble, remove the crust from the freezer and spread the filling evenly over the bottom. Arrange the strawberries over the top. Chill for at least 3 hours before serving.

Covered with plastic wrap and stored in the refrigerator, Mango Pie with Coconut Crust will keep for 3 days.

Per serving: calories: 396, protein: 5 g, fat: 23 g, carbohydrate: 52 g (31 g from sugar), dietary fiber: 7 g, calcium: 54 mg, copper: 610 mcg, iron: 1.5 mg, magnesium: 68 mg, phosphorus: 131 mg, potassium: 490 mg, sodium: 126 mg, zinc: 1.1 mg, thiamin: 0.1 mg, riboflavin: 0.1 mg, niacin: 1.3 mg, vitamin B_6: 0.3 mg, folate: 38 mcg, pantothenic acid: 0.3 mg, vitamin B_{12}: 0 mcg, vitamin A: 27 mcg, vitamin C: 37 mg, vitamin E: 1 mg, vitamin K: 4.5 mcg, omega-6 fatty acids: 7.7g, omega-3 fatty acids: 1.8 g

Percentage of calories from: protein 5%, fat 47%, carbohydrate 48%

If you have a Champion, Green Power, or Green Star juicer, or a sturdy food processor, you can start making the simplest and most delicious fat-free, nondairy ice cream imaginable. This creamy dessert, high in potassium and protective phytochemicals, is sweet without any added sugar. For an extra-special treat, top each serving with chopped nuts, unsweetened shredded dried coconut, or fresh berries.

Tutti-Frutti ICE CREAM

MAKES ABOUT 2½ CUPS (625 ML); 2 TO 3 SERVINGS

2 to 3 ripe bananas, peeled, whole or in chunks, and frozen solid (see sidebar, page 256)

2 cups (500 ml) **frozen fruit** (such as berries, cherries, mangoes, and/or strawberries)

Process the fruit through a Green Power, Green Star, or Champion juicer with the blank attachment, alternating the bananas and other frozen fruit. If your kitchen is warm, chill the attachments in the freezer for about 30 minutes before processing the fruit.

If you do not have the appropriate juicer, put the bananas and other frozen fruit in a food processor. Process until smooth. Serve immediately.

TIP: If there is a lot of airspace in the cup when you measure the frozen fruit (as can occur with strawberries or other large pieces of fruit), use heaping cups.

Carob or Chocolate Ice Cream: Add 1 teaspoon (5 ml) of raw carob or cacao powder for each frozen banana used. For extra sweetness, add a few raisins or pitted soft dates.

Blender Ice Cream: Put the bananas and frozen fruit in a high-speed blender. Add 1 cup (250 ml) of Sunflower-Hemp Milk (page 260). Process on high speed until completely smooth. Serve immediately.

Per one-half recipe: calories: 187, protein: 2 g, fat: 0.6 g, carbohydrate: 48 g (30 g from sugar), dietary fiber: 7 g, calcium: 43 mg, copper: 200 mcg, iron: 2 mg, magnesium: 58 mg, phosphorus: 56 mg, potassium: 768 mg, sodium: 6 mg, zinc: 0.5 mg, thiamin: 0.1 mg, riboflavin: 0.2 mg, niacin: 2 mg, pyridoxine: 0.5 mg, folate: 63 mcg, pantothenic acid: 0.6 mg, vitamin B_{12}: 0 mcg, vitamin A: 4 mcg, vitamin C: 106 mg, vitamin E: 0.8 mg, vitamin K: 1 mcg, omega-6 fatty acids: 0.1 g, omega-3 fatty acids: 0.1 g

Percentage of calories from: protein 3%, fat 4%, carbohydrate 93%

Acceptable Macronutrient Distribution Range (AMDR). The AMDR is the range of intakes for protein, carbohydrates, and fat that is associated with an adequate intake of essential nutrients and a reduced risk of chronic disease. The AMDR, set by the Institute of Medicine, is 10–35 percent of calories from protein, 20–35 percent of calories from fat, and 45–65 percent of calories from carbohydrate.

Adequate intake (AI). When insufficient data is available to set Recommended Dietary Allowances (RDA) for nutrients, adequate intake (AI) is set at levels expected to meet or exceed the amount needed to maintain health in a population.

Alliinase. Alliinase is an enzyme found in *Allium* vegetables, such as garlic and onions. The enzyme alliinase converts the phytochemcial called alliin to allicin, its bioactive metabolite.

Alpha-linolenic acid (ALA). ALA is an essential fatty acid and the "parent" of the omega-3 fatty acid family. It can be converted by the body into longer-chain omega-3 fatty acids. Plant sources of alpha-linolenic acid include walnuts and seeds, such as chia, flax, and hemp.

Amylase. Amylase is a starch-digesting enzyme produced in the salivary glands and the pancreas. It is also produced in plants, especially in germinating seeds.

Anthocyanins. Anthocyanins are water-soluble plant pigments that are blue, purple, red, or orange in color. They are a part of the flavonoid family. Anthocyanins are thought to protect against cancer, diabetes, and inflammation, and may also help to delay the aging process.

Antinutrients. Antinutrients are substances that interfere with the absorption and/or utilization of nutrients.

Antioxidants. Antioxidants are dietary compounds that neutralize reactive and highly destructive molecules called free radicals.

Arachidonic acid (AA). Arachidonic acid is an omega-6 polyunsaturated fatty acid involved in the production of hormonelike substances called eicosanoids. The eicosanoids formed from AA tend to promote inflammation and increase several other risk factors for heart disease, hypertension, immune-inflammatory disorders, type 2 diabetes, neurological disorders, and possibly certain cancers.

Bioavailability. The bioavailability of a nutrient refers to the proportion of that nutrient that is absorbed into the bloodstream relative to the amount consumed.

Body mass index (BMI). The body mass index is a measure of body fatness in adults based on an individual's height and weight. Between two people of the same weight, the taller person will have a lower BMI. The formula for calculating BMI is weight in kilograms (kg) divided by height in meters (m) squared.

Breakdown products. Certain chemical reactions in the body cause larger molecules to be broken down into smaller molecules. The smaller molecules are known as breakdown products.

C-reactive protein (CRP). C-reactive protein is a protein in the plasma that is a marker of inflammation. It is measured with a blood test and is known to be elevated in many medical conditions, including heart disease and advanced cancer.

Caloric density. A food's caloric density is the number of calories (food energy) per gram of that food.

Capsaicin. Capsaicin is the active ingredient in chiles that makes them hot. It is used in some applications for pain control and to reduce inflammation.

Carotenoids. Carotenoids are pigments found in leafy green vegetables and orange, red, and yellow vegetables and fruits. They protect cells and tissues from free radical damage, offering protection to the retina of the eye, enhancing immune function, and defending against heart disease, stroke, and cancer. Common carotenoids are beta-carotene (used to form vitamin A), lycopene, and lutein.

Cholesterol. Cholesterol is the most common steroid in the body and is a component in the structure of every cell. While most of our cholesterol is made by the liver and other body tissues, it also comes from animal products in the diet, especially eggs, organ meats, and shellfish.

Coenzyme Q10. A coenzyme is a substance similar to a vitamin (although, unlike a vitamin, it can be produced by the body) that assists the activity of an enzyme. Coenzyme Q10 works with several enzymes that are essential to the generation of energy in cells. Because it facilitates the transfer of electrons, it often works as an antioxidant.

Conversion enzymes. Conversion enzymes transform substances into different compounds, as with the conversion of omega-6 and omega-3 fatty acids into the highly unsaturated fatty acids.

Dietary Reference Intakes (DRI). The DRI is a system of nutrition recommendations for specific nutrients from the Institute of Medicine of the U.S. National Academy of Sciences. Dietary Reference Intakes include Recommended Dietary Allowances (RDA), Adequate Intakes (AI), and Tolerable Upper Intake Levels (UL). The DRI system is used in the United States and Canada.

Digestive enzymes. Digestive enzymes are enzymes produced by the body to break food into smaller building blocks so that nutrients can be absorbed from the digestive tract into the bloodstream and lymph system.

Digestive leukocytosis. Digestive leukocytosis is the scientific term for the rise in white blood cell count that normally occurs after eating.

Disaccharides. Disaccharides consist of two units of sugar linked together, such as sucrose (common table sugar), maltose, and lactose (milk sugar).

Docosahexaenoic acid (DHA). DHA is a highly unsaturated omega-3 fatty acid that is a critical structural component of cell membranes. It is necessary for the proper development and functioning of the brain and central nervous system.

Eicosapentaenoic acid (EPA). EPA is a highly unsaturated omega-3 fatty acid that is used to create substances called eicosanoids. EPA has the opposite effect of arachidonic acid (AA) in that it forms substances that reduce blood pressure, inflammation, and cell proliferation, as well as markers for heart disease.

Enzyme inhibitors. Enzyme inhibitors are molecules that slow or stop enzyme activity.

Enzymes. Enzymes are substances that enable or increase the rates of chemical reactions.

Essential fatty acids (EFA). Essential fatty acids are fatty acids that cannot be manufactured in the body and must be obtained from the food we eat. There are two essential fatty acids: linoleic acid and alpha-linolenic acid.

Fatty acids. The basic components of fats and oils are called fatty acids. They can be either saturated or unsaturated.

Fecal flora. Microorganisms, such as bacteria, that are found in the feces are known as fecal flora.

Fermentation. Fermentation is a method of food preservation that involves the action of microorganisms to convert sugars and other carbohydrates in foods (such as legumes and vegetables) into organic acids, like lactic acid, or alcohol, as with beer and wine.

Flavonoids. Sometimes known as bioflavonoids, flavonoids are phytochemicals known for their antioxidant, anti-inflammatory, and antiviral properties and activities. Research suggests that flavonoids may assist in fighting allergies, inflammation, harmful microbes, and cancer.

Food enzymes. Enzymes in edible plants that catalyze all the reactions necessary to the life of the plant are called food enzymes. Food enzymes have also been shown to offer advantages for human health.

Free radicals. Free radicals are molecules that have one or more unpaired electrons, making them highly unstable.

Fruitarianism. Fruitarians follow a raw diet that is at least 75 percent or more fruit by weight. High-fruit diets are less restrictive, often containing 50–74 percent of calories from fruits. Fruitarians eat not only sweet fruits but also fruits that are typically used as vegetables, such as avocados, peppers, and tomatoes.

Functional fiber. Fiber that is isolated or extracted from plants and has beneficial physiological effects in humans is known as functional fiber.

Gamma-linoleic acid (GLA). GLA is a highly unsaturated omega-6 fatty acid that the body makes from linoleic acid or obtains directly from black currant, borage, or primrose oil. Substances formed from GLA may be effective in the treatment of skin conditions, asthma, premenstrual conditions, and diabetic neuropathy.

Glycemic index (GI). The glycemic index is a measure of the rise in blood sugar following the consumption of 50 grams of carbohydrate from a food. The higher the number, the greater the rise in blood sugar.

Glycemic load. The glycemic load is also a measure of how food affects blood sugar; however, it factors in the amount of carbohydrate a typical serving of the food contains. It is calculated by multiplying the glycemic index by the grams of carbohydrate provided in a serving of the food and dividing the total by 100.

Glycation. Glycation occurs when a sugar molecule binds to protein, fat, or nucleotides (which are the basic structural units of DNA and RNA), without the action of an enzyme. Glycation is a product of the Maillard reaction. Glycoxidation is a term used for glycation when oxygen is involved. Evidence suggests that the end products of glycation and glycoxidation depress immune-system function, accelerate aging, and contribute to chronic degenerative diseases, such as diabetes, cardiovascular disease, and kidney disease.

Heterocyclic amines (HCAs). Heterocyclic amines are substances that are created when meat, poultry, fish, or eggs are cooked at high temperatures. Evidence suggests that they may increase the risk for cancers of the stomach, colon, pancreas, and breast.

Highly unsaturated fatty acids (HUFA). HUFAs, also known as long-chain fatty acids, are large, biologically active, polyunsaturated fatty acid molecules that are created from the essential fatty acids, alpha-linolenic acid and linoleic acid. They can also be obtained directly from foods in the diet.

Homocysteine. Homocysteine is an amino acid that is not present in the diet but can be made by the body from the dietary amino acid methionine as a by-product and can be toxic. High homocysteine levels can increase risk of disease. Certain B vitamins (folate, B_6, and B_{12}) help rid the body of homocysteine. Shortages of these B vitamins can lead to high homocysteine levels. Consequently, elevated homocysteine is sometimes an indicator of a vitamin B_{12} deficiency.

Indispensable amino acids. Indispensable amino acids (formerly known as essential amino acids) are protein building blocks that can't be made by the body and must be obtained directly from food.

Insoluble fiber. Insoluble fiber is an indigestible dietary substance from plants that does not dissolve in water.

Isoflavones. Isoflavones are phytochemicals related to flavonoids that also are known as phytoestrogens (weak estrogens or antiestrogens). They are most concentrated in soybeans, although they are present in some other legumes and in flaxseeds. Isoflavones may afford protection against certain types of breast and prostate cancer.

Lignans. Lignans are phytochemicals that have estrogen-like properties and also act as antioxidants. The richest known source is flaxseeds.

Linoleic acid (LA). LA is an essential fatty acid and is the "parent" fatty acid of the omega-6 fatty acid family. Highly unsaturated omega-6 fatty acids can be manufactured in the body from LA.

Lipases. Lipases are enzymes that act on fats in the digestive tract to break the fat molecules into smaller fragments so they can be absorbed into the bloodstream and lymph system.

Lipids. Lipids are compounds that do not dissolve in water, such as fats and oils (made up of fatty acids) and sterols (such as cholesterol).

Living-food diet. A living-food diet includes sprouted seeds, fresh fruits and vegetables, soaked nuts and seeds, live vegetable krauts, fermented nut and seed cheeses, and other cultured foods containing acidophilus and other probiotics (friendly bacteria), some sea vegetables, wheatgrass juice, and drinks based on vegetables. Foods dehydrated at low temperatures are eaten on occasion.

Lp(a). Lp(a) is a lipoprotein (a fat-and-protein combination) associated with fatty deposits in arteries and an elevated risk for heart disease.

Metabolic acidosis. Metabolic acidosis is a disturbance in the body's pH balance between acid and alkali that results in the blood becoming too acidic. One contributing factor can be an imbalance between acid- and alkaline-forming foods in the diet.

Metabolic enzymes. Metabolic enzymes are highly specialized molecules that perform a wide variety of tasks necessary to run and maintain the body.

Microflora. Bacteria that exist in the intestines are known as microflora, or gut flora. Occasionally their activity is either neutral or harmful, but microflora often contribute to health by crowding out harmful organisms, stimulating the immune system, or producing vitamins and hormones.

Monosaccharides. The only carbohydrates that can be absorbed directly into the blood stream are single-sugar units known as monosaccharides.

Monounsaturated fat. Monounsaturated fats are composed of fatty acids with one point of unsaturation. They have a neutral or slightly beneficial effect on health, with a modest effect on blood cholesterol levels. Monounsaturated fats are generally liquid at room temperature but thick and cloudy when refrigerated.

Myrosinase. Myrosinase is an enzyme responsible for the conversion of certain phytochemicals in cruciferous vegetables to their more active forms.

Natural hygiene. The philosophy of natural hygiene encompasses a number of health-promoting diets; proponents of vegan natural hygiene base their diets on organically grown fresh fruits, vegetables, nuts, and seeds eaten in their raw, natural state. Those who practice natural hygiene also encourage food combining, exposure to sunshine, exercise, adequate sleep, and other lifestyle components to obtain good health.

Nonstarch polysaccharides (NSP). "Nonstarch polysaccharides" is a term often used interchangeably with "fiber." NSP includes all polysaccharides that are indigestible by humans. While NSP makes up the greatest part of fiber, oligosaccharides, lignins, and some resistant starches are also commonly included in the definition of fiber.

Nutritional intake. Nutritional intake refers to the amount of a nutrient (or other dietary component) consumed in the diet. Supplements may or may not be included.

Nutritional yeast. Nutritional yeast is a yeast grown on molasses for use as a flavorful food ingredient. One particular brand, Red Star Vegetarian Support Formula, contains added vitamin B_{12}, a nutrient commonly lacking in vegan and raw vegan diets.

Oligosaccharides. Relatively small carbohydrates consisting of three to nine molecules of sugar are called oligosaccharides. Many oligosaccharides (also known as prebiotics) are not digested in the small intestine, so they pass through and serve as fuel for beneficial bacteria in the large intestine.

Oxidative damage (oxidative stress). The aging, degeneration, and chronic disease caused by free radicals is known as oxidative damage or oxidative stress.

Phase II enzymes. Phase II enzymes belong to a superfamily of enzymes that the body builds from protein and iron. They are potent anticancer agents that protect cells from DNA damage from carcinogens and free radicals.

Phenolic acids. Phenolic acids are a subclass of phytochemicals in the polyphenol class. They are associated with disease risk reduction and are concentrated in berries and black and green teas.

Phytates. Phytates (also known as phytic acid) are the principal storage form of phosphorus in plants. They are often bound together with calcium, magnesium, iron, and zinc.

Phytochemicals. Phytochemicals are chemicals found in plants, produced by them primarily for their own survival and protection. Some phytochemicals also support human health by reducing the risk of chronic disease and fighting existing disease.

Phytosterols. Sterols (a type of lipid) that are naturally present in plants are known as phytosterols.

Polycyclic aromatic hydrocarbons (PAHs). Polycyclic aromatic hydrocarbons (PAHs) are chemicals that are formed by the incomplete burning of organic substances, such as oil, gas, coal, forests, garbage, tobacco, and food. Food accounts for over 90 percent of PAH exposure. PAHs have been associated with DNA damage and increased cancer risk.

Polyphenols. Polyphenols are a class of phytochemicals with antioxidant, and perhaps anticancer, activity. Anthocyanins, catechins, quercetin, and resveratrol are common polyphenols.

Polysaccharides. Polysaccharides are carbohydrates containing at least ten sugar molecules linked together. (Some contain tens or hundreds of sugar molecules linked together.) They are further divided into two groups called starch and nonstarch polysaccharides (NSP). Starch polysaccharides are the plant's energy stores, while nonstarch polysaccharides provide structure to the plant.

Polyunsaturated fat. A polyunsaturated fat has two or more points of unsaturation on the molecule. Polyunsaturated fats are liquid at room temperature and when refrigerated. They include the omega-6 and omega-3 fatty acid families and generally have favorable effects on health.

Proteases. Proteases are enzymes that break protein molecules into amino acids so they can be absorbed into the bloodstream.

Protein-sparing effect of carbohydrate. When sufficient amounts of carbohydrate are consumed, the body will not need to use protein for energy. This is known as the protein-sparing effect of carbohydrate.

Reactive intermediary compounds. An unstable substance that is formed during a chemical reaction is called a reactive intermediary compound. Those that are formed from the actions of Phase I enzymes can become more dangerous in the body when foods that are smoked or barbecued are consumed.

Recommended Dietary Allowance (RDA). The amount of a nutrient that scientists determine will meet the needs of practically all healthy persons is known as the Recommended Dietary Allowance.

Rejuvelac. Rejuvelac is a drink made from fermented, sprouted grains, particularly soft wheat berries.

Saturated fats. Fatty acids that are completely packed, or saturated, with hydrogen and are generally hard at room temperature are called saturated fats. They are highly stable fats or oils found in all fat-containing foods, although they are concentrated in animal products and tropical oils. Saturated fats have consistently been linked to increased blood cholesterol levels, heart disease, several forms of cancer, and insulin resistance.

Soluble fiber. Soluble fiber is a traditional term that has been used to identify certain types of fiber that will dissolve in water, reduce cholesterol, and help control blood sugar. Recent research has demonstrated that some soluble fiber does not affect blood sugar and cholesterol levels, as would have been expected. For this reason, the use of the term "soluble fiber" may be misleading and is being phased out.

Stearidonic acid (SDA). Stearidonic acid is an omega-3 fatty acid that is formed in the first step of the conversion of ALA to EPA and has been shown to produce many of the favorable effects reported for EPA. While stearidonic acid is not commonly found in food, about 2 percent of the oil in hempseed is SDA, as is 12–14 percent of the fat in echium oil (derived from a member of the borage family called purple viper's bugloss). Small amounts of SDA are also present in blue-green algae.

Sterol. Sterol is a type of lipid that plays multiple roles in the body as a part of cell structure, cell communication, and general metabolism.

Storage carbohydrates. Storage carbohydrates are various starches and oligosaccharides found within a whole seed that are used to feed the seed embryo during germination.

Tolerable upper intake levels (UL). Upper intake levels are the daily intakes of nutrients estimated to be the highest levels of intake that will not pose a health risk for most people. Levels above the UL may be associated with health risks.

Trans-fatty acids. Trans-fatty acids are unsaturated fats formed mainly during the process of hydrogenation, a process that turns liquid oils into solid, stable fats. Gram for gram, trans-fatty acids are considered more damaging to health than any other type of fat. As a result, health authorities recommend that we minimize our intake.

REFERENCES

CHAPTER 1
Becoming Raw for Life

1. Eshel G, Martin PA. Geophysics and nutritional science: toward a novel, unified paradigm. *Am J Clin Nutr.* 2009;89:1710S-1716S.

2. Food and Agriculture Organization (FAO). *Livestock's Long Shadow—Environmental Issues and Options.* Rome, 2006.

3. Carlsson-Kanyama A, González AD. Potential contributions of food consumption patterns to climate change. *Am J Clin Nutr.* 2009;89:1704S-1709S.

4. Marlow HJ, Hayes WK, Soret S, Carter RL, Schwab ER, Sabate J. Diet and the environment: does what you eat matter? *Am J Clin Nutr.* 2009;89:1699S-1703S.

CHAPTER 2 (References and Notes)
A History of the Raw-Food Movement in the United States

1. Boston Medical and Surgical Journal. 1836; XIV(Feb. 10):311.

2. Graham S. *Lectures on the Science of Human Life.* New York: Fowler & Wells, 1873;Vol. II:313-315. Reprint of 1837 edition.

3. Ibid:313-16.

4. Graham S. *Lectures on the Science of Human Life.* New York: Fowler & Wells, 1883;Vol. II:453.

5. Ibid:458.

6. Slotnik BJ. Sylvester Graham. In Smith AF ed. *The Oxford Encyclopedia of Food and Drink in America.* Oxford: Oxford University Press, 2004;Vol. I:573-74.

7. Slotnik writes: "He [Graham] developed an Edenic diet: What Adam and Eve ate was good enough for modern man." That grains, perhaps, soaked and sprouted may also have been a part of the primal couple's diet is indicated by a recent translation of Genesis 29: "I have provided all sorts of grains and all sorts of fruits for you to eat." See *The Good News Bible: Today's English Version.* New York: American Bible Society, 92:2.

8. Day C. *Natural Health Gurus Who Ate Animal Foods, 2.* http://chetday.com/healthgurus.htm.

9. Ibid:85-86. Before encountering Shelton's works, Gandhi had learned a good deal about the art of fasting from an earlier graduate of the Macfadden College of Physical Culture: his friend, Dr. Behramja Madon.

10. Vetrano VV. *Errors in Hygiene: T. C. Fry's Devolution, Demise and Why.* Texas: Proper Precept, 1999:84.

11. Ibid:82-83.

12. Esser WL. *Dictionary of Natural Foods.* Bridgeport CT: Natural Hygiene Press, 1983:viii.

13. Vetrano VV. *Genuine Fruitarianism.* Mt. Vernon Washington: Get Well America, 1992:2.

14. My thanks to William Shurtleff, founder and director of Soyinfo Center in Lafayette, CA, for his permission to use detailed material about Otto Carque from his forthcoming book, *History of the Health Food Movement and Industry in the USA and England (1875-1960).*

15. Ibid.

16. Ibid.

17. The other book was *Uncooked Foods and How to Use Them* (1904) by Eugene and Mallis Christian.

18. See note 15 above.

19. Fathman G and D. *Live Foods: Nature's Perfect System of Human Nutrition.* Tucson AZ: Sun Haven Publishers, 1967:120.

20. Just A. *Return to Nature.* New York: Benedict Lust, 1903L:177.

21. St. Louis A. *Estes, Raw Food and Health.* New York: Estes Raw Food and Health Assn., 1927.

22. It was really the third raw food recipe book, if one counts the Christians' *Uncooked Foods and How to Use Them*, which was more of a dissertation with recipes.

23. This quotation is from an article written by Kathryn Friesen called *My Genealogy Search on Dr. Norman Wardhaugh Walker.* http://chetday.com/normanwalker.htm.

24. See vital data pertaining to the superior efficiency of the Norwalk Juicer at www.nwjcal.com and www.norwalkjuicers.com.

25. Walker NM. *Become Younger*. Prescott AZ: Norwalk Press, 1978:23.

26. Friesen K. *My Genealogy Search on Dr. Norman Wardhaugh Walker*. In Chet Day's *Health & Beyond Weekly* and *Health & Beyond Online*. Her findings may be corroborated by checking the Social Security Death Index at http://ssdi.rootsweb.com and by reading the Walker gravestone at the Cottonwood, AZ, cemetery, which reads "Walker Norman W. 1886-1985 & Helen R. 1905-1993." Helen Ruth was his wife.

27. Bragg.com.

28. *Los Angeles Times*. Son Accuses His Wife and Father in Court. Dec. 21, 1955, and Son Drops His Charge Linking Wife, Father. Jan. 17, 1956.

29. Bragg P. *Cure Yourself*. Hollywood, CA: National Diet and Health Association of America, 1929:78.

30. Bragg P. *Paul Bragg's Health Cookbook*. New York: Alfred Knopf, 1947.

31. Day C. *Natural Health Gurus Who Ate Animal Foods*, 3. http://chetday.com/healthgurus.htm.

32. *Miami Herald*. Friday, Dec. 10, 1976, 10-B.

33. Rodwell J, Eding J eds. *The Complete Book of Raw Food*. New York, 2008:427-28.

34. Gregory D. *Dick Gregory's Natural Diet for Folks Who Eat: Cookin' with Mother Nature*. New York: Harper & Row, 1973:7-23.

35. Kulvinskas V. *Love Your Body*. Fairfield, Iowa: 21st Century Publications, 1974:15.

36. Clement BR. *Hippocrates Life Force: Superior Health and Longevity*. Summertown, TN: Healthy Living Publications, 2007:179.

37. Ibid:12.

38. Interview with Aris LaTham. Aug. 10, 2000.

39. Klein D. *The Fruits of Healing*. Sebastopol CA: Living Nutrition Publications, 1999:11.

40. Josephus F. *Jewish Antiquities Books 15, 10, and 4*.

41. Lovewisdom J. *Spiritualizing Dietetics: Vitarianism*. Kaweah CA, 1953:22.

42. Beskow P. *Strange Tales about Jesus: A Survey of Unfamiliar Gospels*. Philadelphia: Fortress Press, 1983:81-91.

43. Malkmus GH. *Why Christians Get Sick*. Shippensburg, PA: Destiny House, 1989:107-109.

CHAPTER 3
The Raw Report: Scientific Evidence to Date

1. Craig WJ, Mangels AR; American Dietetic Association. Position of the American Dietetic Association: vegetarian diets. *J Am Diet Assoc*. 2009;109(7):1266-82.

2. Agren JJ, Tvrzicka E, Nenonen MT, Helve T, Hanninen O. Divergent changes in serum sterols during a strict uncooked vegan diet in patients with rheumatoid arthritis. *Br J Nutr*. 2001;85:137-39.

3. Hanninen O, Kaartinen K, Rauma A, Nenonen M, Torronen R, Hakkinen S, Adlercreutz H, Laakso J. Antioxidants in vegan diet and rheumatic disorders. *Toxicology*. 2000;155:45-53.

4. Hanninen O, Rauma AL, Kaartinen K, Nenonen M. Vegan diet in physiological health promotion. *Acta Physiol Hung*. 1999;86:171-80.

5. Nenonen MT, Helve TA, Rauma AL, Hanninen O. Uncooked, lactobacilli-rich, vegan food and rheumatoid arthritis. *Br J Rheumatol*. 1998;37:274-81.

6. Peltonen R, Nenonen M, Helve T, Hanninen O, Toivanen P, Eerola E. Faecal microbial flora and disease activity in rheumatoid arthritis during a vegan diet. *Br J Rheumatol*. 1997;36:64-68.

7. Rauma AL, Nenonen M, Helve T, Hanninen O. Effect of a strict vegan diet on energy and nutrient intakes by Finnish rheumatoid patients. *Eur J Clin Nutr*. 1993;47:747-49.

8. Ryhanan EL, Mantere-Alhonen S, Nenonen M, Hanninen O. Modification of faecal flora in rheumatoid arthritis patients by lactobacilli rich vegetarian diet. *Milchwissenschaft*. 1993;48:255-59.

9. Sköldstam L, Brudin L, Hagfors L, Johansson G. Weight reduction is not a major reason for improvement in rheumatoid arthritis from lacto-vegetarian, vegan or Mediterranean diets. *Nutr J*. 2005;4:15.

10. Muller H, de Toledo FW, Resch KL. Fasting followed by vegetarian diet in patients with rheumatoid arthritis: a systematic review. *Scand J Rheumatol*. 2001;30:1-10.

11. Adam O, Beringer C, Kless T, Lemmen C, Adam A, Wiseman M, Adam P, Klimmek R, Forth W. Anti-inflammatory effects of a low arachidonic acid diet and fish oil in patients with rheumatoid arthritis. *Rheumatol Int*. 2003;23:27-36.

12. Hanninen O, Nenonen M, Ling WH, Li DS, Sihvonen L. Effects of eating an uncooked vegetable diet for one week. *Appetite.* 1992;19:243-54.

13. Elkan AC, Sjöberg B, Kolsrud B, Ringertz B , Hafström I, Frostegard, J. Gluten-free vegan diet induces decreased LDL and oxidized LDL levels and raised atheroprotective natural antibodies against phosphorylcholine in patients with rheumatoid arthritis: a randomized study. *Arthritis Res Ther.* 2008;10:R34.

14. McDougall J, Bruce B, Spiller G, Westerdahl J, McDougall M. Effects of a very low-fat, vegan diet in subjects with rheumatoid arthritis. *J Altern Complement Med.* 2002;8:71-75.

15. Hafstrom I, Ringertz B, Spangberg A, von Zweigbergk L, Brannemark S, Nylander I, Ronnelid J, Laasonen L, Klareskog L. A vegan diet free of gluten improves the signs and symptoms of rheumatoid arthritis: the effects on arthritis correlate with a reduction in antibodies to food antigens. *Rheumatology* (Oxford). 2001;40:1175-79.

16. Fujita A, Hashimoto Y, Nakahara K, Tanaka T, Okuda T, Koda M. Effects of a low calorie vegan diet on disease activity and general conditions in patients with rheumatoid arthritis. *Rinsho Byori* (Japanese). 1999;47:554-60.

17. Kjeldsen-Kragh J. Rheumatoid arthritis treated with vegetarian diets. *Am J Clin Nutr.* 1999;70:594S-600S.

18. Kjeldsen-Kragh J, Hvatum M, Haugen M, Forre O, Scott H. Antibodies against dietary antigens in rheumatoid arthritis patients treated with fasting and a one-year vegetarian diet. *Clin Exp Rheumatol.* 1995;13:167-72.

19. Kjeldsen-Kragh J, Haugen M, Borchgrevink CF, Førre O. Vegetarian diet for patients with rheumatoid arthritis—status: two years after introduction of the diet. *Clin Rheumatol.* 1994;13:475-82. Erratum in *Clin Rheumatol.* 1994;13:649.

20. Kjeldsen-Kragh J, Haugen M, Borchgrevink C et al. Controlled trial of fasting and one-year vegetarian diet in rheumatoid arthritis. *Lancet.* 1991:338:899-902.

21. Peltonen R, Kjeldsen-Kragh J, Haugen M et al. Changes of faecal flora in rheumatoid arthritis during fasting and one-year vegetarian diet. *Br J Rheumatol.* 1994;33:638-43.

22. Haugen MA, Kjeldsen-Kragh J, Bjerve KS, Høstmark AT, Førre Ø. Changes in plasma phospholipid fatty acids and their relationship to disease activity in rheumatoid arthritis patients treated with a vegetarian diet. *Br J Nutr.* 1994;72:555-66.

23. Beri D, Malaviya AN, Shandilya R, Singh, RR. Effect of dietary restrictions on disease activity in rheumatoid arthritis. *Ann Rheum Dis.* 1988;47:69-72.

24. Sköldstam L. Fasting and vegan diet in rheumatoid arthritis. *Scand J Rheum.* 1986;15:219-21.

25. Sköldstam L, Larsson L, Lindström FD: Effects of fasting and lactovegetarian diet on rheumatoid arthritis. *Scand J Rheumatol.* 1979;8:249-55.

26. Ebringer A, Rashid T. Rheumatoid arthritis is an autoimmune disease triggered by *Proteus* urinary tract infection. *Clin Dev Immunol.* 2006 Mar;13(1):41-48.

27. Donaldson MS, Speight N, Loomis S. Fibromyalgia syndrome improved using a mostly raw vegetarian diet: an observational study. *BMC Complement Altern Med.* 2001;1:7.

28. Kaartinen K, Lammi K, Hypen M, Nenonen M, Hanninen O, Rauma AL. Vegan diet alleviates fibromyalgia symptoms. *Scand J Rheumatol.* 2000;29:308-13.

29. Hostmark AT, Lystad E, Vellar OD, Hovi K, Berg JE. Reduced plasma fibrinogen, serum peroxides, lipids, and apolipoproteins after a three-week vegetarian diet. *Plant Foods Hum Nutr.* 1993;43:55-61.

30. Azad KA, Alam MN, Haq SA, Nahar S, Chowdhury MA, Ali SM, Ullah AK. Vegetarian diet in the treatment of fibromyalgia. *Bangladesh Med Res Counc Bull.* 2000;26:41-47.

31. Fontana L, Klein S, Holloszy JO. Long-term low-protein, low-calorie diet and endurance exercise modulate metabolic factors associated with cancer risk. *Am J Clin Nutr.* 2006;84:1456-62.

32. Verhagen H, Rauma AL, Torronen R, de Vogel N, Bruijntjes-Rozier GC, Drevo MA, Bogaards JJ, Mykkanen H. Effect of a vegan diet on biomarkers of chemoprevention in females. *Hum Exp Toxicol.* 1996;15:821-25.

33. Ling WH, Hanninen O. Shifting from a conventional diet to an uncooked vegan diet reversibly alters fecal hydrolytic activities in humans. *J Nutr.* 1992;122:924-30.

34. Gaisbauer M, Langosch A. Raw food and immunity. *Fortschr Med* (German). 1990 Jun;108:338-40.

35. Peltonen R, Ling WH, Hanninen O, Eerola E. An uncooked vegan diet shifts the profile of human fecal microflora: computerized analysis of direct stool sample gas-liquid chromatog-

raphy profiles of bacterial cellular fatty acids. *Appl Environ Microbiol*. 1992;58:3660-66.

36. World Cancer Research Fund American Institute for Cancer Research. *Food, Nutrition, Physical Activity and the Prevention of Cancer: A Global Perspective*. Washington DC: AICR, 2007.

37. Steinmetz KA, Potter JD. Vegetables, fruit and cancer prevention: a review. *J Am Diet Assoc*. 1996;96:1027-39.

38. Steinmetz KA, Potter JD. Vegetables, fruit, and cancer. 1: epidemiology. *Cancer Causes Control*. 1991;2:325-57.

39. Link LB, Potter JD. Raw versus cooked vegetables and cancer risk. *Cancer Epidemiol Biomarkers Prev*. 2004;13:1422-35.

40. Bessaoud F, Daurès JP. Dietary factors and breast cancer risk: a case control study among a population in Southern France. *Nutr Cancer*. 2008;60:177-87.

41. Tang L, Zirpoli GR, Guru K, Moysich KB, Zhang Y, Ambrosone CB, McCann SE. Consumption of raw cruciferous vegetables is inversely associated with bladder cancer risk. *Cancer Epidemiol Biomarkers Prev*. 2008;17:938-44.

42. Schouten LJ, Goldbohm RA, van den Brandt PA. Consumption of vegetables and fruits and risk of ovarian carcinoma. *Cancer*. 2005;104:1512-19.

43. Hildenbrand GL, Hildenbrand LC, Bradford K, Cavin SW. Five-year survival rates of melanoma patients treated by diet therapy after the manner of Gerson: a retrospective review. *Altern Ther Health Med*. 1995;1(4):29-37.

44. Lechner P, Kronberger J. Experience with the use of dietary therapy in surgical oncology. *Akt Ernahr-Med* (German). 1990;15:72-78.

45. Austin S, Dale EB, Dekadt S. Long-term follow up of cancer patients using Contreras, Hoxsey and Gerson therapies. *J Naturopath Med*. 1994;5:74-76.

46. Gerson M. Effects of combined dietary regimens on patients with malignant tumors. *Exp Med Surg*. 1949;7:299-317.

47. Gerson, M. Dietary considerations in malignant neoplastic diseases: A preliminary report. *Rev Gastroent*. 1945;12:419-25.

48. Hu FB. Plant-based foods and prevention of cardiovascular disease: an overview. *Am J Clin Nutr*. 2003;78:544S-51S.

49. WHO, Consultation FAO. Diet, Nutrition and the Prevention of Chronic Diseases. WHO Technical Report Series. 2003;916. http://whqlibdoc.who.int/trs/WHO_trs_916.pdf. Accessed July 2009.

50. Esselstyn CB Jr. Resolving the coronary artery disease epidemic through plant-based nutrition. *Prev Cardiol*. 2001;4:171-77.

51. Esselstyn CB Jr. Updating a twelve-year experience with arrest and reversal therapy for coronary heart disease (an overdue requiem for palliative cardiology). *Am J Cardiol*. 1999;84:339-41.

52. Ornish D, Brown SE, Scherwitz LW et al. Can lifestyle changes reverse coronary heart disease: The Lifestyle Heart Trial. *Lancet*. 1990;336:129-33.

53. Ornish D, Scherwitz LW, Billings JH, Gould KL, Merritt TA, Sparler S, Armstrong WT, Ports TA, Kirkeeide RL, Hogeboom C, Brand RJ. Intensive lifestyle changes for reversal of coronary heart disease. *JAMA*. 1998;280:2001-07.

54. Fontana L, Meyer TE, Klein S, Holloszy JO. Long-term low-calorie low-protein vegan diet and endurance exercise are associated with low cardiometabolic risk. *Rejuvenation Res*. 2007;10:225-34.

55. Koebnick C, Garcia AL, Dagnelie PC, Strassner C, Lindemans J, Katz N, Leitzmann C, Hoffmann I. Long-term consumption of a raw food diet is associated with favorable serum LDL cholesterol and triglycerides but also with elevated plasma homocysteine and low serum HDL cholesterol in humans. *J Nutr*. 2005;135:2372-78.

56. Herrmann W, Herrmann M, Obeid R. Hyperhomocysteinaemia: a critical review of old and new aspects. *Curr Drug Metab*. 2007;8:17-31.

57. Krajcovicova-Kudlackova M, Blazicek P, Mislanova C, Valachovicova M, Paukova V, Spustova V. Nutritional determinants of plasma homocysteine. *Bratisl Lek Listy*. 2007;108:510-15.

58. Michos ED, Melamed ML. Vitamin D and cardiovascular disease risk. *Curr Opin Clin Nutr Metab Care*. 2008;11:7-12.

59. Harris WS, Kris-Etherton PM, Harris KA. Intakes of long-chain omega-3 fatty acid associated with reduced risk for death from coronary heart disease in healthy adults. *Curr Atheroscler Rep*. 2008;10:503-09.

60. Saremi A, Arora R. The utility of omega-3 fatty acids in cardiovascular disease. *Am J Ther*. May 19, 2009. Epub ahead of print.

61. Turner-McGrievy GM, Barnard ND, Cohen J, Jenkins DJ, Gloede L, Green AA. Changes in nutrient intake and dietary quality among participants with type 2 diabetes following a low-fat vegan diet or a conventional dia-

betes diet for 22 weeks. *J Am Diet Assoc.* 2008;108:1636-45.

62. Barnard ND, Cohen J, Jenkins DJ, Turner-McGrievy G, Gloede L, Jaster B, Seidl K, Green AA, Talpers S. A low fat vegan diet improves glycemic control and cardiovascular risk factors in a randomized clinical trial in individuals with type 2 diabetes. *Diabetes Care.* 2006;29:1777-83.

63. Redmon BJ, Reck KP; Raatz SK, Swanson JE; Kwong CA, Ji H; Thomas W; Bantle JP. Two-year outcome of a combination of weight loss therapies for type 2 diabetes. *Diabetes Care.* 2005;28:1311-15.

64. Cousens G, Rainoshek G. *There Is a Cure for Diabetes: The Tree of Life 21-day+ Program.* Berkeley CA: North Atlantic Books, 2008.

65. Penckofer S, Kouba J, Wallis DE, Emanuele MA. Vitamin D and diabetes: let the sunshine in. *Diabetes Educ.* 2008;34:939-40, 942, 944.

66. Sahin M, Tutuncu NB, Ertugrul D, Tanaci N, Guvener ND. Effects of metformin or rosiglitazone on serum concentrations of homocysteine, folate, and vitamin B$_{12}$ in patients with type 2 diabetes mellitus. *J Diabetes Complications.* 2007;21:118-23.

67. Sun Y, Lai MS, and Lu CJ. Effectiveness of vitamin B$_{12}$ on diabetic neuropathy: systematic review of clinical controlled trials. *Acta Neurol* (Taiwan). 2005;14:48-54.

68. Pouwer F, Nijpels G, Beekman AT, Dekker JM, van Dam RM, Heine RJ, Snoek FJ. Fat food for a bad mood. Could we treat and prevent depression in type 2 diabetes by means of omega-3 polyunsaturated fatty acids? A review of the evidence. *Diabet Med.* 2005;22:1465-75.

69. Koebnick C, Strassner C, Hoffmann I, Leitzmann C. Consequences of a long-term raw food diet on body weight and menstruation: results of a questionnaire survey. *Ann Nutr Metab.* 1999;43:69-79.

70. Fontana L, Shew JL, Holloszy JO, Villareal DT. Low bone mass in subjects on a long-term raw vegetarian diet. *Arch Intern Med.* 2005;165:684-89.

71. Obeid R, Geisel J, Schorr H, Hübner U, Herrmann W. The impact of vegetarianism on some haematological parameters. *Eur J Haematol.* 2002;69:275-79.

72. Herrmann W, Schorr H, Purschwitz K, Rassoul F, Richter V. Total homocysteine, vitamin B$_{12}$, and total antioxidant status in vegetarians. *Clin Chem.* 2001;47:1094-101.

73. Barr SI, Broughton TM. Relative weight, weight loss efforts and nutrient intakes among health-conscious vegetarian, past vegetarian and nonvegetarian women ages 18 to 50. *J Am Coll Nutr.* 2000;19:781-88.

74. Hokin B, Adams M, Ashton J, Louie H. Comparison of the dietary cobalt intake in three different Australian diets. *Asia Pac J Clin Nutr.* 2004;13:289-91.

75. Crane MG, Sample C, Pathcett S, Register UD. Vitamin B$_{12}$ studies in total vegetarians (vegans). *J Nutr Med.* 1994;4:419-30.

76. Donaldson M. Food and nutrition intake of Hallelujah vegetarians. *Nutr Food Sci.* 2001;31(6):293-303.

77. Donaldson MS. Metabolic vitamin B$_{12}$ status on a mostly raw vegan diet with follow-up using tablets, nutritional yeast, or probiotic supplements. *Ann Nutr Metab.* 2000;44(5-6):229-34.

78. Rauma AL, Torronen R, Hanninen O, Mykkanen H. Vitamin B$_{12}$ status of long-term adherents of a strict uncooked vegan diet ("living food diet") is compromised. *J Nutr.* 1995;125:2511-15.

79. Dong A, Scott SC. Serum vitamin B$_{12}$ and blood cell values in vegetarians. *Ann Nutr Metab.* 1982;26:209-16.

80. Agren JJ, Tormala ML, Nenonen MT, Hanninen O. Fatty acid composition of erythrocyte, platelet, and serum lipids in strict vegans. *Lipids.* 1995;30:365-69.

81. Hoffmann I, Leitzmann C. Raw food diet: health benefits and risks. In Watson RR, ed. *Vegetables, Fruits, and Herbs in Health Promotion.* Boca Raton FL: CRC Press, 2000:293-308.

82. Garcia AL, Koebnick C, Dagnelie PC, Strassner C, Elmadfa I, Katz N, Leitzmann C, Hoffmann I. Long-term strict raw food diet is associated with favourable plasma beta-carotene and low plasma lycopene concentrations in Germans. *Br J Nutr.* 2008;99:1293-300.

83. Rauma AL, Torronen R, Hanninen O, Verhagen H, Mykkanen H. Antioxidant status in long-term adherents to a strict uncooked vegan diet. *Am J Clin Nutr.* 1995;62(6):1221-27.

84. Ganss C, Schlechtriemen M, Klimek J. Dental erosions in subjects living on a raw food diet. *Caries Res.* 1999;33:74-80.

CHAPTER 4

Why Raw Rocks!

1. World Cancer Research Fund American Institute for Cancer Research. *Food, Nutrition, Physical Activity and the Prevention of Cancer: A Global Perspective.* Washington DC: AICR, 2007.

2. Gropper SS, Smith JL, Groff JL. *Advanced Nutrition and Human Metabolism. 5th Edition.* Belmont CA: Wadsworth Cengage Learning, 2009.

3. Denny A, Buttriss J. *Synthesis Report No 4: Plant Foods and Health: Focus on Plant Bioactives.* Norwich, Norfolk UK: British Nutrition Foundation, EuroFIR Institute of Food Research, 2007.

4. Eskin M, Tamir S. *Dictionary of Nutraceuticals and Functional Foods.* Boca Raton FL: CRC Press Taylor and Francis Group, 2005.

5. Liu RH. Potential synergy of phytochemicals in cancer prevention: mechanism of action. *J Nutr.* 2004;134(12 Suppl):3479S-85S.

6. Beliveau R, Gingras, D. *Foods That Fight Cancer: Preventing Cancer through Diet.* Toronto: Molecular medicine laboratory, Sainte-Justine Hospital Research Centre and the University of Quebec at Montreal, 2006.

7. Rao AV. *Anticarcinogenic properties of plant saponins. Second international symposium on the role of soy in preventing and treating chronic disease.* Brussels, Belgium. Sept. 15-18, 1996.

8. Winter C, Davis S. Organic foods: scientific status summary. *J Food Sci.* 2006;71.

9. Zhao X, Carey EE, Wang W, Rajashekar CB. Does organic production enhance phytochemical content of fruit and vegetables? Current knowledge and prospects for research. *Hort Technology.* 2006;16:449-56.

10. Asami DK, Hong YJ, Barrett DM, Mitchell AE. Comparison of the total phenolic and ascorbic acid content of freeze-dried and air-dried marionberry, strawberry, and corn grown using conventional, organic, and sustainable agricultural practices. *J Agric Food Chem.* 2003;51:1237-41.

11. Baxter GJ, Graham AB, Lawrence JR, Wiles D, Paterson JR. Salicylic acid in soups prepared from organically and non-organically grown vegetables. *Eur J Nutr.* 2001;40:289-92.

12. Carbonaro M, Mattera M. Polyphenoloxidase activity and polyphenol levels in organically and conventionally grown peach (Prunus persicaI L., cv. Regina bianca) and pear (Pyrus communis L., cv. Williams). *Food Chem.* 2001;72:419-24.

13. Carbonaro M, Mattera M, Nicoli S, Bergamo P, Cappelloni M. Modulation of antioxidant compounds in organic vs. conventional fruit (peach, Prunus persica L., and pear, Pyrus communis L.). *J Agric Food Chem.* 2002;50:5458-62.

14. Caris-Veyrat C, Amiot MJ, Tyssandier V, Grasselly D, Buret M, Mikolajczak M, Guilland JC, Bouteloup-Demange C, Borel P. Influence of organic versus conventional agricultural practice on the antioxidant microconstituent content of tomatoes and derived purees; consequences on antioxidant plasma status in humans. *J Agric Food Chem.* 2004;52:6503-09.

15. Dani C, Oliboni LS, Vanderlinde R, Bonatto D, Salvador M, Henriques JA. Phenolic content and antioxidant activities of white and purple juices manufactured with organically or conventionally produced grapes. *Food Chem Toxicol.* 2007;45:2574-80.

16. Mitchell AE, Hong YJ, Koh E, Barrett DM, Bryant DE, Denison RF, Kaffka S. Ten-year comparison of the influence of organic and conventional crop management practices on the content of flavonoids in tomatoes. *J Agric Food Chem.* 2007;55:6154-59.

17. Nunez-Delicado E, Sanchez-Ferrer A, Garcia-Carmona FF, Lopez-Nicolas JM. Effect of organic farming practices on the level of latent polyphenoloxidase in grapes. *J Food Sci.* 2005;70:C74-78.

18. Ren H, Endo H, Hayashi T. Antioxidative and antimutagenic activities and polyphenol content of pesticide-free and organically cultivated green vegetables using water-soluble chitosan as a soil modifier and leaf surface spray. *J Sci Food Agric.* 2001;81:1426-32.

19. Tarozzi A, Hrelia S, Angeloni C, Morroni F, Biagi P, Guardigli M, Cantelli-Forti G. Antioxidant effectiveness of organically and non-organically grown red oranges in cell culture systems. *J Nutr.* 2006;45:152-58.

20. Tinttunen S, Lehtonen P. Distinguishing organic wines from normal wines on the basis of concentrations of phenolic compounds and spectral data. *Eur Food Res Technol.* 2001;212:390-94.

21. Veberic R, Trobec M, Herbinger K, Hofer M, Grill D, Stampar F. Phenolic compounds in some apple (Malus domestica Borkh) cultivars of organic and integrated production. *J Sci Food Agric.* 2005;85:1687-94.

22. Young JE, Zhao X, Carey EE, Welti R, Yang SS, Wang W. Phytochemical phenolics in organically grown vegetables. *Mol Nutr Food Res.* 2005;49:1136-42.

23. Briviba K, Stracke BA, Rüfer CE, Watzl B, Weibel FP, Bub A. Effect of consumption of organically and conventionally produced apples on antioxidant activity and DNA damage in humans. *J Agric Food Chem.* 2007;55:7716-21.

24. Hakkinen SH, Torronen AR. Content of flavonols and selected phenolic acids in strawberries and Vaccinium species: influence of cultivar, cultivation site and technique. *Food Res Int.* 2000;33:517-24.

25. Mikkonen TP, Maatta KR, Hukkanen AT, Kokko HI, Torronen AR, Karenlampi SO, Karjalainen RO. Flavonol content varies among black currant cultivars. *J Agric Food Chem.* 2001;49:3274-77.

26. Stracke BA, Rüfer CE, Bub A, Briviba K, Seifert S, Kunz C, Watzl B. Bioavailability and nutritional effects of carotenoids from organically and conventionally produced carrots in healthy men. *Br J Nutr.* 2009;101:1664-72. Epub Nov. 20, 2008.

27. Tarozzi A, Marchesi A, Cantelli-Forti G, Hrelia P. Cold-storage affects antioxidant properties of apples in Caco-2 cells. *J Nutr.* 2004;134:1105-09.

28. Lombardi-Boccia G, Lucarini M, Lanzi S, Aguzzi A, Cappelloni M. Nutrients and antioxidant molecules in yellow plums (Prunus domestics L.) from conventional and organic productions: a comparative study. *J Agric Food Chem.* 2004;52:90-94.

29. Ferracane R, Pellegrini N, Visconti A, Graziani G, Chiavaro E, Miglio C, Fogliano V. Effects of different cooking methods on antioxidant profile, antioxidant capacity, and physical characteristics of artichoke. *J Agric Food Chem.* 2008;56:8601-08.

30. Miglio C, Chiavaro E, Visconti A, Fogliano V, and Pellegrini N. Effects of different cooking methods on nutritional and physicochemical characteristics of selected vegetables. *J Agric Food Chem.* 2008;56:139-47.

31. Fimognari C, Lenzi M, Hrelia P. Chemoprevention of cancer by isothiocyanates and anthocyanins: mechanisms of action and structure-activity relationship. *Curr Med Chem.* 2008;15:440-47.

32. Zhang Y, Callaway EC. High cellular accumulation of sulphoraphane, a dietary anticarcinogen, is followed by rapid transporter-mediated export as a glutathione conjugate. *Biochem J.* 2002;364(Pt 1):301-07.

33. Verkerk R, Dekker M. Glucosinolates and myrosinase activity in red cabbage (Brassica oleracea L. var. Capitata f. rubra DC.) after various microwave treatments. *J Agric Food Chem.* 2004;52:7318-23.

34. Conaway CC, Getahun SM, Liebes LL, Pusateri DJ, Topham DK, Botero-Omary M, Chung FL. Disposition of glucosinolates and sulforaphane in humans after ingestion of steamed and fresh broccoli. *Nutr Cancer.* 2000;38:168-78. Erratum in *Nutr Cancer* 2001;41:196.

35. Rouzaud G, Rabot S, Ratcliffe B, Duncan AJ. Influence of plant and bacterial myrosinase activity on the metabolic fate of glucosinolates in gnotobiotic rats. *Br J Nutr.* 2003;90:395-404.

36. Getahun SM, Chung FL. Conversion of glucosinolates to isothiocyanates in humans after ingestion of cooked watercress. *Cancer Epidemiol Biomarkers Prev.* 1999;8:447-51.

37. Tapiero H, Townsend DM, Tew KD. Organosulfur compounds from alliaceae in the prevention of human pathologies. *Biomed Pharmacother.* 2004;58:183-93.

38. Song K, Milner JA. The influence of heating on the anticancer properties of garlic. *J Nutr.* 2001;131:1054S-57S.

39. Fujisawa H, Suma K, Origuchi K, Seki T, Ariga T. Thermostability of allicin determined by chemical and biological assays. *Biosci Biotechnol Biochem.* 2008;72:2877-83.

40. Vallejo F, Tomás-Barberán FA, Garcia-Viguera C. Glucosinolates and vitamin C content in edible parts of broccoli florets after domestic cooking. *Eur Food Res Technol.* 2002;215:310-16.

41. Galgano F, Favati F, Caruso M, Pietrafesa A, Natella S. The influence of processing and preservation on the retention of health-promoting compounds in broccoli. *J Food Sci.* 2007; 72: S130-35.

42. López-Berenguer C, Carvajal M, Moreno DA, García-Viguera, C. Effects of microwave cooking conditions on bioactive compounds present in broccoli inflorescences. *J Agric Food Chem.* 2007;55:10001-07.

43. Rungapamestry V, Rabot S, Fuller Z, Ratcliffe B, Duncan AJ. Influence of cooking duration of cabbage and presence of colonic microbiota on the excretion of N-acetylcysteine conjugates of allyl isothiocyanate and bioactivity of phase 2 enzymes in F344 rats. *Br J Nutr.* 2008;99:773-81.

44. Micozzi MS, Beecher GR, Taylor PR, Khachik F. Carotenoid analyses of selected raw and cooked foods associated with a lower risk for cancer. *J Natl Cancer Inst.*1990;8:282-85. Erratum in *J Natl Cancer Inst.* 1990;82:715.

45. Rosa EAS, Heaney RK. The effect of cooking and processing on the glucosinolate content: studies on four varieties of Portuguese cabbage and hybrid white cabbage. *J Sci Food Agric.* 1993;62:259-65.

46. Fuller Z, Louis P, Mihajlovski A, Rungapamestry V, Ratcliffe B, Duncan AJ. Influence of cabbage processing methods and prebiotic manipulation of colonic microflora on glucosinolate breakdown in man. *Br J Nutr.* 2007;98:364-72.

47. Volden J, Wicklund T, Verkerk R, Dekker M. Kinetics of changes in glucosinolate concentrations during long-term cooking of white cabbage (Brassica oleracea L. ssp. capitata f. alba). *J Agric Food Chem.* 2008;56:2068-73.

48. Ali M, Thomson M. Consumption of a garlic clove a day could be beneficial in preventing thrombosis. *Prostaglandins Leukot Essentl Fatty Acids.* 1995;53:211-12.

49. Ali M, Bordia T, Mustafa T. Effect of raw versus boiled aqueous extract of garlic and onion on platelet aggregation. *Prostaglandins Leukot Essent Fatty Acids.* 1999;Jan;60(1):43-47.

50. Gorinstein S, Drzewiecki J, Leontowicz H, Leontowicz M, Najman K, Jastrzebski Z, Zachwieja Z, Barton H, Shtabsky B, Katrich E, Trakhtenberg S. Comparison of the bioactive compounds and antioxidant potentials of fresh and cooked Polish, Ukrainian, and Israeli garlic. *J Agric Food Chem.* 2005;53:2726-32.

51. Krishnaswamy K, Raghuramulu N. Bioactive phytochemicals with emphasis on dietary practices. *Indian J Med Res.* 1998;108:167-81.

52. Tarwadi K, Agte V. Potential of commonly consumed green leafy vegetables for their antioxidant capacity and its linkage with the micronutrient profile. *Int J Food Sci Nutr.* 2003; 54:417-25.

53. Rouzaud G, Young SA, Duncan AJ. Hydrolysis of glucosinolates to isothiocyanates after ingestion of raw or microwaved cabbage by human volunteers. *Cancer Epidemiol Biomarkers Prev.* 2004;13:125-31.

54. Lee SU, Lee JH, Choi SH, Lee JS, Ohnisi-Kameyama M, Kozukue N, Levin CE, Friedman M. Flavonoid content in fresh, home-processed, and light-exposed onions and in dehydrated commercial onion products. *J Agric Food Chem.* 2008;56:8541-48.

55. Rohn S, Buchner N, Driemel G, Rauser M, Kroh LW. Thermal degradation of onion quercetin glucosides under roasting conditions. *J Agric Food Chem.* 2007;55:1568-73.

56. Xu B, Chang SK. Total phenolics, phenolic acids, isoflavones, and anthocyanins and antioxidant properties of yellow and black soybeans as affected by thermal processing. *J Agric Food Chem.* 2008;56:7165-75.

57. Andlauer W, Stumpf C, Hubert M, Rings A, Furst P. Influence of cooking process on phenolic marker compounds of vegetables. *Int J Vitam Nutr Res.* 2003;73:152-59.

58. Hedren E, Diaz V, Svanberg U. Estimation of carotenoid accessibility from carrots determined by an in vitro digestion method. *Eur J Clin Nutr.* 2002;56:425-30.

59. Dewanto V, Wu X, Liu RH. Processed sweet corn has higher antioxidant activity. *J Agric Food Chem.* 2002;50(17):4959-64.

60. Truong VD, McFeeters RF, Thompson RT, Dean LL, Shofran B. Phenolic acid content and composition in leaves and roots of common commercial sweet potato (Ipomea batatas L.) cultivars in the United States. *J Food Sci.* 2007;72(6):C343-49.

61. Dewanto V, Wu X, Adom KK, Liu RH. Thermal processing enhances the nutritional value of tomatoes by increasing total antioxidant activity. *J Agric Food Chem.* 2000;50:3010-14.

62. Jiratanan T, Liu RH. Antioxidant activity of processed table beets (Beta vulgaris var, conditiva) and green beans (Phaseolus vulgaris L). *J Agric Food Chem.* 2004;52:2659-70.

63. Gliszczynska-Swiglo A, Ciska E, Pawlak-Lemanska K, Chmielewski E, Borkowski T, Tyrakowska B. Changes in the content of health-promoting compounds and antioxidant activity of broccoli after domestic processing. *Food Addit Contam.* 2006;23:1088-98.

64. Song L, Thornalley PJ. Effect of storage, processing and cooking on glucosinolate content of Brassica vegetables. *Food Chem Toxicol.* 2007;45:216-24.

65. Maiani G, Caston MJP, Catasta G, Toti E, Cambrodon IG, Bysted A, Granado-Lorencio F, Olmedilla-Alonso B, Knuthsen P, Massimo Valoti, Volker B, Mayer-Miebach E, Behsnilian D, Schlemmer U. Carotenoids: actual knowledge on food sources, intakes, stability and bioavailability and their protective role in humans. *Mol Nutr Food Res.* 2008;Nov. 26. Epub ahead of print.

66. Bugianesi R, Salucci M, Leonardi C, Ferracane R, Catasta G, Azzini E et al. Effect of domestic cooking on human bioavailability of naringenin, chlorogenic acid, lycopene and b-carotene in cherry tomatoes. *Eur J Nutr.* 2004;43:360-66.

67. Porrini M, Riso P, Testolin G. Absorption of lycopene from single or daily portions of raw and processed tomato. *Br J Nutr.* 1998;80:353-61.

68. Gartner C, Stahl W, Sies H. Lycopene is more bioavailable from tomato paste than from fresh tomatoes. *Am J Clin Nutr*. 1997;66:116-22.

69. Stahl W, Schwarz W, Sundquist AR, Sies H. Cis-trans isomers of lycopene and beta-carotene in human serum and tissues. *Arch Biochem Biophys*. 1992;294:173-77.

70. Dietz JM, Kantha SS, Erdman JW Jr. Reversed phase HPLC analysis of alpha and beta-carotene from selected raw and cooked vegetables. *Plant Food Hum Nutr*. 1988;38:333-41.

71. Reboul E, Richelle M, Perrot E, Desmoulins-Malezet C, Pirisi V, Borel P. Bioaccessibility of carotenoids and vitamin E from their main dietary sources. *J Agric Food Chem*. 2006;54:8749-55.

72. McEligot AJ, Rock CL, Shanks TG, Flatt SW, Newman V, Faerber S, Pierce JP. Comparison of serum carotenoid responses between women consuming vegetable juice and women consuming raw or cooked vegetables. *Cancer Epidemiol Biomarkers Prev*. 1999;8:227-31.

73. Khachik F, Goli MB, Beecher GR, Holden J, Lusby WR, Tenorio MD, Barrera MR. Effect of food preparation on qualitative and quantitative distribution of major carotenoid constituents of tomatoes and several green vegetables. *J Agric Food Chem*. 1992;40:390-98.

74. Prince MR, Frisoli JK. Beta-carotene accumulation in serum and skin. *Am J Clin Nutr*. 1993;57:175-81.

75. Jalal F, Nesheim MC, Agus Z, Sanjur D, Habicht JP. Serum retinol concentrations in children are affected by food sources of beta-carotene, fat intake, and anthelmintic drug treatment. *Am J Clin Nutr*. 1998;68:623-29.

76. van Het Hof KH, West CE, Weststrate JA, Hautvast JG. Dietary factors that affect the bioavailability of carotenoids. *J Nutr*. 2000;130:503-06.

77. Brown MJ, Ferruzzi MG, Nguyen ML, Cooper DA, Eldridge AL, Schwartz SJ, White WS. Carotenoid bioavailability is higher from salads ingested with full-fat than with fat-reduced salad dressings as measured with electrochemical detection. *Am J Clin Nutr*. 2004;80:396-403.

78. Unlu NZ, Bohn T, Clinton SK, Schwartz SJ. Carotenoid absorption from salad and salsa by humans is enhanced by the addition of avocado or avocado oil. *J Nutr*. 2005;135:431-36.

79. Rock CL, Lovalvo JL, Emenhiser C, Ruffin MT, Flatt SW, Schwartz SJ. Bioavailability of ß-carotene is lower in raw than in processed carrots and spinach in women. *J Nutr*. 1998;128:913-16.

80. Getahun SM, Chung FL. Conversion of glucosinolates to isothiocyanates in humans after ingestion of cooked watercress. *Cancer Epidemiol Biomarkers Prev*. 1999;8(5):447-51.

81. Shapiro TA, Fahey JW, Wade KL, Stephenson KK, Talalay P. Chemoprotecitve clucosinolates and isothiocyanates of broccoli sprouts; metabolism and excretion in humans. *Cancer Epidemiol Biomarkers Prev*. 2001;10:501-08.

82. Vermeulen M, van den Berg R, Freidig AP, van Bladeren PJ, Vaes WH. Association between consumption of cruciferous vegetables and condiments and excretion in urine of isothiocyanate mercapturic acids. *J Agric Food Chem*. 2006;54:5350-58.

83. Chandler LA, Schwartz SJ. HPLC separation of cis-trans carotene isomers in fresh and processed fruits and vegetables. *J Food Sci*. 1987;52:669-72.

84. Yang F, Basu TK, Ooraikul B. Studies on germination conditions and antioxidant contents of wheat grain. *Int J Food Sci Nutr*. 2001;52:319-30.

85. Falcioni G, Fedeli D, Tiano L, Calzuola I, Mancinelli L, Marsili V, Gianfranceschi GL. Antioxidant activity of wheat sprouts extract "in vitro": inhibition of DNA oxidative damage. *J Food Sci*. 2002;67:2918-22.

86. Calzuola, I, Marsili, V, Gianfranceschi, GL. Synthesis of antioxidants in wheat sprouts. *J Agric Food Chem*. 2004;52:5201-06.

87. Marsili V, Calzuola I, Gianfranceschi GL. Nutritional relevance of wheat sprouts containing high levels of organic phosphates and antioxidant compounds. *J Clin Gastroenterol*. 2004;38(6 Suppl):S123-26.

88. Liukkonen KH, Katina K, Wilhelmsson A, Myllymäki O, Lampi AM, Kariluoto S, Piironen V, Heinonen SM, Nurmi T, Adlercreutz H, Peltoketo A, Pihlava JM, Hietaniemi V, Poutanen K. Process-induced changes on bioactive compounds in whole grain rye. *Proc Nutr Soc*. 2003;62:117-22.

89. Osawa T, Ramarathnam N, Kawakishi S, Namiki M, Tashiro T. Antioxidant defense systems in rice hull against damage caused by oxygen radicals. *Agric Biol Chem*. 1985;49:3085-87.

90. Fahey JW, Zhang Y, Talalay P. Broccoli sprouts: an exceptionally rich source of inducers of enzymes that protect against chemical carcinogens. *Proc Natl Acad Sci USA*. 1997;94:10367-72.

91. Galan MV, Kishan AA, Silverman AL. Oral broccoli sprouts for the treatment of Helicobacter pylori infection: a preliminary report. *Dig Dis Sci.* 2004;49:1088-90.

92. Randhir R, Lin YT, Shetty K. Phenolics, their antioxidant and antimicrobial activity in dark germinated fenugreek sprouts in response to peptide and phytochemical elicitors. *Asia Pac J Clin Nutr.* 2004;13:295-307.

93. Katina K, Liukkonen KH, Kaukovirta-Norja A, Adlercreutz H, Heinonen SM, Lampi AM, Pihlava JM, Poutanen K. Fermentation-induced changes in the nutritional value of native or germinated rye. *J Cereal Sci.* 2007;46:348-55.

94. Krajcovicová-Kudláčková M, Dusinská M, Valachovicová M, Blazícek P, Pauková V. Products of DNA, protein and lipid oxidative damage in relation to vitamin C plasma concentration. *Physiol Res.* 2006;55:227-31.

95. Devasagayam TP, Tilak JC, Boloor KK, Sane KS, Ghaskadbi SS, Lele RD. Free radicals and antioxidants in human health: current status and future prospects. *J Assoc Physicians India.* 2004;52:794-804.

96. Blokhina O, Virolainen E, Fagerstedt KV. Antioxidants, oxidative damage and oxygen deprivation stress: a review. *Ann Bot* London. 2003;91 Spec No:179-94.

97. United States Department of Agriculture, Agricultural Research Service. *USDA National Nutrient Database for Standard Reference, Release 21.* 2008. www.nal.usda.gov/fnic/foodcomp/search. Accessed August 2009.

98. ESHA. *The Food Processor, Nutrition and Fitness Software.* 2009. www.esha.com.

99. Carr AC, Frei B. Toward a new recommended dietary allowance for vitamin C based on antioxidant and health effects in humans. *Am J Clin Nutr.* 1999;69:1086-107.

100. López-Berenguer C, Carvajal M, Moreno DA, García-Viguera C. Effects of microwave cooking conditions on bioactive compounds present in broccoli inflorescences. *J Agric Food Chem.* 2007;Nov 28;55(24):10001-07.

101. Kishida E, Maeda T, Nishihama A, Kojo S, Masuzawa Y. Effects of seasonings on the stability of ascorbic acid in a cooking model system. *J Nutr Sci Vitaminol* (Tokyo). 2004;50:431-37.

102. Teucher B, Olivares M, Cori H. Enhancers of iron absorption: ascorbic acid and other organic acids. *Int J Vitam Nutr Res.* 2004;74:403-19.

103. Han JS, Kozukue N, Young KS, Lee KR, Friedman M. Distribution of ascorbic acid in potato tubers and in home-processed and commercial potato foods. *J Agric Food Chem.* 2004;52:6516-21.

104. Nursal B, Yucecan S. Vitamin C losses in some frozen vegetables due to various cooking methods. *Nahrung.* 2000;44:451-53.

105. Steinhart H, Rathjen T. Dependence of tocopherol stability on different cooking procedures of food. *Int J Vitam Nutr* Res. 2003;73:144-51.

106. Thomson CD, Robinson MF. Selenium content of foods consumed in Otago, New Zealand. *N Z Med J.* 1990;103(886):130-35.

107. Higgs DJ, Morris VC, Levander OA. Effect of cooking on selenium content of foods. *J Agric Food Chem.* 1972;20(3):678-80.

108. Peto R. Cancer, cholesterol, carotene, and tocopherol. *Lancet.* 1981;2:97-98.

109. Ziegler RG. A review of epidemiologic evidence that carotenoids reduce the risk of cancer. *J Nutr.* 1989;119:116-22.

110. Ito Y, Kurata M, Hioki R, Suzuki K, Ochiai J, Aoki K. Cancer mortality and serum levels of carotenoids, retinol, and tocopherol: a population-based follow-up study of inhabitants of a rural area of Japan. *Asian Pac J Cancer Prev.* 2005;6:10-15.

111. The ATBC Cancer Prevention Study Group. The alpha-tocopherol, beta-carotene lung cancer prevention study: design, methods, participant characteristics, and compliance. *Ann Epidemiol.* 1994;4:1-10.

112. Hennekens CH, Buring JE, Manson JE et al. Lack of effect of long-term supplementation with beta carotene on the incidence of malignant neoplasms and cardiovascular disease. *N Engl J Med.* 1996;334:1145-49.

113. Omenn GS, Goodman GE, Thornquist MD et al. Risk factors for lung cancer and for intervention effects in CARET, the Beta-Carotene and Retinol Efficacy Trial. *J Natl Cancer Inst.* 1996;88:1550-59.

114. Knekt P, Reunanen A, Jarvinen R, Seppanen R, Heliovaara M, Aromaa A. Antioxidant vitamin intake and coronary mortality in a longitudinal population study. *Am J Epidemiol.* 1994;139:1180-89.

115. Kushi LH, Folsom AR, Prineas RJ, Mink PJ, Wu Y, Bostick RM. Dietary antioxidant vitamins and death from coronary heart disease in postmenopausal women. *N Engl J Med.* 1996;334:1156-62.

116. Rimm EB, Stampfer MJ, Ascherio A, Giovannucci E, Colditz GA, Willett WC. Vitamin E consumption and the risk of coronary heart disease in men. *N Engl J Med.* 1993;328:1450-56.

117. Stampfer MJ, Hennekens CH, Manson JE, Colditz GA, Rosner B, Willett WC. Vitamin E consumption and the risk of coronary disease in women. *N Engl J Med.* 1993;328(20):1444-49.

118. Stephens NG, Parsons A, Schofield PM, Kelly F, Cheeseman K, Mitchinson MJ. Randomised controlled trial of vitamin E in patients with coronary disease: Cambridge Heart Antioxidant Study (CHAOS). *Lancet.* 1996;347:781-86.

119. Lonn E, Bosch J, Yusuf S et al. Effects of long-term vitamin E supplementation on cardiovascular events and cancer: a randomized controlled trial. *JAMA.* 2005;293:1338-47.

120. Yusuf S, Dagenais G, Pogue J, Bosch J, Sleight P. Vitamin E supplementation and cardiovascular events in high-risk patients. The Heart Outcomes Prevention Evaluation Study Investigators. *N Engl J Med.* 2000;342:154-60.

121. Gruppo Italiano per lo Studio della Sopravvivenza nell´Infarto miocardico. Dietary supplementation with n-3 polyunsaturated fatty acids and vitamin E after myocardial infarction: results of the GISSI-Prevenzione trial. *Lancet.* 1999;354:447-55.

122. Miller ER, Pastor-Barriuso R, Dalal D, Riemersma RA, Appel LJ, Guallar E. Meta-analysis: high-dosage vitamin E supplementation may increase all-cause mortality. *Ann Intern Med.* 2005;142:37-46.

123. Eidelman RS, Hollar D, Hebert PR, Lamas GA, Hennekens CH. Randomized trials of vitamin E in the treatment and prevention of cardiovascular disease. *Arch Intern Med.* 2004;164:1552-56.

124. Shekelle PG, Morton SC, Jungvig LK, Udani J, Spar M, Tu W, J Suttorp M, Coulter I, Newberry SJ, Hardy M. Effect of supplemental vitamin E for the prevention and treatment of cardiovascular disease. *J Gen Intern Med.* 2004;19:380-89.

125. Vivekananthan DP, Penn MS, Sapp SK, Hsu A, Topol EJ. Use of antioxidant vitamins for the prevention of cardiovascular disease: meta-analysis of randomized trials. *Lancet.* 2003;361:2017-23. Erratum in *Lancet.* 2004;363:662.

126. Wu X, Beecher GR, Holden JM, Haytowitz DB, Gebhardt SE, Prior RL. Lipophilic and hydrophilic antioxidant capacities of common foods in the United States. *J Agric Food Chem.* 2004;52:4026-37.

127. Femenia A, Selvendran RR, Ring SG, Robertson JA. Effects of heat treatment and dehydration on properties of cauliflower fiber. *J Agric Food Chem.* 1999;47:728-32.

128. Wisker E, Schweizer TF, Daniel M, Feldheim W. Fibre-mediated physiological effects of raw and processed carrots in humans. *Br J Nutr.* 1994;72:579-99.

129. Anderson, NE, Clydesdale, FM. Effect of processing on dietary fiber content of wheat bran, pureed green beans, and carrots. *J Food Sci.* 1980;45:1533-37.

130. Nyman, M. Importance of processing for physic-chemical and physiological properties of dietary fibre. *Proc of the Nutr Society.* 2003;62:187-92.

131. Nyman M, Palsson KE, Asp N-G. Effects of processing on dietary fibre in vegetables. *Lebensmittel Wissenschaft und Technologie.* 1987;20:29-36.

132. Lintas, C, Cappeloni, M. Content and composition of dietary fibre in raw and cooked vegetables. *Hum Nutr Food Sci Nutr.* 1988;42F;117-24.

133. Cummings, JH. The effect of dietary fiber on fecal weight and composition. In Spiller GA, ed. *Handbook of Dietary Fiber in Human Nutrition.* Boca Raton FL: CRC Press, 1980:211-80.

134. Wyman JB, Heaton KW, Manning AP, Wicks ACB. The effect on intestinal transit and the feces of raw and cooked bran in different doses. *Am J Clin Nutr.* 1976;29:1474-9.

135. Groff JL, Gropper SS, Hunt SM. *Advanced Nutrition and Human Metabolism. 2nd ed.* Minneapolis MN: West Publishing Co., 1995.

136. German, JB. Food processing and lipid oxidation. In Jackson et al. ed. *Impact of Processing on Food Safety.* New York: Plenum Publishers, 1999:23-50.

137. WHO, Consultation FAO. *Diet, Nutrition and the Prevention of Chronic Diseases. WHO Technical Report Series.* Geneve: WHO. 2003;916.

138. Messina V, Mangels, R, Messina M. *The Dietitian's Guide to Vegetarian Diets: Issues and Applications. 2nd ed.* Sudbury MA: Jones and Bartlett Publishers, 2004.

139. Donaldson M. Food and nutrition intake of Hallelujah vegetarians. *Nutr Food Sci.* 2001;31:293-303.

140. Trans Fat Task Force (Health Canada and the Heart and Stroke Foundation). *TRANSforming the food supply. Final report submitted to the Minister of Health.* June 2006. www.hc-sc. gc.ca/fn-an/nutrition/gras-trans-fats/tf-ge/tf-gt_rep-rap-eng.php. Accessed July 2009.

141. Mozaffarian D, Katan MB, Ascherio A, Stampfer MJ, Willett WC. Trans fatty acids

and cardiovascular disease. *N Engl J Med.* 2006;354:1601-13.

142. Lopez-Garcia E, Schulze MB, Meigs JB, Manson JE, Rifai N, Stampfer MJ, Willett WC, Hu FB. Consumption of trans fatty acids is related to plasma biomarkers of inflammation and endothelial dysfunction. *J Nutr.* 2005;135:562-66.

143. Institute of Medicine (IOM). *Dietary Reference Intakes for Energy, Carbohydrates, Fiber, Fat, Protein and Amino Acids (Macronutrients).* Washington DC: National Academies Press, 2002.

144. Hu FB, Stampfer MJ, Manson JE, Rimm E, Colditz GA, Rosner BA, Hennekens CH, Willett WC. Dietary fat intake and the risk of coronary heart disease in women. *N Engl J Med.* 1997;337:1491-99.

145. Simin L. Intake of refined carbohydrates and whole grain foods in relation to risk of type 2 diabetes mellitus and coronary heart disease. *J Am Coll Nutr.* 2002;21:298-306.

146. Institute of Medicine Food and Nutrition Board. *Dietary reference intakes for water, potassium, sodium, chloride, and sulfate.* Washington DC: The National Academies Press, 2004.

147. Tsugane S. Salt, salted food intake, and risk of gastric cancer: epidemiologic evidence. *Cancer Sci.* 2005;96:1-6.

148. Harrington M, Cashman KD. High salt intake appears to increase bone resorption in postmenopausal women but high potassium intake ameliorates this adverse effect. *Nutr Rev.* 2003;61(5 Pt 1):179-83.

149. Straub M, Hautmann RE. Developments in stone prevention. *Curr Opin Urol.* 2005;15:119-26.

150. Delvecchio FC, Preminger GM. Medical management of stone disease. *Curr Opin Urol.* 2003;13:229-33.

151. Goldfarb DS, Coe FL. Prevention of recurrent nephrolithiasis. *Am Fam Physician.* 1999; 60:2269-76.

152. Cross AJ, Sinha R. Meat-related mutagens/carcinogens in the etiology of colorectal cancer. *Environ Mol Mutagen.* 2004;44:44-55.

153. Horio F, Youngman LD, Bell RC, Campbell TC. Thermogenesis, low-protein diets, and decreased development of AFB1-induced preneoplastic foci in rat liver. *Nutr Cancer.* 1991;16(1):31-41.

154. Norat T, Lukanova A, Ferrari P, Riboli E. Meat consumption and colorectal cancer risk: dose-response meta-analysis of epidemiological studies. *Int J Cancer.* 2002;98:241-56.

155. Chao A, Thun MJ, Connell CJ, McCullough ML, Jacobs EJ, Flanders WD, Rodriguez C, Sinha R, Calle EE. Meat consumption and risk of colorectal cancer. *JAMA.* 2005;293:172-82.

156. Kuriki K, Hamajima N, Chiba H, Kanemitsu Y, Hirai T, Kato T, Saito T, Matsuo K, Koike K, Tokudome S, Tajima K. Increased risk of colorectal cancer due to interactions between meat consumption and the CD36 gene A52C polymorphism among Japanese. *Nutr Cancer.* 2005;51:170-77.

157. Sinha R, Peters U, Cross AJ, Kulldorff M, Weissfeld JL, Pinsky PF, Rothman N, Hayes RB. Meat, meat cooking methods and preservation, and risk for colorectal adenoma. *Cancer Res.* 2005;65:8034-41.

158. Chan JM, Stampfer MJ, Giovannucci EL. What causes prostate cancer? A brief summary of the epidemiology. *Semin Cancer Biol.* 1998;8:263-73.

159. Kolonel LN. Nutrition and prostate cancer. *Cancer Causes Control.* 1996;7:83-44.

160. Song Y, Manson JE, Buring JE, Liu S. A prospective study of red meat consumption and type 2 diabetes in middle-aged and elderly women: the women's health study. *Diabetes Care.* 2004;27:2108-15.

161. van Dam RM, Willett WC, Rimm EB, Stampfer MJ, Hu FB. Dietary fat and meat intake in relation to risk of type 2 diabetes in men. *Diabetes Care.* 2002;25:417-24.

162. Snowdon DA, Phillips RL. Does a vegetarian diet reduce the occurrence of diabetes? *Am J Public Health.* 1985;75:507-12.

163. Kelemen LE, Kushi LH, Jacobs DR Jr, Cerhan JR. Associations of dietary protein with disease and mortality in a prospective study of postmenopausal women. *Am J Epidemiol.* 2005;161:239-49.

164. Zhan S, Ho SC. Meta-analysis of the effects of soy protein containing isoflavones on the lipid profile. *Am J Clin Nutr.* 2005;81:397-408.

165. Bricarello LP, Kasinski N, Bertolami MC, Faludi A, Pinto LA, Relvas WG, Izar MC, Ihara SS, Tufik S, Fonseca FA. Comparison between the effects of soy milk and non-fat cow milk on lipid profile and lipid peroxidation in patients with primary hypercholesterolemia. *Nutrition.* 2004;20:200-04.

166. Lichtenstein AH, Jalbert SM, Adlercreutz H, Goldin BR, Rasmussen H, Schaefer EJ, Ausman LM. Lipoprotein response to diets high

in soy or animal protein with and without isoflavones in moderately hypercholesterolemic subjects. *Arterioscler Thromb Vasc Biol.* 2002;22:1852-58.

167. Schecter A, Cramer P, Boggess K, Stanley J, Papke O, Olson J, Silver A, Scmitz M. Intake of dioxins and related compounds from food in the U.S. population. *J Toxic Environ Health A.* 2001;63:1-18.

168. Hites RA, Foran JA, Schwager SJ, Knuth BA, Hamilton MC, Carpenter DO. Global assessment of polybrominated diphenyl ethers in farmed and wild salmon. *Environ Sci Technol.* 2004;38:4945-49.

169. Ng PJ, Fleet GH, Heard GM. Pesticides as a source of microbial contamination of salad vegetables. *Int J Food Microbiol.* 2005;101:237-50.

170. Johnsson C, Schutz A, Sallsten G. Impact of consumption of freshwater fish on mercury levels in hair, blood, urine, and alveolar air. *J Toxicol Environ Health.* 2005;68:129-40.

171. FDA/EPA. *Joint Federal Advisory for Mercury in Fish. Backgrounder for the 2004 FDA/EPA Consumer Advisory: What You Need to Know about Mercury in Fish and Shellfish.* 2004. www.epa.gov/fishadvisories/advice/factsheet. html#info. Accessed July 2009.

172. Dufault R, LeBlanc B, Schnoll R, Cornett C, Schweitzer L, Patrick L, Hightower J, Wallinga D, Lukiw W. Mercury from chlor-alkali plants: measured concentrations in food product sugar. *Environ Health.* 2009;8:2.

173. Wallinga D. Sorensen J, Mottl P, Yablon B. *Not So Sweet: Missing Mercury and High Fructose Corn Syrup. Institute for Agriculture and Trade Policy.* Minneapolis, MN. January 2009. www.healthobservatory.org/library. cfm?refid=105026. Accessed July 2009.

174. U.S. Food and Drug Administration Center for Food Safety and Applied Nutrition. *Exploratory Data on Acrylamide in Foods.* 2002. Washington DC: U.S. Food and Drug Administration. www.cfsan.fda.gov/~dms/acrydata. html. Accessed July 2009.

175. Swedish National Food Agency. *Press conference.* Uppsala, April 24, 2002. www.slv.se. Accessed July 2009.

176. Mottram DS, Wedzicha BL, Dodson AT. Acrylamide is formed in the Maillard reaction. *Nature.* 2002;419:448-49.

177. Becalski A, Lau BP, Lewis D, Seaman SW, Hayward S, Sahagian M, Ramesh M, Leclerc Y. Acrylamide in foods: occurrence, sources, and modeling. *J Agric Food Chem.* 2003;51:802-08.

178. Stadler RH, Blank I, Varga N, Robert F, Hau J, Guy PA, Robert MC, Riediker S. Acrylamide from Maillard reaction products. *Nature.* 2002;419:449-50.

179. U.S. Food and Drug Administration. *Acrylamide in Foods.* Washington DC: U.S. Food and Drug Administration. www.cfsan.fda.gov/~lrd/pestadd.html#acrylamide. Accessed July 2009.

180. FAO/WHO. *Joint FAO/WHO Expert Committee on Food Additives. Contaminants.* 64th meeting; Feb. 8-17, 2005. Rome. www.who.int/ipcs/food/jecfa/summaries/summary_report_64_final.pdf. Accessed July 2009.

181. European Commission. *Opinion of the Scientific Committee on Food on New Findings Regarding the Presence of Acrylamide in Food.* 2002. http://europa.eu.int/comm/food/fs/sc/scf/out131_en.pdf. Accessed July 2009.

182. Maza MP, Bravo A, Leiva L, Gattás V, Petermann M, Garrido F, Bunout D, Hirsch S, Barrera G, Fernández M. Fluorescent serum and urinary advanced glycoxidation endproducts in non-diabetic subjects. *Biol Res.* 2007;40:203-12.

183. Miyata T, Kurokawa K, Van Ypersele C. Advanced glycation and lipoxidation end products: role of reactive carbonyl compounds generated during carbohydrate and lipid metabolism. *J Am Soc Nephrol.* 2000;11:1744-52.

184. Vlassara H, Palace MR. Diabetes and advanced glycation end products. *J Intern Med.* 2002;251:87-101.

185. Goldberg T, Cai W, Peppa M, Dardaine V, Suresh Baliga B, Uribarri J, Vlassara H. Advanced glycoxidation end products in commonly consumed foods. *JADA.* 2004;104:1287-91.

186. Zhang Q, Ames JM, Smith RD, Baynes JW, Metz TO. A perspective on the Maillard reaction and the analysis of protein glycation by mass spectrometry: probing the pathogenesis of chronic disease. *J Proteome Res.* 2009;8:754-69.

187. Koschinsky T, He CJ, Mitsuhashi T, Bucala R, Liu C, Buenting C, Heitmann K, Vlassara H. Orally absorbed reactive glycation products (glycotoxins): an environmental risk factor in diabetic nephropathy. *Proc Natl Acad Sci USA.* 1997;94:6474-79.

188. Seiquer I, Díaz-Alguacil J, Delgado-Andrade C, López-Frías M, Muñoz Hoyos A, Galdó G, Navarro MP. Diets rich in Maillard reaction products affect protein digestibility in adolescent males aged 11-14 y. *Am J Clin Nutr.* 2006 May;83(5):1082-88.

189. Trivelli LA, Ranney HM, Lai HT. Hemoglobin components in patients with diabetes mellitus. *N Engl J Med.* 1971;284:353-57.

190. Skog K, Steineck G, Augustsson K, Jagerstad M. Effect of cooking temperature on the formation of heterocyclic amines in fried meat products and pan residues. *Carcinogenesis.* 1995;16:861-67.

191. Layton DW, Bogen KT, Knize MG, Hatch FT, Johnson VM, Felton JS. Cancer risk of heterocyclic amines in cooked foods: an analysis and implications for research. *Carcinogenesis.* 1995;16:39-52.

192. National Cancer Institute. *Heterocyclic Amines in Cooked Meats. Fact Sheet.* www.cancer.gov/cancertopics/factsheet/Risk/heterocyclic-amine. Accessed July 2009.

193. U.S. Department of Health and Human Services, Public Health Service, National Toxicology Program. *11th Report on Carcinogens.* 2005. http://ntp.niehs.nih.gov/ntp/roc/toc11.html. Accessed July 2009.

194. Agency for Toxic Substances and Disease Registry. *Toxicological Profile for Polycyclic Aromatic Hydrocarbons.* Atlanta GA: U.S. Department of Health and Human Services, Public Health Service, 1995.

195. European Commission. *Opinion of the Scientific Committee on Food on the Risks to Human Health of Polycyclic Aromatic Hydrocarbons in Food.* 2002. http://ec.europa.eu/food/fs/sc/scf/out153_en.pdf. Accessed July 2009.

196. D'Mello JPF. *Food Safety: Contaminants and Toxins.* Wallingford Oxon UK: CABI Publishing, 2003.

197. The Government of the Hong Kong Special Administrative Region Risk Assessment Studies, Food and Environmental Hygiene Department. *Report No. 14: Chemical Hazard Evaluation Polycyclic Aromatic Hydrocarbons in Barbecued Meat.* July 2004.

CHAPTER 5
Energy and Power

1. United States Department of Agriculture, Agricultural Research Service. *USDA National Nutrient Database for Standard Reference, Release 21.* 2008. www.nal.usda.gov/fnic/foodcomp/search. Accessed August 2009.

2. ESHA. *The Food Processor, Nutrition and Fitness Software.* 2009. www.esha.com. Accessed August 2009.

3. Institute of Medicine. *Dietary Reference Intakes for Energy, Carbohydrate, Fiber, Fat, Fatty Acids, Cholesterol, Protein, and Amino Acids (Macronutrients).* Washington DC: National Academies Press, 2005:107-264. http://books.nap.edu/openbook.php?record_id=10490&page=107 Accessed August 2009.

4. Trumbo P et al. Dietary reference intakes for energy, carbohydrate, fiber, fat, fatty acids, cholesterol, protein and amino acids. *J Am Diet Assoc.* 2002;102:1621-30.

5. United States Department of Agriculture. *Inside the Pyramid. Discretionary Calories. How Many Discretionary Calories Can I Have?* 2008. www.mypyramid.gov/pyramid/discretionary_calories_amount_print.html Accessed August 2009.

6. Donaldson, MS. Food and nutrient intake of Hallelujah vegetarians. *Nutrition & Food Science.* 2001;31:293-303. www.hacres.com/diet/research/nutrient_intake.pdf. Accessed August 2009.

7. Guenther PM et al. Most Americans eat much less than recommended amounts of fruits and vegetables. *J Am Diet Assoc.* 2006;106:1371-79.

8. Donaldson, MS. *Hallelujah Vegetarians and Nutritional Science: Answering Your Questions.* Personal communication. 2005.

9. Donaldson MS. Metabolic vitamin B_{12} status on a mostly raw vegan diet with follow up using tablets, nutritional yeast, or probiotic supplements. *Ann Nutr Metab.* 2000;44:229-34.

10. Agren JJ et al. Fatty acid composition of erythrocyte, platelet, and serum lipids in strict vegans. *Lipids.* 1995;30:365-69.

11. Fontana L et al. Low bone mass in subjects on a long-term raw vegetarian diet. *Arch Intern Med.* 2005;165:684-89.

12. Fontana L et al. Long-term low-protein, low-calorie diet and endurance exercise modulate metabolic factors associated with cancer risk. *Am J Clin Nutr.* 2006;84:1456-62.

13. Hoffmann I et al. Raw food diet: health benefits and risks. In: Watson RR ed. *Vegetables, Fruits, and Herbs in Health Promotion.* Boca Raton, Fl: CRC Press; 2000:293-308.

14. Koebnick C et al. Long-term consumption of a raw food diet is associated with favorable serum LDL cholesterol and triglycerides but also with elevated plasma homocysteine and low serum HDL cholesterol in humans. *J Nutr.* 2005;135:2372-78.

15. Rauma AL et al. Antioxidant status in long-term adherents to a strict uncooked vegan diet. *Am J Clin Nutr.* 1995;6:1221-27.

16. Ling WH et al. Shifting from a conventional diet to an uncooked vegan diet reversibly alters fecal hydrolytic activities in humans. *J Nutr*. 1992;122:924-30.

17. Koebnick C et al. Consequences of a long-term raw food diet on body weight and menstruation: results of a questionnaire survey. *Ann Nutr Metab*. 1999;43:69-79.

18. Rauma AL. Coumarin 7-hydroxylation in long-term adherents of a strict uncooked vegan diet. *Eur J Clin Pharmacol*. 1996;50(1-2):133-37.

19. Verhagen H et al. Effect of a vegan diet on biomarkers of chemoprevention in females. *Hum Exp Toxicol*. 1996;15:821-25.

20. American Dietetic Association and Dietitians of Canada. Position of the American Dietetic Association and Dietitians of Canada: Vegetarian Diets. *J Am Diet Assoc*. 2003;103:748. www.webdietitians.org/Public/Files/veg.pdf and at http://eatright.org/ada/files/vegnp.pdf. Accessed August 2009. Craig WJ, Mangels AR, American Dietetic Association. Position of the American Dietetic Association: Vegetarian Diets. *J Am Diet Assoc*. 2009 Jul;109(7):1266-82.

21. Messina V et al. *The Dietitian's Guide to Vegetarian Diets. 2nd ed*. Boston: Jones and Bartlett Publishing, 2004.

22. American Dietetic Association and Dietitians of Canada. Position of the American Dietetic Association, Dietitians of Canada, and the American College of Sports Medicine: Nutrition and athletic performance. *J Am Diet Assoc*. 2000;100:1543 and 2009;109:509-527. www.eatright.org/ada/files/Athleticnp.pdf and www.eatright.org/cps/rde/xchg/ada/hs.xsl/advocacy_15986_ENU_HTML.htm. Accessed August 2009.

23. Bordone L et al. Calorie restriction, SIRT1 and metabolism: understanding longevity. *Nat Rev Mol Cell Biol*. 2005;6:298-305.

24. Browner WS et al. The genetics of human longevity. *Am J Med*. 2004;117:851-60.

25. Fontana L et al. Long-term low-calorie low-protein vegan diet and endurance exercise are associated with low cardiometabolic risk. *Rejuvenation Res*. 2007;10:225-34.

26. Pereira MA et al. Effects of a low-glycemic load diet on resting energy expenditure and heart disease risk factors during weight loss. *JAMA*. 2004;292:2482-90.

27. Fontana L et al. Long-term effects of calorie or protein restriction on serum IGF-1 and IGFBP-3 concentration in humans. *Aging Cell*. 2008;7:681-87 and Fontana L et al. IGF-1, nutrition and aging: the big picture. *Aging Cell*. 2008;8:215.

28. Witte AV et al. Caloric restriction improves memory in elderly humans. *Proc Natl Acad Sci USA*. 2009;106:1255-60.

29. Elia M et al. Physiological aspects of energy metabolism and gastrointestinal effects of carbohydrates. *Eur J Clin Nutr*. 2007;61 Suppl 1:S40-74.

30. Groff JL et al. Hunt SM. *Advanced Nutrition and Human Metabolism*. Minneapolis MN: West Publishing Co., 1995.

31. Collins PJ et al. Proximal, distal and total stomach emptying of a digestible solid meal in normal subjects. *Br J Radiol*. 1988;61:12-18.

32. Kalnins D et al. Combining unprotected pancreatic enzymes with pH-sensitive enteric-coated microspheres does not improve nutrient digestion in patients with cystic fibrosis. *J Pediatr*. 2005;146:489-93.

33. Richter C et al. Mechanism of activation of the gastric aspartic proteinases: pepsinogen, progastricsin and prochymosin. *Biochem J*. 1998;335(Pt 3):481-90.

34. Hafström I et al. A vegan diet free of gluten improves the signs and symptoms of rheumatoid arthritis: the effects on arthritis correlate with a reduction in antibodies to food antigens. *Rheumatology* (Oxford). 2001;40:1175-79.

35. Hanninen O et al. Antioxidants in vegan diet and rheumatic disorders. *Toxicology*. 2000;155:45-53.

36. Peltonen R et al. An uncooked vegan diet shifts the profile of human fecal microflora: computerized analysis of direct stool sample gas-liquid chromatography profiles of bacterial cellular fatty acids. *Appl Environ Microbiol*. 1992;58:3660-66.

37. Pettersson J et al. NMR metabolomic analysis of fecal water from subjects on a vegetarian diet. *Biol Pharm Bull*. 2008;31:1192-98.

38. Millward DJ. The nutritional value of plant-based diets in relation to human amino acid and protein requirements. *Proc Nutr Soc*. 1999;58:249-60.

39. Institute of Medicine. *Dietary Reference Intakes for Energy, Carbohydrate, Fiber, Fat, Fatty Acids, Cholesterol, Protein, and Amino Acids (Macronutrients)*. Washington DC, National Academies Press. 2005:589-768. http://books.nap.edu/openbook.php?record_id=10490&page=589. Accessed August 2009.

40. Rand WM et al. Meta-analysis of nitrogen balance studies for estimating protein require-

ments in healthy adults. *Am J Clin Nutr.* 2003;77:109-27.

41. Millward DJ. Sufficient protein for our elders? *Am J Clin Nutr.* 2008;88:1187-88.

42. Craig WJ, Mangels AR; American Dietetic Association. Position of the American Dietetic Association: vegetarian diets. *J Am Diet Assoc.* 2009 Jul;109(7):1266-82.

43. Meade SJ et al. The impact of processing on the nutritional quality of food proteins. *J AOAC Int.* 2005;88:904-22.

44. Gilani GS et al. Effects of antinutritional factors on protein digestibility and amino acid availability in foods. *J AOAC Int.* 2005;88:967-87.

45. Link LB et al. Raw versus cooked vegetables and cancer risk. *Cancer Epidemiol Biomarkers Prev.* 2004;13:1422-35.

46. Millward DJ et al. Protein/energy ratios of current diets in developed and developing countries compared with a safe protein/energy ratio: implications for recommended protein and amino acid intakes. *Public Health Nutr.* 2004;7:387-405.

47. Pellet, P. Personal communication.

48. Ruales J et al. Quinoa (Chenopodium quinoa willd) an important Andean food crop. *Arch Latinoam Nutr.* 1992;42:232-41.

49. Young VR et al. Plant proteins in relation to human protein and amino acid nutrition. *Am J Clin Nutr.* 1994;59:1203S-12S.

50. Young VR. Adult amino acid requirements: the case for a major revision in current recommendations. *J Nutr.* 1994;124(8 Suppl):1517S-23S.

51. Hernot DC et al. In vitro digestion characteristics of unprocessed and processed whole grains and their components. *J Agric Food Chem.* 2008;56:10721-26.

52. Oste RE. Digestibility of processed food protein. *Adv Exp Med Biol.* 1991;289:371-88.

53. Zia-ur-Rehman et al. The effects of hydrothermal processing on antinutrients, protein and starch digestibility of food legumes. *Int J Food Science Technol.* 2005;40:695-700.

54. El-Adawy TA. Nutritional composition and antinutritional factors of chickpeas (Cicer arietinum L.) undergoing different cooking methods and germination. *Plant Foods for Human Nutrition.* 2002;57:83-97.

55. Misas-Villamil JC et al. Enzyme-inhibitor interactions at the plant-pathogen interface. *Curr Opin Plant Biol.* 2008;11:380-88.

56. Savelkoul FHMG et al. The presence and inactivation of trypsin inhibitors, tannins, lectins and amylase inhibitors in legume seeds during germination. A review. *Plant Foods for Human Nutrition.* 1992;42:71-85.

57. Wilson KA. The proteolysis of trypsin inhibitors in legume seeds. *Crit Rev Biotechnol.* 1988;8:197-216.

58. Craig WJ, Mangels AR; American Dietetic Association. Position of the American Dietetic Association: vegetarian diets. *J Am Diet Assoc.* 2009 Jul;109(7):1266-82.

59. Bishnoi S et al. Protein digestibility of vegetables and field peas (Pisum sativum). Varietal differences and effect of domestic processing and cooking methods. *Plant Foods Hum Nutr.* 1994;46:71-76.

60. Chavan JK et al. Nutritional improvement of cereals by sprouting. *Crit Rev Food Sci Nutr.* 1989;28:401-37.

61. Hamilton MJ et al. Germination and nutrient composition of alfalfa seeds. *J Food Science.* 1979;44(2).

62. Rozan P et al. Amino acids in seeds and seedlings of the genus Lens. *Phytochemistry.* 2001;58:281-89.

63. Trugo LC et al. Effect of heat treatment on nutritional quality of germinated legume seeds. *J Agric Food Chem.* 2000;48:2082-86.

64. Dworschák E. Nonenzyme browning and its effect on protein nutrition. *Crit Rev Food Sci Nutr.* 1980;13:1-40.

65. Erbersdobler HF et al. Determination of lysine damage and calculation of lysine bioavailability in several processed foods. *Z Ernahrungswiss.* 1991;30:46-49.

66. Hurrell RF et al. Nutritional significance of cross-link formation during food processing. *Adv Exp Med Biol.* 1977;86B:225-38.

67. Seiquer I et al. Diets rich in Maillard reaction products affect protein digestibility in adolescent males aged 11-14 y. *Am J Clin Nutr.* 2006;83:1082-88.

68. Gorinstein S et al. Comparison of the bioactive compounds and antioxidant potentials of fresh and cooked Polish, Ukrainian, and Israeli garlic. *J Agric Food Chem.* 2005;53:2726-32.

69. Ibrahim SS et al. Effect of soaking, germination, cooking and fermentation on antinutritional factors in cowpeas. *Nahrung.* 2002;46:92-95.

70. Kataria A et al. Contents and digestibility of carbohydrates of mung beans (Vigna radiata L.) as affected by domestic processing and cooking. *Plant Foods Hum Nutr.* 1988;38:51-59.

71. Millward DJ et al. Protein quality assessment: impact of expanding understanding of protein and amino acid needs for optimal health. *Am J Clin Nutr.* 2008;87:1576S-81S.

72. Walsh S. *Plant Based Nutrition and Health.* St Leonards-on-Sea, UK: The Vegan Society, 2003.

73. Rand WM. Meta-analysis of nitrogen balance studies for estimating protein requirements in healthy adults. *Am J Clin Nutr.* 2003 Jan;77(1):109-27.

74. Melina V. Personal communication based on laboratory analysis of Green Giant Juice, kale, and almonds conducted by Cantest Laboratories on April 11-12, 2005.

CHAPTER 6
Carbohydrates in the Raw

1. FAO/WHO. *Carbohydrates in human nutrition. Report of a Joint FAO/WHO Expert Consultation.* 1998;66:1-140.

2. Gray J. Dietary *Fiber: Definition, Analysis, Physiology and Health. ILSI Europe Concise Monograph Series.* Brussels Belgium: ILSI Europe, 2006.

3. Institute of Medicine. *Dietary Reference Intakes for Energy, Carbohydrate, Fiber, Fat, Fatty Acids, Cholesterol, Protein, and Amino Acids (Macronutrients).* Washington DC: National Academies Press, 2002.

4. Cummings JH, Stephen AM. Carbohydrate terminology and classification. *Eur J Clin Nutr.* 2007 Dec;61 Suppl 1:S5-18.

5. Chavan JK, Kadam, SS. Nutritional improvement of cereals by sprouting. *Crit Rev Food Sci Nutr.*1989;28(5):401-437.

6. Kavas A, Sedef NEL. Nutritive value of germinated mung beans and lentils. *J Consumer Studies Home Econ.* 1991;15:357-66.

7. United States Department of Agriculture, Agricultural Research Service. *USDA National Nutrient Database for Standard Reference, Release 21.* 2008. www.nal.usda.gov/fnic/foodcomp/search. Accessed July 2009.

8. World Health Organization. *WHO Technical report series 916. Diet, Nutrition and the Prevention of Chronic Diseases. Report of a joint FAO/WHO Expert Consultation.* 2003.

9. USDA Agricultural Research Service. *Nutrient Intakes from Food: Mean Amounts and Percentages of Calories from Protein, Carbohydrate, Fat, and Alcohol, One Day, 2005-2006.* 2008. www.ars.usda.gov/ba/bhnrc/fsrg. Accessed July 2009.

10. Messina V, Mangels, R, Messina M. *The Dietitian's Guide to Vegetarian Diets: Issues and Applications. 2nd ed.* Sudbury MA: Jones and Bartlett Publishers, 2004.

11. Barnard ND, Gloede L, Cohen J, Jenkins DJ, Turner-McGrievy G, Green AA, Ferdowsian H. A low-fat vegan diet elicits greater macronutrient changes, but is comparable in adherence and acceptability, compared with a more conventional diabetes diet among individuals with type 2 diabetes. *J Am Diet Assoc.* 2009 Feb;109(2):263-72.

12. Garcia AL, Koebnick C, Dagnelie PC, Strassner C, Elmadfa I, Katz N, Leitzmann C, Hoffmann I. Long-term strict raw food diet is associated with favourable plasma beta-carotene and low plasma lycopene concentrations in Germans. *Br J Nutr.* 2008;99:1293-300.

13. Fontana L, Klein S, Holloszy JO. Long-term low-protein, low-calorie diet and endurance exercise modulate metabolic factors associated with cancer risk. *Am J Clin Nutr.* 2006;84:1456-62.

14. Koebnick C, Garcia AL, Dagnelie PC, Strassner C, Lindemans J, Katz N, Leitzmann C, Hoffmann I. Long-term consumption of a raw food diet is associated with favorable serum LDL cholesterol and triglycerides but also with elevated plasma homocysteine and low serum HDL cholesterol in humans. *J Nutr.* 2005;135:2372-78.

15. Donaldson M. Food and nutrition intake of Hallelujah vegetarians. *Nutr Food Sci.* 2001;31:293-303.

16. Agren JJ, Tormala ML, Nenonen MT, Hanninen O. Fatty acid composition of erythrocyte, platelet, and serum lipids in strict vegans. *Lipids.* 1995;30:365-69.

17. Rauma AL, Törrönen R, Hänninen O, Verhagen H, Mykkänen H. Antioxidant status in long-term adherents to a strict uncooked vegan diet. *Am J Clin Nutr.* 1995 Dec;62(6):1221-27.

18. Rauma AL, Nenonen M, Helve T, Hanninen O. Effect of a strict vegan diet on energy and nutrient intakes by Finnish rheumatoid patients. *Eur J Clin Nutr.* 1993;47:747-49.

19. Ling WH and Hanninen O. Shifting from a conventional diet to an uncooked vegan diet reversibly alters fecal hydrolytic activities in humans. *J Nutr.* 1992;122:924-30.

20. Hanninen O, Nenonen M, Ling WH, Li DS, Sihvonen L. Effects of eating an uncooked vegetable diet for one week. *Appetite.* 1992;19:243-54.

21. Graham D, Gianni K. Raw Summit interview with Doug Graham. 2007. www.rawsummit.com/free_download/doug_graham_transcript.pdf. Accessed July 2009.

22. Milton K. Micronutrient intakes of wild primates: are humans different? *Comp Biochem Physiol A Mol Integr Physiol*. 2003;136:47-59.

23. Milton K. Back to basics: why foods of wild primates have relevance for modern human health. *Nutrition*. 2000;16:480-83.

24. Milton K. Nutritional characteristics of wild primate foods: do the diets of our closest living relatives have lessons for us? *Nutrition*. 1999;15:488-98.

25. Popovich DG, Jenkins DJ, Kendall CW, Dierenfeld ES, Carroll RW, Tariq N, Vidgen E. The western lowland gorilla diet has implications for the health of humans and other hominoids. *J Nutr*. 1997;127:2000-05.

26. Joint FAO/WHO Food Standards Programme Codex Alimentarius Commission. *Report of the 30th Session of the Codex Committee on Nutrition and Foods for Special Dietary Uses*. Nov. 3-7, 2008. Cape Town, South Africa.

27. Englyst KN, Liu S, Englyst HN. Nutritional characterization and measurement of dietary carbohydrates. *Eur J Clin Nutr*. 2007 Dec;61 Suppl 1:S19-39.

28. Elia M, Cummings JH. Physiological aspects of energy metabolism and gastrointestinal effects of carbohydrates. *Eur J Clin Nutr*. 2007;61 Suppl 1:S40-S74.

29. Peltonen R, Ling WH, Hanninen O, Eerola E. An uncooked vegan diet shifts the profile of human fecal microflora: computerized analysis of direct stool sample gas-liquid chromatography profiles of bacterial cellular fatty acids. *Appl Environ Microbiol*. 1992;58:3660-66.

30. Peltonen R, Nenonen M, Helve T, Hanninen O, Toivanen P, Eerola E. Faecal microbial flora and disease activity in rheumatoid arthritis during a vegan diet. *Br J Rheumatol*. 1997;36:64-68.

31. Ryhanan EL, Mantere-Alhonen S, Nenonen M, Hanninen O. Modification of faecal flora in rheumatoid arthritis patients by lactobacilli rich vegetarian diet. *Milchwissenschaft*. 1993;48:255-59.

32. Gaisbauer M, Langosch A. Klinik in der Stanggass, Berchtesgaden. (Raw food and immunity). *Fortschr Med* (German). 1990;108:338-40.

33. Peltonen R, Kjeldsen-Kragh J, Haugen M et al. Changes of faecal flora in rheumatoid arthritis during fasting and one-year vegetarian diet. *Br J Rheumatol*. 1994;33:638-43.

34. Kjeldsen-Kragh J. Rheumatoid arthritis treated with vegetarian diets. *Am J Clin Nutr*. 1999;70:594S-600S.

35. Kjeldsen-Kragh J, Rashid T, Dybwad A, Sioud M, Haugen M, Førre O, Ebringer A. Decrease in anti-Proteus mirabilis but not anti-Escherichia coli antibody levels in rheumatoid arthritis patients treated with fasting and a one year vegetarian diet. *Ann Rheum Dis*. 1995 Mar;54(3):221-24.

36. Jenkins, D et al. Glycemic Index of Foods: a Physiological Basis for Carbohydrate Exchange. *Am J Clin Nutr*. 1981;34:362-66.

37. Atkinson FS, Foster-Powell K, Brand-Miller JC. International tables of glycemic index and glycemic load values. *Diabetes Care*. 2008;31(12):2281-83.

38. Gell P. From jelly beans to kidney beans: what diabetes educators should know about the glycemic index. *Diabetes Educ*. 2001 Jul-Aug;27(4):505-08.

39. Studio 34, Wikipedia Project, http://en.wikipedia.org/wiki/File:Glycemic.png. Accessed July 2009.

40. Brand Miller, JC. Importance of glycemic index in diabetes. *Am J Clin Nutr*. 1994;59:747S-752S.

41. Foster-Powell K, Miller JB. International tables of glycemic index. *Am J Clin Nutr*. 1995 Oct;62(4):871S-890S.

42. Foster-Powell K, Holt SH, Brand-Miller JC. International table of glycemic index and glycemic load values: *Am J Clin Nutr*. 2002 Jul;76(1):5-56.

43. Teff KL, Elliott SS, Tschöp M, Kieffer TJ, Rader D, Heiman M, Townsend RR, Keim NL, D'Alessio D, Havel PJ. Dietary fructose reduces circulating insulin and leptin, attenuates postprandial suppression of ghrelin, and increases triglycerides in women. *J Clin Endocrinol Metab*. 2004;89:2963-72.

44. Teff KL, Grudziak J, Townsend RR, Dunn TN, Grant RW, Adams SH, Keim NL, Cummings BP, Stanhope KL, Havel PJ. Endocrine and metabolic effects of consuming fructose- and glucose-sweetened beverages with meals in obese men and women: influence of insulin resistance on plasma triglyceride responses. *J Clin Endocrinol Metab*. 2009;94(5):1562-69.

45. Stanhope KL, Havel PJ. Endocrine and metabolic effects of consuming beverages sweetened with fructose, glucose, sucrose, or high-fructose corn syrup. *Am J Clin Nutr*. 2008;88(6):1733S-37S.

CHAPTER 7

Fat: Friends and Foes

1. Institute of Medicine. *Dietary Reference Intakes for Energy, Carbohydrates, Fiber, Fat, Protein and Amino Acids (Macronutrients).* Washington DC: National Academies Press, 2002. www.nap.edu/catalog.php?record_id=10490. Accessed July 2009.

2. Hu FB, Manson JE, WillettWC. Types of dietary fat and risk of coronary heart disease: a critical review. *J Am Coll Nutr.* 2001;20:5-19.

3. Kris-Etherton PM. Monounsaturated fatty acids and risk of cardiovascular disease. *Circulation.* 1999;100:1253-58.

4. Sacks FM, Katan M. Randomized clinical trials on the effects of dietary fat and carbohydrate on plasma lipoproteins and cardiovascular disease. *Am J Med.* 2002;113 Suppl 9B:13S-24S.

5. Micha R, Mozaffarian D. Trans fatty acids: effects on cardiometabolic health and implications for policy. *Prostaglandins Leukot Essent Fatty Acids.* 2008;79:147-52.

6. Trans Fat Task Force (Health Canada and the Heart and Stroke Foundation). *TRANSforming the Food Supply. Final Report Submitted to the Minister of Health in June 2006.* www.hc-sc.gc.ca/fn-an/nutrition/gras-trans-fats/tf-ge/tf-gt_rep-rap-eng.php. Accessed July 2009.

7. Mozaffarian D, Katan MB, Ascherio A, Stampfer MJ, Willett WC. Trans fatty acids and cardiovascular disease. *N Engl J Med.* 2006;354:1601-13.

8. Ascherio A, Willett WC. Health effects of trans fatty acids. *Am J Clin Nutr.* 1997;66:1006S-10S.

9. Risérus U. Trans fatty acids and insulin resistance. *Atheroscler Suppl.* 2006;7:37-9. Epub May 18, 2006.

10. Graham DN. *The 80:10:10 Diet.* Key Largo FL: FoodSport Press, 2006.

11. Cousens, G. *There is a Cure for Diabetes: The Tree of Life 21-Day+ Program.* Berkeley CA: North Atlantic Books, 2008.

12. Ornish D, Brown SE, Scherwitz LW, Billings JH, Armstrong WT, Ports TA, McLanahan SM, Kirkeeide RL, Brand RJ, Gould KL. Can lifestyle changes reverse coronary heart disease? The Lifestyle Heart Trial. *Lancet.* 1990;336:129-33.

13. McDougall J, Litzau K, Haver E, Saunders V, Spiller GA. Rapid reduction of serum cholesterol and blood pressure by a twelve-day, very low fat, strictly vegetarian diet. *J Am Coll Nutr.* 1995;5:491-96.

14. Esselstyn, CB Jr. Updating a 12 year experience with arrest and reversal therapy of coronary heart disease. *Am J Cardiol.* 1999;84:339-41.

15. Barnard ND, Cohen J, Jenkins DJ, Turner-McGrievy G, Gloede L, Jaster B, Seidl K, Green AA, Talpers S. A low fat vegan diet improves glycemic control and cardiovascular risk factors in a randomized clinical trial in individuals with type 2 diabetes. *Diabetes Care.* 2006;29:1777-83.

16. Ornish D, Scherwitz LW, Billings JH, Gould KL, Merritt TA, Sparler S, Armstrong WT, Ports TA, Kirkeeide RL, Hogeboom C, Brand RJ. Intensive lifestyle changes for reversal of coronary heart disease. *JAMA.* 1998;280:2001-07.

17. Institute of Medicine. *Dietary Reference Intakes for Vitamin A, Vitamin K, Arsenic, Boron, Chromium, Copper, Iodine, Iron, Manganese, Molybdenum, Nickel, Silicon, Vanadium, and Zinc.* Washington DC: National Academies Press, 2000. http://books.nap.edu/books/0309072794/html/1.html. Accessed July 2009.

18. Gartner C., Stahl W., Sies H. Lycopene is more bioavailable from tomato paste than from fresh tomatoes. *Am J Clin Nutr.* 1997;66:116-22.

19. Unlu NZ, Bohn T, Clinton SK, Schwartz SJ. Carotenoid absorption from salad and salsa by humans is enhanced by the addition of avocado or avocado oil. *J Nutr.* 2005;135:431-436.

20. Willet WC. *Eat, Drink, and Be Healthy. The Harvard Medical School Guide to Healthy Eating.* New York: Simon and Schuster Source, 2001.

21. Keys A. Wine, garlic, and CHD in seven countries. *Lancet.* 1980;1:145-46.

22. Keys A, Menotti A, Toshima H. The diet and 15-year death rate in the Seven Countries Study. *Am J Epidemiol.* 1986;124:903-15.

23. Sarri K, Kafatos A. The Seven Countries Study in Crete: olive oil, Mediterranean diet or fasting? *Public Health Nutr.* 2005;8:666.

24. WHO, Consultation FAO. *Diet, nutrition and the prevention of chronic diseases. WHO Technical Report Series.* 2003:916. http://whqlibdoc.who.int/trs/WHO_trs_916.pdf. Accessed July 2009.

25. World Cancer Research Fund American Institute for Cancer Research. *Food, Nutrition, Physical Activity and the Prevention of Cancer: A Global Perspective.* Washington DC: AICR, 2007.

26. Bladbjerg EM, Marckmann P, Sandström B, Jespersen J. Non-fasting factor VII coagulant

activity (FVII:C) increased by high fat diet. *Thromb Haemost*. 1994;71:755-58.

27. Larsen LF, Bladbjerg EM, Jespersen J, Marckmann P. Effects of dietary fat quality and quantity on postprandial activation of blood coagulation factor VII. *Arterioscler Thromb Vasc Biol*. 1997;17:2904-09.

28. Chow, CK. *Fatty Acids in Foods and Their Health Implications*. 3rd ed. Boca Raton FL: CRC Press, 2007.

29. Bolton GE, Sanders TH. Effect of roasting oil composition on the stability of roasted high-oleic peanuts. *JAOCS*. 2002;79:129-132.

30. Raatz SK, Bibus D, Thomas W, Kris-Etherton P. Total fat intake modifies plasma fatty acid composition in humans. *J Nutr*. 2001;131:231-34.

31. Lichtenstein AH, Appel LJ, Brands M, Carnethon M, Daniels S, Franch HA, Franklin B, Kris-Etherton P, Harris WS, Howard B, Karanja N, Lefevre M, Rudel L, Sacks F, Van Horn L, Winston M, Wylie-Rosett J. Diet and lifestyle recommendations revision 2006: a scientific statement from the American Heart Association Nutrition Committee. *Circulation*. 2006;114;82-96.

32. American Diabetes Association. Nutrition Recommendations and Interventions for Diabetes. A position statement of the American Diabetes Association. *Diabetes Care*. 2008;31:S61-78.

33. Messina V, Mangels R, Messina M. *The Dietitian's Guide to Vegetarian Diets: Issues and Applications*. Sudbury MA: Jones and Bartlett Publishers, 2004.

34. U.S. Department of Agriculture, Agricultural Research Service. *Nutrient Intakes from Food: Mean Amounts and Percentages of Calories from Protein, Carbohydrate, Fat, and Alcohol, One Day, 2005-2006*. 2008. www.ars.usda.gov/ba/bhnrc/fsrg. Accessed July 2009.

35. Fontana L, Klein S, Holloszy JO. Long-term low-protein, low-calorie diet and endurance exercise modulate metabolic factors associated with cancer risk. *Am J Clin Nutr*. 2006;84:1456-62.

36. Agren JJ, Tvrzicka E, Nenonen MT, Helve T, Hanninen O. Divergent changes in serum sterols during a strict uncooked vegan diet in patients with rheumatoid arthritis. *Br J Nutr*. 2001;85:137-139.

37. Rauma AL, Torronen R, Hanninen O, Verhagen H, Mykkanen H. Antioxidant status in long-term adherents to a strict uncooked vegan diet. *Am J Clin Nutr*. 1995;6:1221-07.

38. Ågren J, Törmalä M, Nenonen M, Hänninen O. Fatty acid composition of erythrocyte, platelet, and serum lipids in strict vegans. *Lipids*. 1995;30:365-69.

39. Das UN. Essential fatty acids and their metabolites could function as endogenous HMG-CoA reductase and ACE enzyme inhibitors, anti-arrhythmic, anti-hypertensive, anti-atherosclerotic, anti-inflammatory, cytoprotective, and cardioprotective molecules. *Lipids Health Dis*. 2008;7:37.

40. Simopoulos AP. The importance of the ratio of omega-6/omega-3 essential fatty acids. *Biomed Pharmacother*. 2002;56:365-79.

41. Simopoulos AP. Essential fatty acids in health and chronic disease. *Am J Clin Nutr*. 1999;70 Suppl:560S-69S.

42. Das UN. Essential fatty acids: biochemistry, physiology, and pathology. *Biotech J*. 2006;1:420-39.

43. Doughman SD, Krupanidhi S, Sanjeevi CB. Omega-3 fatty acids for nutrition and medicine: considering microalgae oil as a vegetarian source of EPA and DHA. *Curr Diabetes Rev*. 2007;3(3):198-203.

44. Berti M, Johnson BL, Dash S, Fischer S, Wilckens R, Hevia F. Echium: a source of stearidonic acid adapted to the Northern Great Plains in the US. In Janick J, Whipkey A eds. *Issues in New crops and New Uses*. Alexandria VA: ASHS Press, 2007:120-25.

45. Bailey N. Current choices in omega 3 supplementation. *Nutr Bull*. 2009;34:85-91.

46. Davis B., Kris-Etherton P. Achieving optimal essential fatty acid status in vegetarians: current knowledge and practical implications. *Am J Clin Nutr*. 2003:78 suppl;640S-46S.

47. Indu M, Ghafoorunissa SA. N-3 fatty acids in Indian diets—comparison of the effects of precursor (alpha-linolenic acid) vs. product (long-chain n-3 polyunsaturated fatty acids). *Nutr Res*. 1992;12:569-82.

48. Masters C. Omega-3 fatty acids and the peroxisome. *Mol Cell Biochem*. 1996;165:83-93.

49. Harnack K, Andersen G, Somoza V. Quantitation of alpha-linolenic acid elongation to eicosapentaenoic and docosahexaenoic acid as affected by the ratio of n6/n3 fatty acids. *Nutr Metab* (London). 2009;6:8.

50. Krajcovicova-Kudlackova M, Simoncic R, Bederova A, Klvanova J. Plasma fatty acid profile and alternative nutrition. *Ann Nutr Metab*. 1997;41:365-70.

51. Reddy S, Sanders TAB, Obeid O. The influence of maternal vegetarian diet on the essential fatty acid status of the newborn. *Euro J Clin Nutr*. 1994;48:358-68.

52. Sanders TAB, Ellis FR, Dickerson JWT. Studies of vegans: the fatty acid composition of plasma choline phosphoglycerides and some indicators of susceptibility to ischemic heart disease in vegan and omnivore control. *Am J Clin Nutr.* 1978;31:805-13.

53. Sanders TAB, Roshanai F. Platelet phospholipid fatty acid composition and function in vegan compared with age- and sex-matched omnivore controls. *Euro J Clin Nutr.* 1992;46:823-31.

54. Melchert HU, Limsathayourat N, Mibajlovic H, Eichber J, Thefeld W, Rottkea H. Fatty acid patterns in triglycerides, diglycerides, free fatty acids, cholesterol esters and phosphatidlycholine in serum from vegetarians and non-vegetarians. *Atherosclerosis.* 1987;65:159-66.

55. Donaldson M. Food and nutrition intake of Hallelujah vegetarians. *Nutr Food Sci.* 2001;31:293-303.

56. Emken EA, Adlof RO, Gulley RM. Dietary linoleic acid influences desaturation and acylation of deuterium-labeled linoleic and ALAs in young adult males. *Biochim Biophys Acta.* 1994;1213:277-88.

57. Gerster H. Can adults adequately convert alpha-linolenic acid (18:3 n-3) to eicosapentaenoic acid (20:5 n-3) and docosahexaenoic acid (22:6 n-3)? *Int J Vit Nutr Res.* 1998;68:159-73.

58. Koebnick C, Strassner C, Hoffmann I, Leitzmann C. Consequences of a long-term raw food diet on body weight and menstruation: results of a questionnaire survey. *Ann Nutr Metab.* 1999;43:69-79.

59. Siguel EN, Lerman RH. Altered fatty acid metabolism in patients with angiographically documented coronary artery disease. *Metabolism.* 1994;43:982-93.

60. Horrobin DF. Nutritional and medical importance of gamma-linolenic acid. *Prog Lipid Res.* 1992;31:163-94.

61. Callaway JC. Hempseed as a nutritional resource: an overview. *Euphytica.* 2004;140:65-72.

62. Burge GC, Wootton SA. Conversion of alpha-linolenic acid to eicosapentaenoic, docosapentaenoic and docosahexaenoic acids in young women. *Br J Nutr.* 2002;88:411-20.

63. Ghafoorunissa SA. Requirements of dietary fats to meet nutritional needs and prevent the risk of atherosclerosis—an Indian perspective. *Indian J Med Res.* 1998;108:191-202.

64. Burge GC, Jones AE, Wootton SA. Eicosapentaenoic and docosapentaenoic acids are the principal products of alpha-linolenic acid metabolism in young men. *Br J Nutr.* 2002;88:355-63.

65. Innis SM. Polyunsaturated fatty acids in human milk: an essential role in infant development. *Adv Exp Med Biol.* 2004;554:27-43.

66. Uauy R, Hoffman DR, Peirano P, Birch DG, Birch EE. Essential fatty acids in visual and brain development. *Lipids.* 2001;36:885-95.

67. Harper CR, Edwards MJ, DeFilippis AP, Jacobson TA. Flaxseed oil increases the plasma concentrations of cardioprotective (n-3) fatty acids in humans. *J Nutr.* 2006;136:83-87.

68. United States Department of Agriculture, Agricultural Research Service. *USDA National Nutrient Database for Standard Reference, Release 21.* 2008. www.nal.usda.gov/fnic/foodcomp/search. Accessed July 2009.

69. Sanders T, Lewis F. *Review of Nutritional Attributes of Good Oil (Cold Pressed Hemp Seed Oil).* King's College London: Nutritional Sciences Division, 2008. www.goodwebsite.co.uk/kingsreport.pdf. Accessed July 2009.

70. Marckmann P, Gronbaek M. Fish consumption and coronary heart disease mortality. A systematic review of prospective cohort studies. *Eur J Clin Nutr.* 1999;53:585-90.

71. Doughman SD, Krupanidhi S, Sanjeevi CB. Omega-3 fatty acids for nutrition and medicine: considering microalgae oil as a vegetarian source of EPA and DHA. *Curr Diabetes Rev.* 2007 Aug;3(3):198-203.

72. Kusbak R., Drapeau C., van Cott E., and Winter H. *Blue-Green Algaaphanizomenon Flos-aquae as a Source of Dietary Polyunsaturated Fatty Acids and a Hypocholesterolemic Agent.* Annual Meeting of the American Chemical Society, Chemistry, and Nutrition of Highly Unsaturated Fatty Acids. March 21-25, 1999. Anaheim CA.

73. Hu FB, Stampfer MJ. Nut consumption and risk of coronary heart disease: a review of the epidemiologic evidence. *Curr Atheroscler Rep.* 1999;1:204-09.

74. Sabaté J, Ang Y. Nuts and health outcomes: new epidemiologic evidence. *Am J Clin Nutr.* 2009;89:1643S-48S. Epub March 25, 2009.

75. Albert CM, Gaziano JM, Willett WC, Manson JE. Nut consumption and decreased risk of sudden cardiac death in the Physicians' Health Study. *Arch Intern Med.* 2002;162:1382-87.

76. Fraser GE, Sabate J, Beeson WL, Strahan TM. A possible protective effect of nut consumption on risk of coronary heart disease. The Adventist Health Study. *Arch Intern Med.* 1992;152:1416-24.

77. Fraser GE. Nut consumption, lipids, and risk of a coronary event. *Clin Cardiol.* 1999;22(7 Suppl):III11-15.

78. Fraser GE, Lindsted KD, Beeson WL. Effect of risk factor values on lifetime risk of and age at first coronary event. The Adventist Health Study. *Am J Epidemiol.* 1995;142:746-58.

79. Hu, FB, Stampfer MJ, Manson JE, Rimm EB, Colditz GA, Rosner BA, Speizer FE, Hennekens, CH, Willett WC. Frequent nut consumption and risk of coronary heart disease in women: prospective cohort study. *BMJ.* 1998;317:1341-45.

80. Ellsworth JL, Kushi LH, Folsom AR. Frequent nut intake and risk of death from coronary heart disease and all causes in postmenopausal women: the Iowa Women's Health Study. *Nutr Metab Cardiovasc Dis.* 2001;11:372-77.

81. Brown L, Sacks F, Rosner B, Willett WC. Nut consumption and risk of coronary heart disease in patients with myocardial infarction. *FASEB J.* 1999;13:A4332.

82. Kushi LH, Folsom AR, Prineas RJ, Mink PJ, Bosick RM. Dietary antioxidant vitamins and death from coronary heart disease in postmenopausal women. *N Engl J Med.* 1996;334:1156-62.

83. Mukuddem-Petersen J, Oosthuizen W, Jerling JC. A systematic review of the effects of nuts on blood lipid profiles in humans. *J Nutr.* 2005;135:2082-89.

84. Lamarche B, Desroche S, Jenkins DJ et al. Combined effects of a dietary portfolio of plant sterols, vegetable protein, viscous fiber and almonds on LDL particle size. *Br J Nutr.* 2004;92:654-63.

85. Yochum LA, Folsom AR, Kushi LH. Intake of antioxidant vitamins and risk of death from stroke in post-menopausal women. *Am J Clin Nutr.* 2000;72:476-83.

86. Jiang R, Manson JE, Stampher MJ, Liu S, Willet WC, Hu FB. Nut and peanut butter consumption and risk of type 2 diabetes in women. *JAMA.* 2002;288:2554-60.

87. Zhang SM, Hernan MA, Chen H, Spiegelman D, Willett WC, Ascherio A. Intakes of vitamins E and C, carotenoids, vitamin supplements, and PD risk. *Neurology.* 2002;59:1161-69.

88. Seddon JM, Cote J, Rosner B. Progression of age-related macular degeneration: association with dietary fat, transunsaturated fat, nuts and fish intake. *Arch Ophthal.* 2003;121:1728-37.

89. Tsai CJ, Leitzmann MF, Hu FB, Willet WC, Giovannucci EL. Frequent nut consumption and decreased risk of cholecystectomy in women. *Am J Clin Nutr.* 2004;80:76-81.

90. Hu FB, Stampfer MJ, Manson JE et al. Dietary saturated fats and their food sources in relation to the risk of coronary heart disease in women. *Am J Clin Nutr.* 1999;70:1001-08.

91. Fraser GE, Shavik, DJ. Ten years of life: is it a matter of choice? *Arch Int Med.* 2001;161:1645-52.

92. Sabaté J. Nut consumption, vegetarian diets, ischemic heart disease risk, and all-cause mortality: evidence from epidemiologic studies. *Am J Clin Nutr.* 1999;70(3 Suppl):500S-03S.

93. Mattes RD, Kris-Etherton PM, Foster GD. Impact of peanuts and tree nuts on body weight and healthy weight loss in adults. *J Nutr.* 2008;138(9):1741S-45S.

94. Rainey C, Nyquist L. Nuts—nutrition and health benefits of daily use. *Nutr Today.* 1997;32:157-63.

95. Hu, FB. Plant-based foods and prevention of cardiovascular disease: an overview. *Am J Clin Nutr.* 2003;78:544S-51S.

96. Yaacoub R, Saliba R, Nsouli B, Khalaf G, Birlouez-Aragon I. Formation of lipid oxidation and isomerization products during processing of nuts and sesame seeds. *J Agric Food Chem.* 2008;56:7082-90.

97. Lukac H, Amrein TM, Perren R, Conde-Petit B, Amado R, Escher F. Influence of roasting conditions on the acrylamide content and the color of roasted almonds. *J Food Sci.* 2006;72:c033-38.

98. World Intellectual Property Organization (WO/2005/039322). *Edible Testa-On (Skin-On) Cashew Nuts and Methods for Preparing Same.* 2005. www.wipo.int/pctdb/en/wo.jsp ?IA=IB2003005287&DISPLAY=DESC. Accessed July 2009.

99. Hotz C, Gibson RS. Traditional food-processing and preparation practices to enhance the bioavailability of micronutrients in plant-based diets. *J Nutr.* 2007 Apr;137(4):1097-100.

100. Gibson RS, Perlas L, Hotz C. Improving the bioavailability of nutrients in plant foods at the household level. *Proc Nutr Soc.* 2006 May;65(2):160-68.

101. Visioli F, Bellomo G, Galli C. Free radical scavenging properties of olive oil polyphenols. *Biochem Biophys Res Commun.* 1998;247:60-64.

102. Stupans I, Kirlich A, Tuck KL, Hayball PJ. Comparison of radical scavenging effect, inhibition of microsomal oxygen free radical generation, and serum lipoprotein oxidation of several natural antioxidants. *J Agric Food Chem.* 2002;50:2464-69.

103. Kremastinos DT. Olive and oleuropein. *Hellenic J Cardiol.* 2008;49:295-96.

104. Owen RW, Haubner R, Würtele G, Hull E, Spiegelhalder B, Bartsch H. Olives and olive oil in cancer prevention. *Eur J Cancer Prev.* 2004;13:319-26.

105. Cunnane SC, Hamadeh MJ, Liede AC et al. Nutritional attributes of traditional flaxseed in healthy young adults. *Am J Clin Nutr.* 1995;61:62-68.

106. Manda escu S, Mocanu V, D scali a AM, Haliga R, Nestian I, Stitt PA, Luca V. Flaxseed supplementation in hyperlipidemic patients. *Rev Med Chir Soc Med Nat Iasi.* 2005;109:502-06.

107. Lucas EA, Wild RD, Hammond LJ et al. Flaxseed improves lipid profile without altering biomarkers of bone metabolism in postmenopausal women. *J Clin Endocrinol Metab.* 2002;87:1527-32.

108. Jenkins DJA, Kendall CWC, Vidgen E et al. Health aspects of partially defatted flaxseed, including effects on serum lipids, oxidative measures, and ex vivo androgen and progestin activity: A controlled crossover trial. *Am J Clin Nutr.* 1999;69:395-402.

109. Thompson LU, Li T, Chen J, Goss PE. Biological effects of dietary flaxseed in patients with breast cancer (abstract). *Breast Cancer Res Treatment.* 2000;64:50.

110. Sung MK, Lautens M, Thompson LU. Mammalian lignans inhibit the growth of estrogen-independent human colon tumor cells. *Anticancer Res.* 1998;18:1405-08.

111. Ayerza R, Coates W. *Chia.* Tucson AZ: The University of Arizona Press, 2005.

112. Connor WE. Harbingers of coronary heart disease: dietary saturated fatty acids and cholesterol. Is chocolate benign because of its stearic acid content? *Am J Clin Nutr.* 1999;70:951-52.

113. de Roos NM, Schouten EG, Katan MB. Consumption of a solid fat rich in lauric acid results in a more favorable serum lipid profile in healthy men and women than consumption of a solid fat rich in trans-fatty acids. *J Nutr.* 2001;131:242-45.

114. Mensink RP, Zock PL, Kester AD, Katan MB. Effects of dietary fatty acids and carbohydrates on the ratio of serum total to HDL cholesterol and on serum lipids and apolipoproteins: a meta-analysis of 60 controlled trials. *Am J Clin Nutr.* 2003;77:1146-55.

115. Ng TK, Hassan K, Lim JB, Lye MS, Ishak R. Nonhypercholesterolemic effects of a palm-oil diet in Malaysian volunteers. *Am J Clin Nutr.* 1991;53(4 Suppl):1015S-20S.

116. Prior IA, Davidson F, Salmond CE, Czochanska Z. Cholesterol, coconuts, and diet on Polynesian atolls: a natural experiment: the Pukapuka and Tokelau island studies. *Am J Clin Nutr.* 1981;34:1552-61.

117. Lipoeto NI, Mmedsci, Agus Z, Oenzil F, Masrul M, Wattanapenpaiboon N. Contemporary Minangkabau food culture in West Sumatra, Indonesia. *Asia Pac J Clin Nutr.* 2001;10:10-16.

118. Lipoeto NI, Agus Z, Oenzil F, Wahlqvist M, Wattanapenpaiboon N. Dietary intake and the risk of coronary heart disease among the coconut-consuming Minangkabau in West Sumatra, Indonesia. *Asia Pac J Clin Nutr.* 2004;13:377-84.

119. Ogbolu DO, Oni AA, Daini OA, Oloko AP. In vitro antimicrobial properties of coconut oil on Candida species in Ibadan, Nigeria. *J Med Food.* 2007;10:384-87.

120. Erguiza GS, Jiao AG, Reley M, Ragaza S. The effect of virgin coconut oil supplementation for community-acquired pneumonia in children aged 3 to 60 months admitted at the Philippine Children's Medical Center: a single blinded randomized controlled trial. *Chest.* 2008;134:139001.

121. Hierholzer JC, Kabara JJ. In vitro effects of monolaurin compounds on enveloped RNA and DNA viruses. *J Food Safety.* 1982;4:1-12.

122. Carpo BG, Verallo-Rowell VM, Kabara J. Novel antibacterial activity of monolaurin compared with conventional antibiotics against organisms from skin infections: an in vitro study. *J Drugs Dermatol.* 2007;6:991-98.

123. Nevin KG, Rajamohan T. Beneficial effects of virgin coconut oil on lipid parameters and in vitro LDL oxidation. *Clin Biochem.* 2004;37:830-35.

124. Marina AM, Man YB, Nazimah SA, Amin I. Antioxidant capacity and phenolic acids of virgin coconut oil. *Int J Food Sci Nutr.* 2008; Dec 29:1-10. Epub ahead of print.

CHAPTER 8
Vitamins: Inviting Vitality

1. Institute of Medicine. *Dietary Reference Intakes for Calcium, Phosphorus, Magnesium, Vitamin D, and Fluoride.* Washington DC: National Academies Press, 1997. http://books.nap.edu/openbook.php?record_id=5776&chapselect=yo&page=R1. Accessed July 2009.

2. Institute of Medicine. *Dietary Reference Intakes for Vitamin C, Vitamin E, Selenium, and Carotenoids (2000) Panel on Dietary Antioxidants and Related Compounds*. Washington DC: National Academies Press, 2000. www.nap.edu/catalog.php?record_id=9810#toc. Accessed September 2009.

3. Institute of Medicine. *Dietary Reference Intakes for Vitamin A, Vitamin K, Arsenic, Boron, Chromium, Copper, Iodine, Iron, Manganese, Molybdenum, Nickel, Silicon, Vanadium, and Zinc*. Washington DC: National Academies Press, 2000. http://books.nap.edu/books/0309072794/html/1.html. Accessed September 2009.

4. Hoffmann I et al. Raw food diet: health benefits and risks. In Watson RR ed. *Vegetables, Fruits, and Herbs in Health Promotion*. Boca Raton, FL: CRC Press, 2000:293-308.

5. Koebnick C et al. Long-term consumption of a raw food diet is associated with favorable serum LDL cholesterol and triglycerides but also with elevated plasma homocysteine and low serum HDL cholesterol in humans. *J Nutr*. 2005;135:2372-78.

6. Donaldson, MS. Food and nutrient intake of Hallelujah vegetarians. *Nutrition & Food Science*. 2001;31:293-303. www.hacres.com/diet/research/nutrient_intake.pdf.

7. Rauma AL et al. Coumarin 7-hydroxylation in long-term adherents of a strict uncooked vegan diet. *Eur J Clin Pharmacol*. 1996;50:133-37.

8. Rauma AL et al. Effect of a strict vegan diet on energy and nutrient intakes by Finnish rheumatoid patients. *Eur J Clin Nutr*. 1993 Oct;47(10):747-49.

9. Peltonen R et al. An uncooked vegan diet shifts the profile of human fecal microflora: computerized analysis of direct stool sample gas-liquid chromatography profiles of bacterial cellular fatty acids. *Appl Environ Microbiol*. 1992;58:3660-66.

10. Fontana L et al. Low bone mass in subjects on a long-term raw vegetarian diet. *Arch Intern Med*. 2005;165:684-89.

11. Garcia AL et al. Long-term strict raw food diet is associated with favourable plasma beta-carotene and low plasma lycopene concentrations in Germans. *Br J Nutr*. 2008;99:1293-300.

12. Adzersen KH et al. Raw and cooked vegetables, fruits, selected micronutrients, and breast cancer risk: a case-control study in Germany. *Nutr Cancer*. 2003;46:131-37.

13. Bland JS. Oxidants and antioxidants in clinical medicine: past, present and future potential. *J Nutr Environ Med*. 1995;5:255-80.

14. Liska DJ. The detoxification enzyme systems. *Altern Med Rev*. 1998;3:187-98.

15. Randhir R et al. Phenolics, their antioxidant and antimicrobial activity in dark germinated fenugreek sprouts in response to peptide and phytochemical elicitors. *Asia Pac J Clin Nutr*. 2004;13:295-307.

16. Rauma AL et al. Antioxidant status in long-term adherents to a strict uncooked vegan diet. *Am J Clin Nutr*. 1995;62:1221-27.

17. Szeto YT et al. Total antioxidant and ascorbic acid content of fresh fruits and vegetables: implications for dietary planning and food preservation. *Br J Nutr*. 2002;87:55-59.

18. Takaya Y et al. Antioxidant constituents of radish sprout (Kaiware-daikon), Raphanus sativus L. *J Agric Food Chem*. 2003;51:8061-66.

19. Yang F et al. Studies on germination conditions and antioxidant contents of wheat grain. *Int J Food Sci Nutr*. 2001;52:319-30.

20. Maiani G et al. Carotenoids: actual knowledge on food sources, intakes, stability and bioavailability and their protective role in humans. *Mol Nutr Food Res*. 2009;53.

21. Milner JA. Incorporating basic nutrition science into health interventions for cancer prevention. *J Nutr*. 2003;133(11 Suppl 1):3820S-26S.

22. Takaya Y et al. Antioxidant constituents of radish sprout (Kaiware-daikon), Raphanus sativus L. *J Agric Food Chem*. 2003 Dec 31;51(27):8061-66.

23. Bland J. Managing biotransformation: introduction and overview. *Altern Ther Health Med*. 2007;13:S85-87.

24. Murray M. Altered CYP expression and function in response to dietary factors: potential roles in disease pathogenesis. *Curr Drug Metab*. 2006;7:67-81.

25. Stipanuk MH. Detoxification and Protective Functions of Nutrients. In Stipanuk MH ed. *Biochemical and Physiological Aspects of Human Nutrition*. Philadelphia: WB Saunders Company, 2000:909-12.

26. Beecher CW. Cancer preventive properties of varieties of Brassica oleracea: a review. *Am J Clin Nutr*. 1994;59(5 Suppl):1166S-70S.

27. Gill CI et al. Watercress supplementation in diet reduces lymphocyte DNA damage and alters blood antioxidant status in healthy adults. *Am J Clin Nutr*. 2007;85:504-10.

28. Pool-Zobel B et al. Modulation of xenobiotic metabolising enzymes by anticarcinogens—focus on glutathione S-transferases and their role as targets of dietary chemoprevention in colorectal carcinogenesis. *Mutat Res.* 2005;591:74-92.

29. Calzuola I et al. Synthesis of antioxidants in wheat sprouts. *J Agric Food Chem.* 2004;52:5201-06.

30. Sheweita SA et al. Cancer and phase II drug-metabolizing enzymes. *Curr Drug Metab.* 2003;4:45-58.

31. Wargovich MJ et al. Diet, individual responsiveness and cancer prevention. *J Nutr.* 2003;133(7 Suppl):2400S-03S.

32. Kapiszewska M. A vegetable to meat consumption ratio as a relevant factor determining cancer preventive diet. The Mediterranean versus other European countries. *Forum Nutr.* 2006;59:130-53.

33. Link LB et al. Raw versus cooked vegetables and cancer risk. *Cancer Epidemiol Biomarkers Prev.* 2004;13:1422-35.

34. Nestle M. Broccoli sprouts as inducers of carcinogen-detoxifying enzyme systems: clinical, dietary, and policy implications. *Proc Natl Acad Sci USA.* 1997;94:11149-51.

35. Pereira MA et al. Effects of a low-glycemic load diet on resting energy expenditure and heart disease risk factors during weight loss. *JAMA.* 2004;292:2482-90.

36. Martínez-Sánchez A et al. A comparative study of flavonoid compounds, vitamin C, and antioxidant properties of baby leaf Brassicaceae species. *J Agric Food Chem.* 2008;56:2330-40.

37. Wigmore A. *The Sprouting Book.* Wayne NJ: Avery, 1986.

38. van Het Hof KH et al. Dietary factors that affect the bioavailability of carotenoids. *J Nutr.* 2000;130:503-06.

39. Calzuola I et al. Synthesis of antioxidants in wheat sprouts. *J Agric Food Chem.* 2004 Aug 11;52(16):5201-06.

40. Adzersen KH et al. Raw and cooked vegetables, fruits, selected micronutrients, and breast cancer risk: a case-control study in Germany. *Nutr Cancer.* 2003;46(2):131-37.

41. Brown MJ et al. Carotenoid bioavailability is higher from salads ingested with full-fat than with fat-reduced salad dressings as measured with electrochemical detection. *Am J Clin Nutr.* 2004;80:396-403. www.ajcn.org/cgi/reprint/80/2/396.

42. Messina V et al. *The Dietitian's Guide to Vegetarian Diets. 2nd ed.* Boston: Jones and Bartlett Publishing, 2004.

43. Hänninen O et al. Antioxidants in vegan diet and rheumatic disorders. *Toxicology.* 2000;155:45-53.

44. Verhagen H et al. Effect of a vegan diet on biomarkers of chemoprevention in females. *Hum Exp Toxicol.* 1996;15:821-25.

45. Clemens R et al. Detox diets provide empty promises. *Food Technology.* 2005;59:18.

46. Matsufuji H et al. Antioxidant content of different coloured sweet peppers, white green, yellow, orange and red (Capsicum annum L.). *Int J Food Science and Technol.* 2007;42:1482-88.

47. Niizu PY et al. New data on the carotenoids composition of raw salad vegetables. *J Food Composition and Analysis.* 2005;18:739-49.

48. Sun T et al. Antioxidant activities of different colored sweet bell peppers (Capsicum annuum L.). *J Food Science* 2007;72:S98-102.

49. Agte V et al. Vitamin profile of cooked foods: how healthy is the practice of ready-to-eat foods? *Int J Food Sci Nutr.* 2002;53:197-208.

50. Edwards AJ et al. Alpha- and beta-carotene from a commercial puree are more bioavailable to humans than from boiled-mashed carrots, as determined using an extrinsic stable isotope reference method. *J Nutr.* 2002;132:159-67.

51. Gliszczy ska-Swigło A et al. Changes in the content of health-promoting compounds and antioxidant activity of broccoli after domestic processing. *Food Addit Contam.* 2006;23:1088-98.

52. Khachik F. Effect of food preparation on qualitative and quantitative distribution of major carotenoid constituents of tomatoes and several green vegetables. *J Agric Food Chem.* 1992;40:390-98.

53. Livny O et al. Beta-carotene bioavailability from differently processed carrot meals in human ileostomy volunteers. *Eur J Nutr.* 2003;42:338-45.

54. McEligot AJ et al. Comparison of serum carotenoid responses between women consuming vegetable juice and women consuming raw or cooked vegetables. *Cancer Epidemiol Biomarkers Prev.* 1999;8:227-31.

55. Rock CL et al. Bioavailability of beta-carotene is lower in raw than in processed carrots and spinach in women. *J Nutr.* 1998;128:913-16.

56. Ruiz-Cruz S et al. Sanitation procedure affects biochemical and nutritional changes of shredded carrots. *J Food Sci.* 2007;72:S146-52.

57. Reboul E et al. Bioaccessibility of carotenoids and vitamin E from their main dietary sources. *J Agric Food Chem.* 2006;54:8749-55.

58. Porrini M et al. Factors influencing the bioavailability of antioxidants in foods: a critical appraisal. *Nutr Metab Cardiovasc Dis.* 2008;18:647-50.

59. Layrisse M et al. Measurement of the total daily dietary iron absorption by the extrinsic tag model. *Am J Clin Nutr.* 1974;27:152-62.

60. Naidu KA. Vitamin C in human health and disease is still a mystery? An overview. *Nutr J.* 2003;2:7.

61. USDA, Agricultural Research Service. *USDA National Nutrient Database for Standard Reference, Release 21.* 2005. www.ars.usda.gov/Services/docs.htm?docid=8964 or www.nal.usda.gov/fnic/foodcomp/search. Accessed September 2009.

62. Topuz A et al. Assessment of carotenoids, capsaicioids, and ascorbic acid composition of some selected pepper cultivars (Caprsicum annum L.) grown in Turkey. *J Food Composition and Analysis.* 2007;20:596-602.

63. Hamilton MJ et al. Germination and nutrient composition of alfalfa seeds. *J Food Science.* 1979;44:443-45.

64. Moriyama M et al. Comparative study on the vitamin C contents of the food legume seeds. *J Nutr Sci Vitaminol* (Tokyo). 2008;54:1-6.

65. Wunderlich SM et al. Nutritional quality of organic, conventional, and seasonally grown broccoli using vitamin C as a marker. *Int J Food Sci Nutr.* 2008;59:34-45.

66. Galgano F et al. The influence of processing and preservation on the retention of health-promoting compounds in broccoli. *J Food Sci.* 2007;72:S130-35.

67. Donaldson, MS. *Hallelujah vegetarians and nutritional science: answering your questions.* Personal communication. 2005.

68. Miyazawa T et al. Antiangiogenic and anti-cancer potential of unsaturated vitamin E (tocotrienol). *J Nutr Biochem.* 2009;20:79-86.

69. Miller ER et al. Meta-analysis: high-dosage vitamin E supplementation may increase all-cause mortality. *Ann Intern Med.* 2005;142:37-46.

70. Ruales J et al. Quinoa (Chenopodium quinoa willd) an important Andean food crop. *Arch Latinoam Nutr.* 1992;42:232-41.

71. Simopoulos et al. Common purslane: a source of omega-3 fatty acids and antioxidants. *J Am Coll Nutr.* 1992;11:374-82.

72. Steinhart H et al. Dependence of tocopherol stability on different cooking procedures of food. *Int J Vitam Nutr Res.* 2003;73:144-51.

73. McLean RR et al Association of dietary and biochemical measures of vitamin K with quantitative ultrasound of the heel in men and women. *Osteoporos Int.* 2006;17(4):600-07.

74. Chan J et al. Serum 25-hydroxyvitamin D status of vegetarians, partial vegetarians, and nonvegetarians: the Adventist Health Study-2. *Am J Clin Nutr.* 2009;89:1686S-92S.

75. Grant WB et al. Estimated benefit of increased vitamin D status in reducing the economic burden of disease in western Europe. *Prog Biophys Mol Biol.* Epub March 4, 2009.

76. Kimlin M et al. Does a high UV environment ensure adequate vitamin D status? *J Photochem Photobiol B.* 2007;89:139-47.

77. Nowson CA et al. Vitamin D intake and vitamin D status of Australians. *Med J Aust.* 2002;177:149-52.

78. Schoenmakers I et al. Abundant sunshine and vitamin D deficiency. *Br J Nutr.* 2008;99:1171-73.

79. Yetley EA et al. Dietary reference intakes for vitamin D: justification for a review of the 1997 values. *Am J Clin Nutr.* 2009;89:719-27.

80. Yetley EA. Assessing the vitamin D status of the U.S. population. *Am J Clin Nutr.* 2008;88:558S-64S.

81. Aloia JF et al. Vitamin D intake to attain a desired serum 25-hydroxyvitamin D concentration. *Am J Clin Nutr.* 2008;87:1952-58.

82. Holick MF et al. Vitamin D_2 is as effective as vitamin D_3 in maintaining circulating concentrations of 25-hydroxyvitamin D. *J Clin Endocrinol Metab.* 2008;93:677-81.

83. Davis CD. Vitamin D and cancer: current dilemmas and future research needs. *Am J Clin Nutr.* 2008;88:565S-69S.

84. Heaney RP et al. 25-Hydroxylation of vitamin D_3: relation to circulating vitamin D_3 under various input conditions. *Am J Clin Nutr.* 2008 Jun;87(6):1738-42.

85. Chaplin G et al. Vitamin D and the evolution of human depigmentation. *Am J Phys Anthropol.* 2009 Aug;139(4):451-61.

86. American Dietetic Association and Dietitians of Canada. Position of the American Dietetic Association and Dietitians of Canada: vegetarian diets. *J Am Diet Assoc.* 2003;103:748. www.webdietitians.org/Public/Files/veg.pdf.

87. Craig WJ, Mangels AR; American Dietetic Association. Position of the American Dietetic

Association: vegetarian diets. *J Am Diet Assoc.* 2009 Jul;109(7):1266-82.

88. Binkley N et al. Low vitamin D status despite abundant sun exposure. *J Clin Endocrinol Metab.* 2007;92:2130-35.

89. Jacobs ET et al. Vitamin D insufficiency in southern Arizona. *Am J Clin Nutr.* 2008 Mar;87(3):608-13.

90. Berger KJ et al. Mycotoxins revisited: Part I. *J Emerg Med.* 2005;28:53-62. Berger KJ et al. Mycotoxins revisited: Part II. *J Emerg Med.* 2005;28:175-83.

91. Erguven M et al. Mushroom poisoning. *Indian J Pediatr.* 2007;74:847-52.

92. Hanada K et al. Flagellate mushroom (shiitake) dermatitis and photosensitivity. *Dermatology.* 1998;197:255-57.

93. Koyyalamudi SR et al. Vitamin D_2 formation and bioavailability from Agaricus bisporus button mushrooms treated with ultraviolet irradiation. *J Agric Food Chem.* 2009;57:3351-55.

94. Nakamura K et al. Fish as a major source of vitamin D in the Japanese diet. *Nutrition.* 2002;18:415-16.

95. Outila TA et al. Bioavailability of vitamin D from wild edible mushrooms (Cantharellus tubaeformis) as measured with a human bioassay. *Am J Clin Nutr.* 1999;69:95-98.

96. Ozzard A et al. Vitamin D deficiency treated by consuming UVB-irradiated mushrooms. *Br J Gen Pract.* 2008;58:644-45.

97. Sasaki H et al. Sugihiratake mushroom (angel's wing mushroom)-induced cryptogenic encephalopathy may involve vitamin D analogues. *Biol Pharm Bull.* 2006;29:2514-18.

98. Smith AG et al. Plants need their vitamins too. *Curr Opin Plant Biol.* 2007;10:266-75.

99. Pieper JR et al. Effects of organic and conventional production systems on quality and nutritional parameters of processing tomatoes. *J Sci Food Agric.* 2009;89:177-94.

100. Worthington V. Nutritional quality of organic versus conventional fruits, vegetables, and grains. *J Altern Complement Med.* 2001;7:161-73.

101. Dangour AD et al. Nutritional quality of organic foods: a systematic review. *Am J Clin Nutr.* 2009 Sep;90(3):680-85.

102. Institute of Medicine. *Dietary Reference Intakes for Thiamin, Riboflavin, Niacin, Vitamin B_6, Folate, Vitamin B_{12}, Pantothenic Acid, Biotin, and Choline.* Washington DC: National Academies Press, 1998. www.nap.edu/catalog.php?record_id=6015#toc. Accessed July 2009.

103. Melina V. Personal communication based on laboratory analysis of Green Giant Juice, kale, and almonds conducted by Cantest Laboratories on April 11-12, 2005.

104. ESHA. *The Food Processor, Nutrition and Fitness Software.* 2005. www.esha.com/foodpro.htm.

105. Kylen AM et al. Nutrients in seeds and sprouts of alfalfa, lentils, mung beans, and soybeans. *J Food Science.* 1975;40:1008-09.

106. Donaldson MS et al. Fibromyalgia syndrome improved using a mostly raw vegetarian diet: an observational study. *BMC Complement Altern Med.* 2001;1:7.

107. Rauma A. Some algae are potentially adequate sources of vitamin B_{12} for vegans. *J Nutr.* 1995;125:2511-15.

108. Rauma AL et al. Vitamin B_{12} status of long-term adherents of a strict uncooked vegan diet ("living food diet") is compromised. *J Nutr.* 1995;125:2511-15.

109. Davis DR. *J Nutr.* 1997;127:378; author reply 380. Comment on Rauma AL. Some algae are potentially adequate sources of vitamin B_{12} for vegans. *J Nutr.* 1995;125:2511-15.

110. Dagnelie PC. *J Nutr.* 1997 Feb;127:379; author reply 380. Comment on Rauma AL. Some algae are potentially adequate sources of vitamin B_{12} for vegans. *J Nutr.* 1995 Oct;125:2511-15.

111. Ling WH et al. Shifting from a conventional diet to an uncooked vegan diet reversibly alters fecal hydrolytic activities in humans. *J Nutr.* 1992;122:924-30.

112. Katinaa K et al. Fermentation-induced changes in the nutritional value of native or germinated rye. *J Cereal Science.* 2007;46:348-55.

113. McKillop DJ et al. The effect of different cooking methods on folate retention in various foods that are amongst the major contributors to folate intake in the UK diet. *Br J Nutr.* 2002;88:681-88.

114. USDA. *Database for the Choline Content of Common Foods, Release 2.* www.nal.usda.gov/fnic/foodcomp/Data/Choline/Choln02.pdf. 2008. Accessed July 2009.

115. Stabler SP et al. Vitamin B_{12} deficiency as a worldwide problem. *Annu Rev Nutr.* 2004;24:299-326.

116. Aaron S et al. Clinical and laboratory features and response to treatment in patients presenting with vitamin B_{12} deficiency-related neurological syndromes. *Neurol India.* 2005;53:55-58.

117. Molloy AM et al. Maternal vitamin B_{12} status and risk of neural tube defects in a popula-

tion with high neural tube defect prevalence and no folic acid fortification. *Pediatrics.* 2009;123:917-23.

118. Walsh S. *Plant Based Nutrition and Health.* St Leonards-on-Sea U.K.: The Vegan Society, 2003.

119. Donaldson MS. Metabolic vitamin B_{12} status on a mostly raw vegan diet with follow-up using tablets, nutritional yeast, or probiotic supplements. *Ann Nutr Metab.* 2000;44:229-34.

120. Herrmann W et al. Functional vitamin B_{12} deficiency and determination of holotranscobalamin in populations at risk. *Clin Chem Lab Med.* 2003;41:1478-88.

121. Green R. Is it time for vitamin B_{12} fortification? What are the questions? *Am J Clin Nutr.* 2009 Feb;89(2):712S-16S.

122. Mørkbak AL et al. Effect of vitamin B_{12} treatment on haptocorrin. *Clin Chem.* 2007;53:367-68.

123. Norris J. *Vitamin B_{12}: Are You Getting It?* Vegan Outreach. 2009. www.veganhealth.org/b12. Accessed 2009.

124. Albert MJ et al. Vitamin B_{12} synthesis by human small intestinal bacteria. *Nature.* 1980;283:781-82.

125. Baroni L et al. Effect of a Klamath algae product ("AFA-B_{12}") on blood levels of vitamin B_{12} and homocysteine in vegan subjects: a pilot study. *Intl J Vitamin and Nutrition Research* (REF 08/596). In press at time of printing. 2009.

126. Walsh S. *Vegetarian Myths: Things "Everyone Knows" Which Are Not True.* Presentation at the 38th World Vegetarian Congress in Dresden. July 31, 2008. www.ivu.org/congress/2008/texts/Dresden2.pdf. Accessed July 2009.

127. Watanabe F et al. Characterization and bioavailability of vitamin B_{12}-compounds from edible algae. *J Nutr Sci Vitaminol* (Tokyo). 2002;48:325-31.

128. Dong A et al. Serum vitamin B_{12} and blood cell values in vegetarians. *Ann Nutr Metab.* 1982;26:209-16.

129. Andrès E et al. Clinical aspects of cobalamin deficiency in elderly patients. Epidemiology, causes, clinical manifestations, and treatment with special focus on oral cobalamin therapy. *Eur J Intern Med.* 2007;18:456-62.

130. Allen LH. How common is vitamin B_{12} deficiency? *Am J Clin Nutr.* 2009;89:693S-96S.

131. Chen JH et al. Determination of cobalamin in nutritive supplements and chlorella foods by capillary electrophoresis-inductively coupled plasma mass spectrometry. *J Agric Food Chem.* 2008;56:1210-15.

132. Hoffmann I. Long-term strict raw food diet is associated with favourable plasma beta-carotene and low plasma lycopene concentrations in Germans. *Br J Nutr.* 2008;99:1293-300.

133. Holick MF et al. Vitamin D and skin physiology: a D-lightful story. *J Bone Miner Res.* 2007;22 Suppl 2:V28-33.

134. Kittaka-Katsura H et al. Purification and characterization of a corrinoid compound from Chlorella tablets as an algal health food. *J Agric Food Chem.* 2002;50:4994-97.

135. Pratt R et al. Deficiency of vitamin B_{12} in Chlorella. *J Pharm Sci.* 1968;57:1040-41.

136. Saleh AM et al. The nutritional quality of drum-dried algae produced in open door mass culture. *Z Ernahrungswiss.* 1985;24:845-63.

137. Melina V, Melina D. Personal communication. 2009.

138. Reddy MB et al. The impact of food processing on the nutritional quality of vitamins and minerals. *Adv Exp Med Biol.* 1999;459:99-106.

139. Hajslová J et al. Quality of organically and conventionally grown potatoes: four-year study of micronutrients, metals, secondary metabolites, enzymic browning and organoleptic properties. *Food Addit Contam.* 2005;22:514-34.

140. Lester GE. Organic versus conventionally grown produce: quality differences and guidelines for comparison studies. *Hort Science.* 2006;41:296-300.

141. Pérez-López AJ et al. Effects of agricultural practices on color, carotenoids composition, and minerals contents of sweet peppers, cv. Almuden. *J Agric Food Chem.* 2007;55:8158-64.

142. Woese K et al. A comparison of organically and conventionally grown foods. Results of a review of the relevant literature. *J Sci Food Agric.* 1997;74:281-293.

143. Smith S et al. Efficacy of a commercial produce wash on bacterial contamination of lettuce in a food service setting. *J Food Prot.* 2003;66:2359-61.

144. Miyamoto E et al. Characterization of vitamin B_{12} compounds from Korean purple laver (Porphyra sp.) products. *J Agric Food Chem.* 2009 Apr 8;57(7):2793-96.

CHAPTER 9

Acid-Base Balance, Bones, and Minerals

1. Clancy J et al. Short-term regulation of acid-base homeostasis of body fluids. *Br J Nurs.* 2007;16:1016-21.

2. Clancy J et al. Intermediate and long-term regulation of acid-base homeostasis. *Br J Nurs.* 2007;16:1076-79.

3. Remer T et al. Potential renal acid load of foods and its influence on urine pH. *J Am Diet Assoc.* 1995;95:791-97.

4. Remer T. Influence of diet on acid-base balance. *Semin Dial.* 2000;13:221-26.

5. Milton K. Micronutrient intakes of wild primates: are humans different? *Comp Biochem Physiol A Mol Integr Physiol.* 2003;136:47-59.

6. Milton K. Nutritional characteristics of wild primate foods: do the diets of our closest living relatives have lessons for us? *Nutrition.* 1999;15:488-98.

7. Kuhnlein HV et al. Composition of traditional Hopi foods. *J Am Diet Assoc.* 1979;75:37-41.

8. Smith BD et al. Initial formation of an indigenous crop complex in eastern North America at 3800 B.P. *Proc Natl Acad Sci USA.* 2009;106:6561-66.

9. Frassetto L et al. Diet, evolution and aging—the pathophysiologic effects of the post-agricultural inversion of the potassium-to-sodium and base-to-chloride ratios in the human diet. *Eur J Nutr.* 2001;40:200-13.

10. Milton K. The critical role played by animal source foods in human (Homo) evolution. *J Nutr.* 2003;133(11 Suppl 2):3886S-92S.

11. Milton K. Back to basics: why foods of wild primates have relevance for modern human health. *Nutrition.* 2000;16:480-83.

12. Milton K. Hunter-gatherer diets—a different perspective. *Am J Clin Nutr.* 2000;71:665-67.

13. Minich DM et al. Acid-alkaline balance: role in chronic disease and detoxification. *Altern Ther Health Med.* 2007;13:62-65.

14. Sebastian A et al. Estimation of the net acid load of the diet of ancestral preagricultural Homo sapiens and their hominid ancestors. *Am J Clin Nutr.* 2002;76:1308-16.

15. Frassetto LA et al. Standardizing terminology for estimating the diet-dependent net acid load to the metabolic system. *J Nutr.* 2007;137:1491-92.

16. Welch A et al. Calcaneum broadband ultrasound attenuation relates to vegetarian and omnivorous diets differently in men and women: an observation from the European Prospective Investigation into Cancer in Norfolk (EPIC-Norfolk) population study. *Osteoporos Int.* 2005;16:590-96.

17. Macdonald HM et al. Low dietary potassium intakes and high dietary estimates of net endogenous acid production are associated with low bone mineral density in premenopausal women and increased markers of bone resorption in postmenopausal women. *Am J Clin Nutr.* 2005;81:923-33.

18. Wiederkehr M et al. Metabolic and endocrine effects of metabolic acidosis in humans. *Swiss Med Wkly.* 2001;10:127-32.

19. Alexy U et al. Potential renal acid load in the diet of children and adolescents: impact of food groups, age and time trends. *Public Health Nutr.* 2008;11:300-06.

20. Andrews RD. *Athletes and Alkalinity. Vegetarian Nutrition Update.* 2008. XVII(2):1, 8-9. Vegetarian Dietary Practice Group of the American Dietetic Association. www.vegetariannutrition.net.

21. Frassetto L et al. Potassium bicarbonate reduces urinary nitrogen excretion in postmenopausal women. *J Clin Endocrinol Metab.* 1997;82:254-59.

22. Welbourne TC et al. Enteral glutamine spares endogenous glutamine in chronic acidosis. *J Parenter Enteral Nutr.* 1994;18:243-47.

23. Berkemeyer S et al. Renal net acid excretion capacity is comparable in prepubescence, adolescence, and young adulthood but falls with aging. *J Am Geriatr Soc.* 2008;56:1442-48.

24. New SA. Nutrition Society Medal lecture. The role of the skeleton in acid-base homeostasis. *Proc Nutr Soc.* 2002;61:151-64.

25. Buclin T et al. Diet acids and alkalis influence calcium retention in bone. *Osteoporos Int.* 2001;12:493-99.

26. Dawson-Hughes B et al. Treatment with potassium bicarbonate lowers calcium excretion and bone resorption in older men and women. *J Clin Endocrinol Metab.* 2009;94:96-102.

27. Maurer M et al. Neutralization of Western diet inhibits bone resorption independently of K intake and reduces cortisol secretion in humans. *Am J Physiol Renal Physiol.* 2003;284:F32-40.

28. Frassetto LA et al. Worldwide incidence of hip fracture in elderly women: relation to consumption of animal and vegetable foods. *J Gerontol A Biol Sci Med Sci.* 2000;55:M585-92.

29. World Health Organization/Food and Agriculture Organization. *Diet, Nutrition and the Prevention of Chronic Disease.* Geneva: WHO, 2003. http://whqlibdoc.who.int/trs/WHO_trs_916.pdf.

30. Schönau E. The peak bone mass concept: is it still relevant? *Pediatr Nephrol.* 2004;19:825-31.

31. Frassetto LA et al. Adverse effects of sodium chloride on bone in the aging human population resulting from habitual consumption of typical American diets. *J Nutr*. 2008;138:419S-22S.

32. Heaney RP. Role of dietary sodium in osteoporosis. *J Am Coll Nutr*. 2006;25(3 Suppl):271S-76S.

33. Heaney RP et al. Amount and type of protein influences bone health. *Am J Clin Nutr*. 2008;87:1567S-70S.

34. Sebastian A. Dietary protein content and the diet's net acid load: opposing effects on bone health. *Am J Clin Nutr*. 2005;82:921-22.

35. Prentice A et al. Nutrition and bone growth and development. *Proc Nutr Soc*. 2006;65:348-60.

36. Groff JL et al. *Advanced Nutrition and Human Metabolism*. Minneapolis MN: West Publishing Co., 1995.

37. Weaver CM et al. Biomarkers of bone health appropriate for evaluating functional foods designed to reduce risk of osteoporosis. *Br J Nutr*. 2002;88 Suppl 2:S225-32.

38. Sandberg AS. Bioavailability of minerals in legumes. *Br J Nutr*. 2002;88 Suppl 3:S281-85.

39. Gilani GS et al. Effects of antinutritional factors on protein digestibility and amino acid availability in foods. *J AOAC Int*. 2005;88:967-87.

40. Garcia AL et al. Long-term strict raw food diet is associated with favourable plasma beta-carotene and low plasma lycopene concentrations in Germans. *Br J Nutr*. 2008;99:1293-300.

41. Kies CV. Mineral utilization of vegetarians: impact of variation in fat intake. *Am J Clin Nutr*. 1988;48(3 Suppl):884-87.

42. Benway DA et al. Assessing chemical form of calcium in wheat, spinach, and kale. *J Food Science*. 1993;58:605-08.

43. Heaney RP et al. Calcium absorption from kale. *Am J Clin Nutr*. 1990;51:656-57.

44. Heaney RP et al. Calcium absorbability from spinach. *Am J Clin Nutr*. 1988;47:707-09.

45. Weaver CM et al. Choices for achieving adequate dietary calcium with a vegetarian diet. *Am J Clin Nutr*. 1999;70(3 Suppl):543S-48S.

46. Fine KD et al. Intestinal absorption of magnesium from food and supplements. *J Clin Invest*. 1991;88:396-402.

47. Hotz C et al. Traditional food-processing and preparation practices to enhance the bioavailability of micronutrients in plant-based diets. *J Nutr*. 2007;137:1097-100.

48. Weaver, C. *Dietary Calcium*. Unpublished article. Personal communication.

49. Kimura M et al. Cooking losses of minerals in foods and its nutritional significance. *J Nutr Sci Vitaminol* (Tokyo). 1990;36 Suppl 1:S25-32, discussion S33.

50. Brandt K et al. Organic agriculture: does it enhance or reduce the nutritional value of plant foods? *J Sci Food Agric*. 2001;81:924-931.

51. Dangour AD et al. Nutritional quality of organic foods: a systematic review. *Am J Clin Nutr*. 2009 Sep;90(3):680-85.

52. Györéné KG et al. A comparison of chemical composition and nutritional value of organically and conventionally grown plant derived foods. *Orv Hetil*. 2006;147:2081-90.

53. Lundegardh B et al. Organically produced plant foods: evidence of health benefits. *Acta Agric Scand Sec B Soil Plant Sci*. 2003;53:3-15.

54. Magkos F et al. Organic food: Nutritious food or food for thought? A review of the evidence. *Int J Food Sci Nutr*. 2003;54:357-71.

55. Pérez-López AJ et al. Effects of agricultural practices on color, carotenoids composition, and minerals contents of sweet peppers, cv. Almuden. *J Agric Food Chem*. 2007;55:8158-64.

56. Woese K et al. A comparison of organically and conventionally grown foods: Results of a review of the relevant literature. *J Sci Food Agric*. 1997;74:281-93.

57. Worthington V. Nutritional quality of organic versus conventional fruits, vegetables, and grains. *J Altern Complement Med*. 2001;7:161-73.

58. United States Department of Agriculture. *Oxalic Acid Content of Selected Vegetables*. www.ars.usda.gov/Services/docs.htm?docid=9444.

59. Chai W et al. Effect of different cooking methods on vegetable oxalate content. *J Agric Food Chem*. 2005;53:3027-30.

60. Genannt Bonsmann SS et al. Oxalic acid does not influence nonhaem iron absorption in humans: a comparison of kale and spinach meals. *Eur J Clin Nutr*. 2008;62:336-41.

61. Gibson RS et al. Improving the bioavailability of nutrients in plant foods at the household level. *Proc Nutr Soc*. 2006;65:160-68.

62. Massey LK. Food oxalate: factors affecting measurement, biological variation, and bioavailability. *J Am Diet Assoc*. 2007;107:1191-94.

63. Viadel B et al. Effect of cooking and legume species upon calcium, iron and zinc uptake by Caco-2 cells. *J Trace Elem Med Biol*. 2006;20:115-20.

64. Chitra U et al. Phytic acid, in vitro protein digestibility, dietary fiber, and minerals of pulses

as influenced by processing methods. *Plant Foods Hum Nutr*. 1996;49:307-16.

65. Fredlund K et al. Absorption of zinc and calcium: dose dependent inhibition by phytate. *J Applied Microbiology*. 2002;93:197-204.

66. Sandberg AS. The effect of food processing on phytate hydrolysis and availability of iron and zinc. *Adv Exp Med Biol*. 1991;289:499-508.

67. Urbano G et al. The role of phytic acid in legumes: antinutrient or beneficial function? *J Physiol Biochem*. 2000 Sep;56(3):283-94.

68. Institute of Medicine. *Dietary Reference Intakes for Calcium, Phosphorus, Magnesium, Vitamin D, and Fluoride*. Washington DC: National Academies Press, 1997. http://books.nap.edu/openbook.php?record_id=5776&chapselect=yo&page=R1.

69. Institute of Medicine. *Dietary Reference Intakes for Vitamin A, Vitamin K, Arsenic, Boron, Chromium, Copper, Iodine, Iron, Manganese, Molybdenum, Nickel, Silicon, Vanadium, and Zinc*. Washington DC: National Academies Press, 2000. http://books.nap.edu/books/0309072794/html/1.html.

70. Institute of Medicine. *Dietary Reference Intakes for Water, Potassium, Sodium, Chloride, and Sulfate*. Washington DC: National Academies Press, 2004. www.nap.edu/books/0309091691/html.

71. Hoffmann I et al. Raw food diet: health benefits and risks. In: Watson RR ed. *Vegetables, Fruits, and Herbs in Health Promotion*. Boca Raton FL: CRC Press, 2000:293-308.

72. Donaldson, MS. Food and nutrient intake of Hallelujah vegetarians. *Nutrition & Food Science*. 2001;31:293-303. www.hacres.com/diet/research/nutrient_intake.pdf.

73. Rauma AL et al. Coumarin 7-hydroxylation in long-term adherents of a strict uncooked vegan diet. *Eur J Clin Pharmacol*. 1996;50:133-37.

74. Rauma AL et al. Antioxidant status in long-term adherents to a strict uncooked vegan diet. *Am J Clin Nutr*. 1995;62:1221-27.

75. Rauma AI et al. Iodine status in vegans consuming a living food diet. *Nutr Res*. 1994;14:1789-95.

76. Rauma AL et al. Effect of a strict vegan diet on energy and nutrient intakes by Finnish rheumatoid patients. *Eur J Clin Nutr*. 1993;47:747-49.

77. Ling WH et al. Shifting from a conventional diet to an uncooked vegan diet reversibly alters fecal hydrolytic activities in humans. *J Nutr*. 1992;122:924-30.

78. Peltonen R et al. An uncooked vegan diet shifts the profile of human fecal microflora: computerized analysis of direct stool sample gas-liquid chromatography profiles of bacterial cellular fatty acids. *Appl Environ Microbiol*. 1992;58:3660-66.

79. Fontana L et al. Low bone mass in subjects on a long-term raw vegetarian diet. *Arch Intern Med*. 2005;165:684-89.

80. Fontana L et al. Long-term low-calorie low-protein vegan diet and endurance exercise are associated with low cardiometabolic risk. *Rejuvenation Res*. 2007;10:225-34.

81. Eaton SB et al. Paleolithic nutrition. A consideration of its nature and current implications. *N Engl J Med*. 1985;312:283-89.

82. Linus Pauling Institute. *Micronutrient Information Center*. http://lpi.oregonstate.edu/infocenter. Accessed July 2009.

83. Martin BR et al. Calcium absorption from three salts and CaSO4-fortified bread in premenopausal women. *J Agric Food Chem*. 2002;50:3874-76.

84. Lukaski HC. Chromium as a supplement. *Annu Rev Nutr*. 1999;19:279-302.

85. Messina V et al. *The Dietitian's Guide to Vegetarian Diets. 2nd ed*. Boston: Jones and Bartlett Publishing, 2004.

86. Fields C et al. Iodine-deficient vegetarians: a hypothetical perchlorate-susceptible population? *Regul Toxicol Pharmacol*. 2005;42:37-46.

87. Miller D. Extrathyroidal benefits of iodine. *J Amer Physicians Surgeons*. 2006;119:106-10.

88. New SA. Intake of fruit and vegetables: implications for bone health. *Proc Nutr Soc*. 2003;62:889-99. Erratum in *Proc Nutr Soc*. 2004;63:187.

89. New SA. Do vegetarians have a normal bone mass? *Osteoporos Int*. 2004;15:679-88.

90. Geelhoed GW. Health care advocacy in world health. *Nutrition*. 1999;15:940-43.

91. Geelhoed GW. Metabolic maladaptation: individual and social consequences of medical intervention in correcting endemic hypothyroidism. *Nutrition*. 1999;15:908-32, discussion 939.

92. Cunnane SC. Hunter-gatherer diets—a shore-based perspective. *Am J Clin Nutr*. 2000;72:1584-88. Comment on *Am J Clin Nutr*. 2000;71:665-67 and *Am J Clin Nutr*. 2000;71:682-92.

93. Crohn DM. Perchlortae controversy calls for improving iodine nutrition. *Vegetarian Nutrition Update*. 2005;XIV(2)1:6-8. Vegetar-

ian Nutrition Dietary Practice Group of the American Dietetic Association. http://vegetariannutrition.net.

94. Teas J et al. Variability of iodine content in common commercially available edible seaweeds. *Thyroid*. 2004;14:836-41.

95. Walsh S. *Plant Based Nutrition and Health*. St Leonards-on-Sea U.K.: The Vegan Society, 2003.

96. Rose M et al. Arsenic in seaweed—forms, concentration and dietary exposure. *Food Chem Toxicol*. 2007 Jul;45(7):1263-67.

97. Amster E et al. Case report: potential arsenic toxicosis secondary to herbal kelp supplement. *Environ Health Perspect*. 2007;115:606-08. *Environ Health Perspect*. 2007;115:A574; author reply A576-77. *Environ Health Perspect*. 2007;115:A575-76; author reply A576-77. *Environ Health Perspect*. 2007;115:A575; author reply A576-77.

98. Davis TA et al. A review of the biochemistry of heavy metal biosorption by brown algae. *Water Res*. 2003;37:4311-30.

99. Phaneuf D et al. Evaluation of the contamination of marine algae (seaweed) from the St. Lawrence River and likely to be consumed by humans. *Environ Res*. 1999;80(2 Pt 2):S175-82.

100. Eden Foods. www.edenfoods.com or contact the company.

101. ESHA. *The Food Processor, Nutrition and Fitness Software*. 2005. www.esha.com/foodpro.htm.

102. Koebnick C et al. Long-term consumption of a raw food diet is associated with favorable serum LDL cholesterol and triglycerides but also with elevated plasma homocysteine and low serum HDL cholesterol in humans. *J Nutr*. 2005;135:2372-78.

103. Donaldson, MS. *Hallelujah vegetarians and nutritional science: answering your questions*. Personal communication. 2005.

104. Cook JD et al. Assessment of the role of non-heme-iron availability in iron balance. *Am J Clin Nutr*. 1991;54:717-22.

105. Craig WJ, Mangels AR; American Dietetic Association. Position of the American Dietetic Association: vegetarian diets. *J Am Diet Assoc*. 2009 Jul;109(7):1266-82.

106. Simpson RJ et al. Regulation of intestinal iron absorption: the mucosa takes control? *Cell Metab*. 2009 Aug;10(2):84-87.

107. Bergman C et al. What is next for the Dietary Reference Intakes for bone metabolism related nutrients beyond calcium: phosphorus, magnesium, vitamin D, and fluoride? *Crit Rev Food Sci Nutr*. 2009;49:136-44.

108. Fox TE et al. Bioavailability of selenium from fish, yeast and selenate: a comparative study in humans using stable isotopes. *Eur J Clin Nutr*. 2004;58:343-49.

109. Institute of Medicine. *Dietary Reference Intakes for Vitamin C, Vitamin E, Selenium, and Carotenoids (2000) Panel on Dietary Antioxidants and Related Compounds*. Washington DC: National Academies Press, 2000. www.nap.edu/catalog.php?record_id=9810#toc. Accessed September 2009.

110. Schomburg L et al. On the importance of selenium and iodine metabolism for thyroid hormone biosynthesis and human health. *Mol Nutr Food Res*. 2008;52:1235-46.

111. Eaton SB et al. Calcium in evolutionary perspective. *Am J Clin Nutr*. 1991;54(1 Suppl):281S-87S.

112. Health and Welfare Canada. *Nutrition Recommendations. The Report of the Scientific Review Committee. Minister of Supply and Services*. Ottawa, ON. 1990.

113. Donaldson MS. Metabolic vitamin B_{12} status on a mostly raw vegan diet with follow up using tablets, nutritional yeast, or probiotic supplements. *Ann Nutr Metab*. 2000;44:229-34.

114. USDA, Agricultural Research Service. 2005. *USDA National Nutrient Database for Standard Reference, Release 21*. www.ars.usda.gov/Services/docs.htm?docid=8964. Accessed July 2009.

115. Thomas K. Arsenic in seaweed—forms, concentration and dietary exposure. *Food Chem Toxicol*. 2007;45:1263-67.

CHAPTER 10
The Great Enzyme Controversy

1. Heinzelman P, Snow CD, Wu I, Nguyen C, Villalobos A, Govindarajan S, Minshull J, Arnold FH. A family of thermostable fungal cellulases created by structure-guided recombination. *PNAS*. 2009;106:5610-15.

2. Jiang L, Althoff EA, Clemente FR, Doyle L, Röthlisberger D, Zanghellini A, Gallaher JL, Betker JL, Tanaka F, Barbas CF, Hilvert D, Houk KN, Stoddard BL, Baker D. De novo computational design of retro-aldol enzymes. *Science*. 2008;319:1387-91.

3. Baum, SJ. *Introduction to Organic and Biological Chemistry. 2nd ed*. New York: Macmillan Publishing Co., 1978.

4. Liebow, C, Rothman, SS. Enteropancreatic circulation of digestive enzymes. *Science.* 1975;189:472-74.

5. Gotze H, Rothman SS. Enteropancreatic circulation of digestive enzymes as a conservative mechanism. *Nature.* 1975;257:607-09.

6. Rothman S, Liebow C, Isenman L. Conservation of digestive enzymes. *Physiol Rev.* 2002;82:1-18.

7. Fontana L. Calorie restriction and cardiometabolic health. *Eur J Cardiovasc Prev Rehabil.* 2008;15:3-9.

8. Bordone L, Guarente L. Calorie restriction, SIRT1 and metabolism: understanding longevity. *Nat Rev Mol Cell Biol.* 2005;6:298-305.

9. Pottenger, FM. The effect of heat-processed foods and metabolized vitamin D milk on the dentofacial structures of experimental animals. *Am J Orthod Oral Surg.* 1946;32:467-85.

10. Pottenger, FM. *Pottenger's Cats.* La Mesa, CA: Price-Pottenger Nutrition Foundation, 1995.

11. Hayes KC, Carey RE, Schmidt SY. Retinal degeneration associated with taurine deficiency in the cat. *Science.* 1975;188:949-51.

12. Schmidt SY, Berson EL, Hayes KC. Retinal degeneration in cats fed casein. I. Taurine deficiency. *Invest Ophthalmol.* 1976;15:47-52.

13. Rabin B, Nicolosi RJ, Hayes KC. Dietary influence on bile acid conjugation in the cat. *J Nutr.* 1976;106:1241-56.

14. Knopf K, Sturman JA, Armstrong M, Hayes KC. Taurine: an essential nutrient for the cat. *J Nutr.* 1978;108:773-78.

15. Sturman JA, Gargano AD, Messing JM, Imaki H. Feline maternal taurine deficiency: effect on mother and offspring. *J Nutr.* 1986;116:655-67.

16. Sturman JA, Moretz RC, French JH, Wisniewski HM. Taurine deficiency in the developing cat: persistence of the cerebellar external granule cell layer. *Prog Clin Biol Res.* 1985;179:43-52.

17. Palackal T, Moretz R, Wisniewski H, Sturman J. Abnormal visual cortex development in the kitten associated with maternal dietary taurine deprivation. *J Neurosci Res.* 1986;15:223-39.

18. Hickman MA, Rogers QR, Morris JG. Effect of processing on fate of dietary [14C] taurine in cats. *J Nutr.* 1990;120:995-1000.

19. Kim SW, Rogers QR, Morris JG. Maillard reaction products in purified diets induce taurine depletion in cats which is reversed by antibiotics. *J Nutr.* 1996;126:195-201.

20. Spitze AR, Wong DL, Rogers QR, Fascetti AJ. Taurine concentrations in animal feed ingredients; cooking influences taurine content. *J Anim Physiol Anim Nutr.* 2003;87:251-62.

21. Garrey WE, Butler V. The digestive leucocytosis question. *Am J Physiol.* 1932;100:351-56.

22. Bykov KM. The effect of food stimuli on leukocytosis in man communication I. the significance of various foods in the characteristics of conditioned and complex reflex food-induced leukocytosis. *Bull Exp Biol Med.* 1958;46:774-78.

23. Author not stated. Previous investigations of 12 hourly and 24 hourly variations of the leukocytes. *Acta Psychiatr Scand.* 1946;21:42-73.

24. Kouchakoff P. The influence of food on the blood formula of man. First International Congress of Microbiology, Paris, 1930. Serologie et Immunite. Masson and Cie, eds. Section IV. Paris:1932:490-93.

25. Kouchakoff P. Nouvelles lois de l'alimentation humaine basées sur la leucocytose digestive. *Mémoires de la Société Vaudoise des Sciences Naturelles.* 1937;39:319-48.

26. Toole S, Toole Sue. *Essential A2 Biology for OCR. III ed.* London: Nelson Thornes, 2004.

27. Hui YH. *Handbook of Food Science, Technology, and Engineering. Volume III.* Boca Raton FL: Taylor & Francis/CRC Press, 2006.

28. Howell E. Enzyme Nutrition. WaWe NJ: Avery Publishing, 1985.

29. Kong F, Singh RP. Disintegration of solid foods in the human stomach. *J Food Sci.* 2008;73:R67-80.

30. Collins PJ, Horowitz M, Chatterton BE. Proximal, distal and total stomach emptying of a digestible solid meal in normal subjects. *Br J Radiol.* 1988;61:12-18.

31. Collins PJ, Houghton LA, Read NW, Horowitz M, Chatterton BE, Heddle R, Dent J. Role of the proximal and distal stomach in mixed solid and liquid meal emptying. *Gut.* 1991;32:615-19.

32. Horowitz Ml, Maddox A, Wishart J, Vernon-Roberts J, Chatterton B, Shearman D. Effect of dexfenfluramine on gastric emptying of a mixed solid-liquid meal in obese subjects. *Br J Nutr.* 1990;63:447-55.

33. Hodge C, Lebenthal E, Lee PC, Topper W. Amylase in the saliva and in the gastric aspirates of premature infants: its potential role in glucose polymer hydrolysis. *Pediatr Res.* 1983;17:998-1001.

34. Fried M, Abramson S, Meyer JH. Passage of salivary amylase through the stomach in humans. *Dig Dis Sci.* 1987;32:1097-103.

35. Sundd M, Kundu S, Pal GP, Medicherla JV. Purification and characterization of a highly stable cysteine protease from the latex of

Ervatamia coronaria. *Biosci Biotechnol Biochem.* 1998;62:1947-55.

36. Araki J, Hirasawa Y, Kitada M, Shiratori K, Moriyoshi Y, Watanabe S, Takeuchi T. Influence of gastric juice on human amylase activity. *Rinsho Byori* (Japanese). 1990;38:1155-60.

37. Donaldson MS. Personal correspondence. June 2005.

38. Chatterton TR, Vogelsong MK, Lu Y, Ellman BA, Hudgens AG. Salivary alpha-amylase as a measure of endogenous adrenergic activity. *Clin Physiol.* 1996;16:433-48.

39. Kalnins D, Corey M, Ellis L, Durie PR, Pencharz PB. Combining unprotected pancreatic enzymes with pH-sensitive enteric-coated microspheres does not improve nutrient digestion in patients with cystic fibrosis. *J Pediatr.* 2005;146:489-93.

40. Gardner MLG. Gastrointestinal absorption of intact proteins. *Annu Rev Nutr.* 1988;8:329-50.

41. Prochaska LJ, Piekutowski WV. On the synergistic effects of enzymes in food with enzymes in the human body. A literature survey and analytical report. *Med Hypotheses.* 1994;42:355-362.

42. Prochaska LJ, Nguyen XT, Donat N, Piekutowski WV. Effects of food processing on the thermodynamic and nutritive value of foods: literature and database survey. *Med Hypotheses.* 2000;54:254-62.

43. Savaiano DA, Levitt MD. Milk intolerance and microbe-containing dairy foods. *J Dairy Sci.* 1987;70:397-406.

44. Martini MC, Bollweg GL, Levitt MD, Savaiano DA. Lactose digestion by yogurt beta-galactosidase: influence of pH and microbial cell integrity. *Am J Clin Nutr.* 1987;45:432-36.

45. Kotz CM, Furne JK, Savaiano DA, Levitt MD. Factors affecting the ability of a high beta-galactosidase yogurt to enhance lactose absorption. *J Dairy Sci.* 1994;77:3538-44.

46. Martini MC, Kukielka DA, Savaiano. Lactose digestion from yogurt: influence of a meal and additional lactose. *Am J Clin Nutr.* 1991;53:1253-1258.

47. National Enzyme Company, TNO Nutrition and Food Research. *The First Quantitative Evidence Proving the Efficacy of Supplemental Enzymes.* 2004. www.nationalenzyme.com. Accessed July 2009.

48. Sandberg AS, Andersson H, Kivistö B, Sandström B. Extrusion cooking of a high-fibre cereal product. 1. Effects on digestibility and absorption of protein, fat, starch, dietary fibre and phytate in the small intestine. *Br J Nutr.* 1986;55:245-54.

49. Sandberg AS, Andersson H, Carlsson NG, Sandström B. Degradation products of bran phytate formed during digestion in the human small intestine: effect of extrusion cooking on digestibility. *J Nutr.* 1987;117:2061-65.

50. Sandberg AS, Hulthén LR, Türk M. Dietary Aspergillus niger phytase increases iron absorption in humans. *J Nutr.* 1996 Feb;126(2):476-80.

51. Sandberg AS. Bioavailability of minerals in legumes. *Br J Nutr.* 2002 Dec;88 Suppl 3:S281-85.

52. Krogdahl A, Holm H. Soybean proteinase inhibitors and human proteolytic enzymes: selective inactivation of inhibitors by treatment with human gastric juice. *J Nutr.* 1981;111:2045-2051.

CHAPTER 11
Food Safety: Raw Case Files

1. Arbour G. Are buckwheat greens toxic? *Townsend Letter for Doctors and Patients.* June 2004. www.gillesarbour.com/buckwheat_assets/Buckwheat%20Greens.pdf. Accessed July 2009.

2. Hagels H, Wagenbreth D, Schilcher H. Phenolic compounds of buckwheat herb and influence of plant and agricultural factors (Fagopyrum esculentum Moench and Fagopyrum tataricum Gartner). *Curr Adv Buckwheat Res.* 1995:801-09.

3. Lee EH, Him CJ. Nutritional changes of buckwheat during germination. *Korean Medical Database.* 2008;23:121-29. http://kmbase.cedric.or.kr/Main.aspx?d=KMBASE&m=VIEW&i=0665420080230010121. Accessed July 2009.

4. Cousens, G. *Conscious Eating.* Patagonia AZ: Essene Vision Books, 1992.

5. Akaogi J, Barker T, Kuroda Y, Nacionales DC, Yamasaki Y, Stevens BR, Reeves WH, Satoh M. Role of non-protein amino acid L-canavanine in autoimmunity. *Autoimmun Rev.* 2006;5:429-35.

6. Malinow MR, Bardana EJ Jr, Goodnight SH Jr. Pancytopenia during ingestion of alfalfa seeds. *Lancet.* 1981;1:615.

7. Roberts JL, Hayashi JA. Exacerbation of SLE associated with alfalfa ingestion. *N Engl J Med.* 1983;308(22):1361.

8. Alcocer-Varela J, Alarcon-Segovia D. Reply. *Arthritis Rheum.* 1985;28:1200.

9. Petri M, Thompson E, Abusuwwa R, Huang J, Garret E. BALES: the Baltimore Lupus Environmental Study. *Arthritis Rheum.* 2001;44:S331.

10. Bengtsson AA, Rylander L, Hagmar L, Nived O, Sturfelt G. Risk factors for developing systemic lupus erythematosus: a case control study in southern Sweden. *Rheumatol* (Oxford). 2002:41:563-71.

11. Kasai T, Sakamura S. Reexamination of canavanine disappearance during germination of alfalfa (Medicago Sativa). *J Nutr Sci Vitaminol* (Tokyo). 1986;32:77-82.

12. Thompson LU, Rea RL, Jenkins DJA. Effect of heat processing on hemagglutinin activity in red kidney beans. *J Food Sci*. 1983;48:235-36.

13. el-Adawy TA. Nutritional composition and antinutritional factors of chickpeas (Cicer arietinum L.) undergoing different cooking methods and germination. *Plant Foods Hum Nutr*. 2002;57;83-97.

14. Mubarak AE. Nutritional composition and antinutritional factors of mung bean seeds (Phaseolus aureus) as affected by some home traditional processes. *Food Chem*. 2005;89:489-95.

15. Chen LH, Thacker RR. Pan SH. Effect of germination on hemagglutinating activity of pea and bean seeds. *J Food Sci*. 1977:42;1666.

16. Sudhir S, Deshpande SS, Singh RK. Hemagglutinating activity of lectins in selected varieties of raw and processed dry beans. *J Food Proc Pres*. 1991;15;81-87.

17. Ologhobo AD, Fetuga BL. Pathological observations on rats dosed with limabean and cowpea hemagglutinins. *Toxicol Lett*. 1983;18:301-06.

18. Belitz HD, Grosch W, Schieberle P. *Food Chemistry. 4th ed*. Illustrated. Translated by Burghagen MM. Springer, 2009.

19. Frias J, Diaz-Pollan C, Hedley CL, Vidal-Valverde C. Evolution of trypsin inhibitor activity during germination of lentils. *J Agric Food Chem*. 1995;43;2231-34.

20. Deshpande SS. *Handbook of Food Toxicology*. Illustrated ed. New York: Marcel Dekker, 2002.

21. Liener IE. Possible adverse effects of soybean anticarcinogens. *J Nutr*. 1995;125(3 Suppl):744S-50S.

22. Champ MM. Non-nutrient bioactive substances of pulses. *Br J Nutr*. 2002;88 Suppl 3:S307-19.

23. Lajolo FM, Genovese MI. Nutritional significance of lectins and enzyme inhibitors from legumes. *J Agric Food Chem*. 2002;50:6592-98.

24. Gilani GS, Cockell KA, Sepehr E. Effects of antinutritional factors on protein digestibility and amino acid availability in foods. *J AOAC Int*. 2005;88(3):967-87.

25. Savelkoul FH, van der Poel AF, Tamminga S. The presence and inactivation of trypsin inhibitors, tannins, lectins and amylase inhibitors in legume seeds during germination. A review. *Plant Foods Hum Nutr*. 1992;42:71-85.

26. Khattab RY, Arntfield SD. Nutritional quality of legume seeds as affected by some physical treatments 2. Antinutritional factors. *Food Sci Tech*. 2009;42:1113-18.

27. Vidal-Valverde C, Frias J, Prodanov M, Tabera J, Ruiz R, Bacon J. Effect of natural fermentation on carbohydrates, riboflavin and trypsin inhibitor activity of lentils. *Z Lebensm Unters Forsch*. 1993;197:449-52.

28. Ibrahim SS, Habiba RA, Shatta AA, Embaby HE. Effect of soaking, germination, cooking and fermentation on antinutritional factors in cowpeas. *Nahrung*. 2002;46(2):92-5.

29. Losso JN. The biochemical and functional food properties of the bowman-birk inhibitor. *Crit Rev Food Sci Nutr*. 2008;48:94-118. Erratum in *Crit Rev Food Sci Nutr*. 2008;48:798.

30. Khalil MM. Effect of soaking, germination, autoclaving and cooking on chemical and biological value of guar compared with faba bean. *Nahrung*. 2001;45:246-50.

31. Liu KS. *Soybeans: Chemistry, Technology and Utilization*. New York: Chapman & Hall, 1997.

32. Sharma A, Sehgal S. Effect of domestic processing, cooking and germination on the trypsin inhibitor activity and tannin content of faba bean (Vicia faba). *Plant Foods Hum Nutr*. 1992;42:127-33.

33. Alonso R, Aguirre A, Marzo F. Effects of extrusion and traditional processing methods on antinutrients and in vitro digestibility of protein and starch in faba and kidney beans. *Food Chem*. 2000;68:159-65.

34. Sathe SK, Deshpande SS, Reddy NR, Goll DE, Salunkhe DK. Effects of germination on proteins, raffinose oligosaccharides, and antinutritional factors in the Great Northern Beans. *J Food Sci*. 1983;48:1796-800.

35. Neves VA, Lourenço EJ. Changes in protein fractions, trypsin inhibitor and proteolytic activity in the cotyledons of germinating chickpea. *Arch Latinoam Nutr*. 2001;51:269-75.

36. Osman, MA. Effect of different processing methods on nutrient composition, antinutritional factors and in vitro protein digestibility of Dolichos lablab bean [Lablab purpuresus (L) Sweet]. *Pak. J Nutr*. 2007;6:299-303.

37. Sangronis E, Machado CJ. Influence of germination on the nutritional quality of Phaseolus

vulgaris and Cajanus cajan. *Food Sci Tech*. 2007;40:116-20.

38. Torres A, Frias J, Granito M and Vidal-Valverde C. Germinated Cajanus cajan seeds as ingredients in pasta products: chemical, biological and sensory evaluation. *Food Chem*. 2007;101:202-11.

39. El-Hag N, Haard NF, Morse RE. Influence of sprouting on the digestibility coefficient, trypsin inhibitor and globulin proteins of red kidney beans. *J Food Sci*. 1978;43:1874-75.

40. Collins JL, Sanders GG. Changes in trypsin inhibitory activity in some soybean varieties during maturation and germination. *J Food Sci*. 1976;41:168-72.

41. Andersson HC, Gry J. Phenylhydrazines in the cultivated mushroom (Agaricus bisporus)—occurrence, biological properties, risk assessment and recommendations. *TemaNord*. 2004;558:123.

42. Schulzová V, Hajslova J, Peroutkay R, Gry J, Andersson HC. Influence of storage and household processing on the agaritine content of the cultivated Agaricus mushroom. *Food Addit Contam*. 2002;19:853-62.

43. Toth B, Erickson J. Cancer induction in mice by feeding of the uncooked cultivated mushroom of commerce Agaricus bisporus. *Cancer Res*. 1986;46:4007-11.

44. Kondo K, Watanabe A, Akiyama H, Maitani T. The metabolisms of agaritine, a mushroom hydrazine in mice. *Food Chem Toxicol*. 2008;46:854-62.

45. Oikawa S, Ito T, Iwayama M, Kawanishi S. Radical production and DNA damage induced by carcinogenic 4-hydrazinobenzoic acid, an ingredient of mushroom Agaricus bisporus. *Free Radic Res*. 2006;40:31-39.

46. Shephard SE, Gunz D, Schlatter C. Genotoxicity of agaritine in the lacI transgenic mouse mutation assay: evaluation of the health risk of mushroom consumption. *Food Chem Toxicol*. 1995;33:257-64.

47. Chen S, Oh SR, Phung S, Hur G, Ye JJ, Kwok SL, Shrode GE, Belury M, Adams LS, Williams D. Anti-aromatase activity of phytochemicals in white button mushrooms (Agaricus bisporus). *Cancer Res*. 2006;66:12026-34.

48. Grube BJ, Eng ET, Kao YC, Kwon A, Chen S. White button mushroom phytochemicals inhibit aromatase activity and breast cancer cell proliferation. *J Nutr*. 2001;131:3288-93.

49. Adams LS, Phung S, Wu X, Ki L, Chen S. White button mushroom (Agaricus bisporus) exhibits antiproliferative and proapoptotic properties and inhibits prostate tumor growth in athymic mice. *Nutr Cancer*. 2008;60:744-56.

50. Zhang M, Huang J, Xie X, Holman CD. Dietary intakes of mushrooms and green tea combine to reduce the risk of breast cancer in Chinese women. *Int J Cancer*. 2009;124:1404-08.

51. Hajslová J, Hájková L, Schulzová V, Frandsen H, Gry J, Andersson HC. Stability of agaritine—a natural toxicant of Agaricus mushrooms. *Food Addit Contam*. 2002;19:1028-33.

52. Centre for Food Safety, Government of Hong Kong. 2009. www.cfs.gov.hk/english/programme/programme_rafs/programme_rafs_fa_02_09.html. Accessed July 2009.

53. Mason DJ, Sykes MD, Panton SW, Rippon EH. Determination of naturally occurring formaldehyde in raw and cooked Shiitake mushrooms by spectrophotometry and liquid chromatography-mass spectrometry. *Food Addit Contam*. 2004;21(11):1071-82.

54. Hanada K, Hashimoto I. Flagellate mushroom (Shiitake) dermatitis and photosensitivity. *Dermatology*. 1998;197:255-57.

55. Nakamura, T. Shiitake (Lentinus edodes) dermatitis. *Contact Dermatitis*. 1992;27:65-70.

56. Levy AM, Kita H, Phillips SF et al. Eosinophilia and gastrointestinal symptoms after ingestion of shiitake mushrooms. *J Allergy Clin Immunol*. 1998;101:613-20.

57. Hyry H, Kariniemi AL. Shiitake dermatitis: shiitake mushrooms must be cooked before their use. *Duodecim* (Finnish). 1998;114:555-57.

58. Stamets P. *Growing Gourmet and Medicinal Mushrooms*. 3rd ed. Illustrated, revised. Berkeley CA: Ten Speed Press, 2000.

59. Campbell, D. On eating raw mushrooms. *The Mycena News*. 2008;59:4-5.

60. Hobbs C. *Medicinal Mushrooms, 3rd ed*. Loveland CO: Interweave Press, 1996.

61. Ng ML, Yap AT. Inhibition of human colon carcinoma development by lentinan from shiitake mushrooms (Lentinus edodes). *J Altern Complement Med*. 2002;8:581-89.

62. Ngai PH, Ng TB. Lentin, a novel and potent antifungal protein from shiitake mushroom with inhibitory effects on activity of human immunodeficiency virus-1 reverse transcriptase and proliferation of leukemia cells. *Life Sci*. 2003;73:3363-74.

63. Memorial Sloan-Kettering Cancer Center. *Lentinan*. 2007. www.mskcc.org/mskcc/html/69279.cfm. Accessed July 2009.

64. WHO. *Environmental Health Criteria No 18: Arsenic*. Geneva: WHO, 1981:43-102. www.inchem.org/documents/ehc/ehc/ehc018. htm#SubSectionNumber:1.1.6.

65. WHO, Consultation FAO. Evaluation of certain food additives and contaminants. *WHO Technical Report Series*. 1989:776.

66. FSANZ. Inorganic arsenic in hijiki seaweed. *Food Standards News 52*. 2004. www.nzfsa. govt.nz/consumers/chemicals-nutrients-additives-and-toxins/hijiki-seaweed/index.htm. Accessed July 2009.

67. Government of Hong Kong. Food and Environmental Hygiene Department. *Risk in Brief. Issue No. 17: Hijiki and Arsenic*. 2005. www.fehd.gov. hk/safefood/report/hijiki/. Accessed July 2009.

68. CFIA. *Inorganic Arsenic and Hijiki Seaweed Consumption*. 2001. www.inspection.gc.ca/ english/fssa/concen/specif/arsenice.shtml. Accessed July 2009.

69. UK Food Standards Agency. *Arsenic in Seaweed*. 2004. www.food.gov.uk/science/surveillance/ fsis2004branch/fsis6104.

70. Hamano-Nagaoka M, Hanaoka K, Usui M, Nishimura T, Maitani T. Nitric acid-based partial-digestion method for selective determination of inorganic arsenic in hijiki and application to soaked hijiki. *Shokuhin Eiseigaku Zasshi*. 2008;49:88-94.

71. Nakajima Y, Endo Y, Inoue Y, Yamanaka K, Kato K, Wanibuchi H, Endo G. Ingestion of Hijiki seaweed and risk of arsenic poisoning. *Appl Organometal Chem*. 2006;20:557-64.

72. Amster E, Tiwary A, Schenker MB. Case report: potential arsenic toxicosis secondary to herbal kelp supplement. *Environ Health Perspect*. 2007;115:606-08.

73. Almela C, Clemente MJ, Vélez D, Montoro R. Total arsenic, inorganic arsenic, lead and cadmium contents in edible seaweed sold in Spain. *Food Chem Toxicol*. 2006;44:1901-08.

74. Rose M, Lewis J, Langford N, Baxter M, Origgi S, Barber M, MacBain H, Thomas K. Arsenic in seaweed—forms, concentration and dietary exposure. *Food Chem Toxicol*. 2007;45:1263-67.

75. FDA. *Foodborne Pathogenic Microorganisms and Natural Toxins Handbook*. www.foodsafety.gov/~mow/intro.html. Accessed July 2009.

76. Mead PS, Slutsker L, Dietz V et al. Food-related illness and death in the United States. *Emerg Infect Dis*. 1999;5:607-25.

77. Center for Science in the Public Interest. *Food Safety (includes outbreak database)*. www. cspinet.org/foodsafety. Accessed July 2009.

78. Burkholder J, Libra B, Weyer P, Heathcote S, Kolpin D, Thorne PS, Wichman M. Impacts of waste from concentrated animal feeding operations on water quality. *Environ Health Perspect*. 2007;115:308-12.

79. Department of Health and Human Services. Centers for Disease Control and Prevention. *Foodborne Illness*. 2005. www.cdc.gov/ncidod/dbmd/diseaseinfo/foodborneinfections_g. htm#riskiestfoods. Accessed July 2009.

80. USDA. *Factsheets: Safe Food Handling: Basics for Handling Foods Safely*. www.fsis.usda.gov/ Factsheets/Basics_for_Handling_Food_Safely/ index.asp. Accessed July 2009.

81. Lynch, Michael. Produce Related Foodborne Infections: Review of the Centers for Disease Control Foodborne Outbreak Surveillance. FDA Public Meeting on Produce Safety March 20, 2007. http://www.fda.gov/ohrms/ dockets/dockets/07n0051/07n-0051-ts00001. pdf. Accessed December 2009.

82. U.S. Food and Drug Administration. *Consumers Advised of Risks Associated With Raw Sprouts*. 1999. www.cfsan.fda.gov/~lrd/ hhssprts.html.

83. Health Canada. *Risks Associated with Sprouts*. 2007. www.hc-sc.gc.ca/hl-vs/iyh-vsv/ food-aliment/sprouts-germes-eng.php.

84. Gill CJ, Keene WE, Mohle-Boetani JE, Farrar JA, Waller PL, Hahn CG et al. Alfalfa seed decontamination in Salmonella outbreak. *Emerg Infect Dis*. 2003;9:474-79. www.cdc. gov/ncidod/EID/vol9no4/02-0519.htm. Accessed July 2009.

85. U.S. Food and Drug Administration. National Advisory Committee on Microbiological Criteria for Food. Microbiological Safety Evaluations and Recommendations on Sprouted Seeds. *Int J Food Microbiol*. 1999;52(3):123-53.

86. Sproutpeople. *Sprouts Are Safer Than They Want You to Think*. www.sproutpeople.com/ Political/fda.html. Accessed July 2009.

87. Hu H, Churey JJ, Worobo RW. Heat treatments to enhance the safety of mung bean seeds. *J Food Prot*. 2004;67:1257-60.

88. Bari ML, Inatsu, Y, Isobe S, Kawamoto S. Hot water treatments to inactivate Escherichia coli 0157:H7 and Salmonella in mung bean seeds. *J Food Protection*. 2008;71(4):830-34.

89. Society for General Microbiology. *A Hot Solution to Bean Sprout Safety*. SGM meeting release, March 2009. www.alphagalileo.org/

ViewItem.aspx?ItemId=56557&CultureCode= en. Accessed July 2009.

90. University of California at Davis. *Growing Seed Sprouts at Home*. www.postharvest. ucdavis.edu/datastorefiles/234-412.pdf. Accessed July 2009.

CHAPTER 12 (Resources)

Nutrition Guidelines and Menus

1. American Dietetic Association, Dietitians of Canada. Position of the American Dietetic Association and Dietitians of Canada: vegetarian diets. *J Am Diet Assoc*. 2003;103:748. www.webdietitians.org/Public/Files/veg.pdf.

2. Craig WJ, Mangels AR. American Dietetic Association. Position of the American Dietetic Association: vegetarian diets. *J Am Diet Assoc*. 2009 Jul;109(7):1266-82.

3. Davis B, Melina V. *Becoming Vegan*. Summertown TN: Book Publishing Company, 2000.

4. Golay A, Allaz AF, Ybarra J, Bianchi P, Saraiva S, Mensi N, Gomis R, de Tonnac N. Similar weight loss with low-energy food combining or balanced diets. *Int J Obes Relat Metab Disord*. 2000;24:492-96.

5. McCarty MF. The origins of western obesity: a role for animal protein? *Med Hypotheses*. 2000;54:488-94.

Raw Products and Sources

New and exciting raw products are finding their way to natural food stores, online stores and local markets. The following is a short list of products and sources that we have found to be particularly helpful. A quick search online will uncover many more!

Living Light Marketplace and Online Store

301-B North Main Street
Fort Bragg, CA 95437
800-816-2319
rawfoodchef.com/store/marketplace.html

Retail and online store for an outstanding selection of raw foods, culinary supplies, videos, books, and personal care products

Mail Order Catalog

800-695-2241
healthy-eating.com/sproutman.html

A large selection of quality sprouting seeds, sprouting books, and other sprouting supplies

The Raw Food World

866-729-3438
therawfoodworld.com

An extensive supply of raw lifestyle products and foods

Vega

866-839-8863
shop.sequelnaturals.com

An exceptional, predominately raw line of bars, smoothie infusions, and meal replacements

Page references to graphics and sidebars appear in *italics*.

Recipe titles appear in *green italicized* typeface.

Brenda Davis did her undergraduate studies at the University of Guelph, Ontario, and her internship with Health Canada and several hospitals in Ottawa, Ontario. Brenda is a past chair of the Vegetarian Nutrition Dietetic Practice Group of the American Dietetic Association. In 2007, she was inducted into the North American Vegetarian Society's Vegetarian Hall of Fame. Brenda has worked as a public health nutritionist, clinical nutrition specialist, nutrition consultant, and academic nutrition instructor. She is currently the lead dietitian in a diabetes intervention research project in Majuro, Marshall Islands.

Brenda is the coauthor of *The New Becoming Vegetarian* (with Vesanto Melina), *Becoming Vegetarian* (with Vesanto Melina), *Becoming Vegan* (with Vesanto Melina), *The Raw Food Revolution Diet* (with Cherie Soria and Vesanto Melina), *Defeating Diabetes* (with Tom Barnard, MD), and *Dairy-Free and Delicious* (with Bryanna Clark Grogan and Jo Stepaniak).

Vesanto Melina did her undergraduate and graduate work at the University of Toronto and the University of London, England. She has taught nutrition at the University of British Columbia and at Seattle's Bastyr University. She is a coauthor of the Dietitians of Canada and the American Dietetic Association's position paper on vegetarian diets and is a consultant to the Government of British Columbia. She has been vegetarian for over thirty years and vegan for sixteen years, and was introduced to a raw diet through Cherie Soria's excellent chef training program at the Living Light Culinary Arts Institute. Vesanto's website is www.nutrispeak.com.

Vesanto is the author of *Healthy Eating for Life: To Prevent and Treat Cancer* and is the coauthor of *The New Becoming Vegetarian* (with Brenda Davis), *Becoming Vegetarian* (with Brenda Davis), *Becoming Vegan* (with Brenda Davis), *The Raw Food Revolution Diet* (with Cherie Soria and Brenda Davis), *Food Allergy Survival Guide* (with Jo Stepaniak and Dina Aronson), and *Raising Vegetarian Children* (with Jo Stepaniak).

Rynn Berry did his undergraduate and graduate work at the University of Pennsylvania and Columbia University. He is the historical advisor to the North American Vegetarian Society and the author of *The New Vegetarians*, *Famous Vegetarians*, *Food for the Gods: Vegetarianism and the World's Religions*, *Hitler: Neither Vegetarian Nor Animal Lover*, and *The Vegan Guide to New York City*, as well as numerous articles on vegetarian food history for the *Oxford Companion to American Food and Drink*.

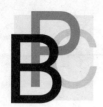
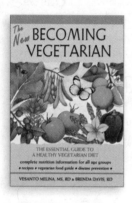
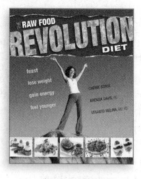
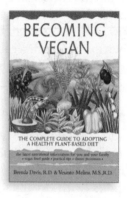
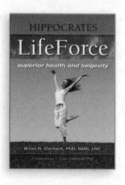
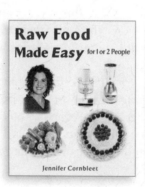
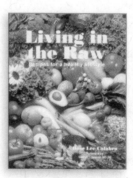
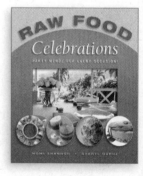